SYNOPSIS OF PATHOLOGY
FOR THE
ALLIED HEALTH PROFESSIONS

SYNOPSIS OF PATHOLOGY FOR THE ALLIED HEALTH PROFESSIONS

By

ALVIN F. GARDNER, Ph.D.
*Bureau of Drugs, Food and Drug Administration
Department of Health, Education and Welfare
Washington, D.C.
Formerly, Associate Professor of Pathology
University of Maryland
Baltimore, Maryland
Formerly, Consultant in Pathology
U.S. Public Health Service and Veteran's Administration
Baltimore, Maryland*

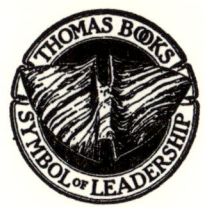

CHARLES C THOMAS • PUBLISHER
Springfield • Illinois • U.S.A.

Published and Distributed Throughout the World by
CHARLES C THOMAS • PUBLISHER
BANNERSTONE HOUSE
301-327 East Lawrence Avenue, Springfield, Illinois, U.S.A.

This book is protected by copyright. No part of it may be reproduced in any manner without written permission from the publisher.

© 1979, by CHARLES C THOMAS • PUBLISHER
ISBN 0-398-03884-8
Library of Congress Catalog Card Number: 78-25766

With THOMAS BOOKS *careful attention is given to all details of manufacturing and design. It is the Publisher's desire to present books that are satisfactory as to their physical qualities and artistic possibilities and appropriate for their particular use.* THOMAS BOOKS *will be true to those laws of quality that assure a good name and good will.*

Printed in the United States of America
N-11

Library of Congress Cataloging in Publication Data

Gardner, Alvin F
    Synopsis of pathology for the allied health professions.

    Bibliography: p.
    Includes index
    1. Pathology.   2. Allied health personnel.   I. Title. [DNLM:
1. Health occupations.   2. Pathology. QZ4.3 G226s]
RB111.G37 1979   616.07'02'4613   78-25766
ISBN 0-398-03884-8

*This book is dedicated to my wife,
Esther Vita
for nobility of thought
and whose constant love and support
enabled me to complete this book.*

PREFACE

Synopsis of Pathology for the Allied Health Professions advances new knowledge of general pathology while providing a basic medical science background to aid the allied health professions in their current progress. Success in the modern allied health professions is dependent upon pathologic as well as clinical considerations. The interdependence of the allied health professions on general pathology is so vital that allied health professionals require knowledge of general pathology to understand the local and systemic basis of disease in their patients. Various pathologic processes are currently becoming very sound and vital foundations for the allied health professions. This textbook prepared for the allied health students is charged with a striving ardor of pathologic knowledge and is prepared *de rigueur* with new insights. *Entscheidungs-problem* are discussed. A tradition will be established throughout this textbok of offering the allied health student comprehensive coverage of recent developments in the various aspects of general pathology, while the author presents self-contained chapters directed to the allied health student. This textbook is, therefore, charged with providing the most current knowledge in general pathology, particularly for the allied health student.

It is the author's hope that *Synopsis of Pathology for the Allied Health Professions* will truly assist allied health students in fulfilling their responsibility to their patients and to their physicians through sound judgments based upon pathologic knowledge and proper technical knowledge. The author has focused attention, in succinct fashion, on those aspects of general pathology causing the allied health student the greatest concern and difficulty. This textbook of general pathology will, therefore, help the allied health student to meet the challenges of his courses in the basic sciences and also those of clinical practice. The knowledge discussed here should become extremely beneficial to all allied health students seeking to attain the best treatment and diagnostic procedures for the medical patient. It is our hope that this book will provide an important link of communication between general pathology and the allied health professions and result in better holistic patient care. This textbook thus attempts to put the written current concepts in general pathology into clinical practice and combat obsolescence for modern-day allied health students.

The purpose of the monograph is to advance the opportunity to publish the latest concepts, ideas, and thoughts on the most advanced fronts of general pathology. Each chapter reflects advanced viewpoints while incorporating unique and significantly different concepts not previously considered by allied health students.

The importance of readability by the allied health student cannot be overemphasized. The problem of communication of a vast area of pathologic knowledge has been resolved by summarizing frontiers of thought and research in each area of general pathology. The goals of the author have been dictated by those current concepts and advances useful to the allied health student in moving forward in his undergraduate education. In turn, the goal of *Synopsis of Pathology for the Allied Health Professions* is to present a well-balanced view of the entire field of general pathology, with no specialty of pathology excluded.

Washington, D.C., 1979 ALVIN F. GARDNER

No official support or endorsement by the Food and Drug Administration or the Department of Health, Education and Welfare is intended or should be inferred.

CONTENTS

	Page
Preface	vii

Chapter

1. INTRODUCTION TO PATHOLOGY FOR THE ALLIED HEALTH PROFESSIONS 3
2. CONGENITAL ANOMALIES AND HEREDITARY DISEASES 16
3. PATHOLOGY OF CELL INJURY 24
4. RETROGRADE CELLULAR ALTERATIONS AND INFILTRATIONS (CELL DEATH) 30
5. DISSEMINATION OF DISEASE AND SECONDARY IMPAIRMENTS .. 46
6. DISTURBANCES OF BODY WATER AND ELECTROLYTES AND CIRCULATION OF BLOOD 53
7. INFLAMMATION 94
8. RESOLUTION, ORGANIZATION, REPAIR, AND REGENERATION . 109
9. DISEASES OF AGING 118
10. ACUTE INFECTIOUS DISEASES 124
11. SPECIFIC GRANULOMATOUS INFLAMMATIONS 130
12. VIRAL AND RICKETTSIAL DISEASES 154
13. DISEASES DUE TO PHYSICAL INJURIES, CHEMICAL POISONS, AND THERMAL AND IRRADIATION INJURIES 160
14. NUTRITIONAL DEFICIENCY 180
15. DISTURBANCES IN GROWTH AND NEOPLASIA 197
16. HYPERSENSITIVITY (ALLERGY) AND DISEASES OF CONNECTIVE TISSUES 215
17. HEART AND BLOOD VESSELS 225
18. THE RESPIRATORY SYSTEM 246
19. KIDNEYS AND LOWER URINARY TRACT 257
20. THE GASTROINTESTINAL TRACT 267

Chapter		Page
21.	THE LIVER AND BILIARY TRACT	279
22.	THE LYMPH NODES AND SPLEEN	291
23.	BLOOD AND BONE MARROW	298
24.	THE ENDOCRINE SYSTEM	309
25.	FEMALE GENITAL TRACT	318
26.	THE BREAST	354
27.	MALE GENITAL SYSTEM	368
28.	THE SKIN	385
29.	THE MUSCULOSKELETAL SYSTEM	400
30.	THE NERVOUS SYSTEM	414

Index 441

SYNOPSIS OF PATHOLOGY
FOR THE
ALLIED HEALTH PROFESSIONS

CHAPTER 1

INTRODUCTION TO PATHOLOGY FOR THE ALLIED HEALTH PROFESSIONS

THE PURPOSE OF THIS SYNOPSIS of pathology is to give the student of the allied health professions a general framework of pathology, introduce him or her to a general vocabulary of disease terminology, clarify definitions used in pathology, emphasize major problems of disease, and discuss interrelationships that have direct significance for the allied health professional. The allied health student must realize that, because of the magnitude of general pathology, only a framework will be presented in this synopsis. The allied health student should fill in this framework of general pathology with additional pertinent details obtained from other courses, textbooks, and teaching materials and future clinical experience in the allied health profession. The purpose of this synopsis is to eliminate the problems presented by verbose and detailed pathology books, which are impossible to comprehend during the relatively short period of didactic study available to the allied health student. One problem facing the allied health student is that different allied health disciplines frequently use certain terms with slightly different meanings. The allied health student may learn a half-true definition for a term, i.e. the definition is correct as far as it goes, but it fails to adequately delineate the entire meaning of the term. These problems must be solved by the individual student.

SCOPE OF PATHOLOGY FOR THE ALLIED HEALTH PROFESSION

Pathology is defined as the study of disease and injury plus the body's response, i.e., inflammation and repair. Disease is caused by some demonstrable agent of injury. Invisible living agents, i.e., bacteria and viruses, can produce disease. Physical violence and poisons produce injury and death. Negative factors are also responsible for causing disease. The absence of various vitamins plays a role in the production of diseases such as rickets and scurvy. Finally, the causes of a number of common and very important diseases, such as arteriosclerosis, cancer, hypertension, and even the common cold, are still obscure, and the cause or causes must be revealed through future research. However, disease involves an agent of injury and the response of living cells and tissue to that harmful influence. Thus, disease is defined as the interaction between an agent of injury and living cells resulting in physiology under duress.

The noxious influences that produce disease are referred to as the etiological agents or factors of disease. Etiological factors are congenital if acquired by an injury that takes place during gestation, or hereditary defects if transmitted through the germ plasm from prior generations. Etiological factors of disease may be inanimate or animate. The inanimate factors cause disease by physical force(s) and thus are referred to as traumatic etiological factors. Inanimate factors such as chemicals or poisons are referred to as chemotoxic etiological factors. The absence of foods, vitamins, air, or essential metabolites produces deprivation diseases due to the withholding of chemicals. Burns are referred to as thermoradiation injuries.

The animate factors of disease are the result of infections of the tissues by living pathogenic organisms and are referred to as pathogens. The injurious organisms produce disease by elaborating biologically toxic materials into the tissues. The animate diseases of man are due to invasion by bacteria, fungi, viruses, rickettsiae, parasites, and zootic forms of life. The etiologic agents of animate diseases have the following in common: they produce damage to tissues and organs by either destroying or decreasing the normal functions of living cells, tissues, and organs. The normal physiologic capacity of cells is either reduced or completely eliminated in the involved tissues and organs.

Human disease results from the total of all affected physiologic processes within the human body. Disease is initiated by damage or death of living cells and tissues, i.e. (1) the agent of injury plus the human living tissue results in damage and (2) the physiologic response of living tissue minus the damage induced results in the body's response. The damage (1) plus the body's response (2) equals human disease.

The pathologist determines the degree of damage to the organs and tissues based upon the amount of alteration imposed on normal anatomical structures in man. Structural alterations of normal anatomy are described in pathology as degenerations and necroses. The degenerations and necroses include abscesses, blisters due to burns, ulcerations of body surfaces and nonhealed wounds of the skin, plus coagulation of cell proteins and precipitation of mineral components of cells and tissues. The pathologist determines where possible, the amount of tissue destruction or alteration by using a variety of biochemical and laboratory tests in the clinical pathology laboratory. For instance, the pathologist uses clinical and laboratory tests to describe any alterations of the blood and urine, the capacity of the lungs and heart, renal clearance, and liver function. The pathologist's primary purpose is to determine the degree of loss of physiologic capacity induced by the damage (impairment or death) to living cells and tissues.

Human disease is concerned with two factors: (1) the noxious agents or pathogens and (2) the response of the affected tissue plus the susceptibility of the organs to injury and their powers of recovery. The individual possesses modifying factors that make him predisposed or susceptible to certain diseases. The individual may fight off disease by means of his natural resistance. On the other hand, the individual may suffer disease because his or her health is generally below normal. Susceptibility to disease(s) is an important predisposing factor, since it sets the groundwork for the initiation of the attack of disease. Along with susceptibility to disease are such factors as age, sex, and race, which are added to other influences, responsible for initiating disease processes. Susceptibility means the ability of the individual to respond to the noxious agents or pathogens in a positive or negative or average manner.

Humans have a tendency to inherit certain traits and are susceptible to specific infections to which animals may be resistant. For instance, the American Indians have a high susceptibility to tuberculosis. The black race has less susceptibility to solar radiation than the white race. Pigmentations present in Caucasians have been correlated to a tendency to develop certain diseases. The sexes differ in their tendency to develop diseases. The male is more prone to develop gout, peptic ulcer, skin cancer, lung cancer, and larynx cancer. The female is more prone to develop hypertension, scleroderma, cholecystitis, and pyelitis.

Age is an important predisposing factor to disease. The aged are more prone to develop osteoarthritis, cataracts, arteriosclerosis, diabetes mellitus, cancer, and emphysema of the lungs. Infants and children are more prone to develop poliomyelitis, acute rheumatic fever, and vitamin deficiencies.

Reaction to Injury

Disease means a reaction of the human tissue to injury. The pathologist is, therefore, primarily interested in the response of tissues to injury. Injured tissues, whether from trauma, living organisms, and poisons, can only react with the following major responses:

1. the affected tissue(s) may die;
2. the affected tissue(s) may resist alterations; and
3. the affected tissue(s) may heal after the injury.

If the noxious agent injures the tissue but does not produce immediate death, the tissue responds as a unit to the injury. The unit of response is composed of three factors, i.e., impairment of the tissue, defense of the tissue, and repair of the tissue. Impairment of the tissue means both reversible and irreversible alterations in cells. Defense of the tissue means a variety of protections such as blood clots, inflammatory exudate, endocrine response, and immunity. Repair of the tissue means several steps in the healing process. The impairment, defense, and repair processes (triad) follow each other, but generally there is an overlapping so that two processes are existing at any one time as viewed in histopathologic specimens in the general pathology laboratory. The triad of impairment, defense, and repair is an excess of normal physiology. Impairment may result in the death or destruction of living tissues. The student should remember that impairment occurs in normal individuals, i.e. millions of red blood cells, white blood cells, and epithelial cells lining body surfaces succumb and are eliminated daily without any deleterious effect on the human body. Blood platelets protect blood vessels against leakage, and when they are decreased from the normal, bruises (hemorrhages) develop.

Impairment encompasses everything from the normal tissue to the debilitated cells, to the dead or devitalized cells, and to the decay and dissolution of cells. All tissues in the human body may undergo impairment involving debility, death, and decay of cells. In histopathologic specimens, the student of pathology can visualize debility as degenerative (regressive) alterations in cells; death and decay are viewed as various types of necrosis of cells. Necrosis in general pathology means death plus subsequent decay of tissue during the life of the host.

Defensive Responses

Local resistance to tissue injury encompasses the coagulation of blood and the formation of an inflammatory exudate (both are local vascular responses to injury). The local resistance is reinforced by the endocrine and reticuloendothelial systems, which have the capacity to increase blood platelets during severe hemorrhages, modify fluid and electrolyte balance after trauma, and increase leukocytes during severe infections. The cells that take part in the defense of the injured tissues are destroyed during the process. The initial local tissue damage spreads to the adjacent tissues and structures so that these structures undergo secondary impairment. The adjacent vascular endothelium, mobile reticuloendothelial cells, and stromal cells of the adjacent tissue are impaired during the defense process.

Healing follows the defense processes. Healing occurs by repair or regeneration. Repair means that the original tissue has been replaced by fibrous tissue that is actually substituting for the lost cells. Repair terminates in a scar. Regeneration means that the lost tissue has been replaced by the same kind of cells that were originally present. Regeneration occurs by division and differentiation of reserve cells present before the injury took place. Regeneration is possible in most tissues and organs but not in all of them. Repair or regeneration may occur along with the defense processes. Repair may lead to contractures and deformities.

Impairment

When tissues are injured, the alterations are termed *degeneration* and *necrosis*. Degeneration means that the tissues are partially devitalized and are capable of recovering from the reversible damage present. Necrosis of tissue means death of the affected tissue while the body as a whole is living. Necrosis or disintegration of cells and tissues is an irreversible process.

Impairment of tissues may result either in abnormal pigmentations or in precipitation of calcium salts. When human tissues are impaired by injury, a sequence of responses occurs, i.e. impairment of local primary focus of tissue, impairment of adjacent tissues, defense, and repair, regardless of the organ or tissue involved and regardless of the form or type of the injury. Impairment becomes the only tissue response in sudden death. In sudden death, the alterations to the tissues may be highly incipient, causing suppression of vital physiologic processes. When the disease occurs in a less rapid and less progressive state, the damage has time to spread to the adjacent tissues and involve an interrelated organ, causing its impairment. Significant damage to tissue in a primary focus will spread to anatomically and physiologically related organs and structures. The primary damage commonly involves the most highly specialized tissues of an organ, i.e. parenchymatous tissue of the particular organ. The more highly specialized cells of the organ are the most susceptible to the irreversible damage compared to the stroma during irreversible necrosis. The vascular tissues and the loose connective tissues of the impaired organ are also highly susceptible and show reversible damage. The arterioles, capillaries, and venules are the first tissue elements to demonstrate alterations in both form and function due to the impairment of the adjacent tissue. Healing and defensive processes counteract the vascular changes in impairment of adjacent tissues.

Defensive Mechanisms of the Body

Thrombosis

The primary local reactions involved in defense of the injured tissue are clotting of blood, inflammation, and resolution. Thrombosis means the clotting of blood during life. Thrombosis prevents loss of blood from the damaged vessels by concentrating blood platelets and fibrin at the site of injury. Thrombosis also produces retraction and constriction of injured vessels. Thrombosis is characterized by the following features: vasoconstriction, fusion of blood platelets with the thrombocytes adhering to the surface of the damaged endothelial cells and uniting together to form columns projecting into the lumen, precipitation of strands of fibrin by the action of thrombin or fibrinogen in the plasma. Fibrin produces a network or meshlike structure between the columns of blood platelets. Red blood cells and leukocytes are caught up in the meshwork of fused platelets, and fibrin aids in producing the adherent clot. Thrombosis may interfere with the blood supply.

The death of tissues caused by an interruption of their blood supply is termed an *infarction*. The thrombosis in a large blood vessel or in the heart chamber may produce a dislodged fragment from the central clotted material. This dislodged fragment is termed an *embolus*. The embolus may be propelled about in the circulation and eventually block some distant vessel.

Inflammation

Inflammation is a pathologic process that localizes, neutralizes, or dilutes the toxic effects of tissue injuries. Inflammation is a defensive process characterized by capillary dilatation and increased permeability of capillaries, resulting in an exudate of plasma at the local site of injury. Large numbers of migrating leukocytes are present in the affected tissue. The initial vascular response during inflammation is leakage from the blood vessels. Note that the initial response of inflammation is the reverse of the response during defense, i.e. thrombosis. The leakage produces extravasated fluid, the purpose of which is to neutralize and dilute the damage caused by the noxious agent. The extravasated fluid also increases the lymphatic damage in the affected part. The leukocytes migrate to and accumulate in the injured tissue in order to engulf particulate matter by phagocytosis. The accumulated leukocytes also provide digestive ferments to the injured tissue. The function of the exudate during inflammation is to dispose of harmful matter and decontaminate the impaired tissue. Inflamed tissues have the following four clinical features first recognized by Celsus: color (heat); rubor (redness); tumor (swelling); and dolor (pain).

Serum, leukocytes, and immune bodies move or shift to the local site of infection with the exudate of inflammation. Injuries that allow the survival and local defense of tissues provoke the migration of fluid and cells to the local area of damage. The shift of fluid involves portions of the blood and lymph. The shift of mobile cells involves cellular components of the reticuloendothelial system. When moderate blood vessels are injured, there is a shift of the platelets and fibrin to form a thrombus (blood clot) within the lumen of the damaged vessels. Thrombosis, therefore, is an intraluminal blood clot formed as a defensive mechanism. In defense of the damaged tissue there is a shift of both cells and fluid. The cells and fluid mobilize at the site of injury; however, they are mobile and expendable. The highly mobile and expendable elements are vascular endothelial cells, loose connective tissue, circulating fluids and reticuloendothelial cells. All are derivatives of the reticuloendothelial system responsible for defense. Only a small number of derivatives of mesenchymal tissues take part in the defensive response of the tissues during thrombosis, inflammation, resolution, and immunity. Injury to the vascular endothelial cells is responsible for triggering the response of the local tissues since any alteration in the form and function of endothelial cells is enough to stimulate the first phase of thrombosis and inflammation.

The defense of impaired tissues is prompt, and the body responds with speed as if an emergency existed. The fluid and mobile cells present in inflammation are drawn from local areas. The injured tissue in the area of impairment is lost and now must be replaced during complete recovery. Three separate processes are involved: (1) loss of tissue following injury; (2) borrowing fluid and mobile cells for defense from adjacent areas; (3) replacement of tissue during recovery.

Resolution

The dead and dying cells present during inflammation are being constantly removed by phagocytes. Monocytes from the blood stream plus histiocytes from the adjacent stroma migrate as phagocytes to the area of inflammation. The tissue debris is shifted to organs of the reticuloendothelial system, where they are eliminated. Disposal takes place in the spleen, lymph nodes, and liver sinusoids. The noxious agent has now been localized and neutralized. Resolution is the removal of damaged and inflamed tissues with a return of the area to a normal state. It is accomplished by phagocytic activity that is responsible for the demobilization of the inflammation. Resolution with phagocytosis of debris is truly the end of the defense mechanism of the impaired tissues and the beginning of the healing process (repair and regeneration). Severe injury with death of tissues requires the healing or repair process before the impaired tissues may return to a physiologic state. Resolution thus is dependent on the major healing response.

Repair

Repair (healing) of injured tissues requires the following processes: (1) organization, (2) fibrosis, and (3) regeneration. Organization of the impaired site means that there is an ingrowth of fibroblasts and new blood vessels into areas of inflammation. The latter ingrowth is, however, either preceded or accompanied by resolution. Therefore, the student can readily see that defense of tissue and repair (healing) represent overlapping processes. The process of resolution and phagocytosis of debris either becomes the terminal phase of the defensive mechanism or the initial phase of the repair (healing) mechanism.

Inflammation is reversed when the injury and damage are neutralized. This permits fibroblasts to proliferate and migrate along with migration and proliferation of endothelial buds from capillaries into the previous damaged tissue. As the fibroblasts mature they produce a collagen fiber network, which holds together the site of repair. Subsequently, a scar forms by means of fibrosis. The repair has occurred by replacement or substitution of the lost or damaged tissue by a dense scar. Repair (healing) of damaged brain tissue is accomplished by glial tissue or astrocytes rather than by fibroblasts, and the healing is termed *gliosis of the brain.*

Regeneration

In organs capable of undergoing regeneration, the loss of epithelial cells or epithelial lining and covering surfaces is restored by proliferation and migration of reserve epithelial cells. Therefore, regeneration is replacement of lost cells by an identical new reserve epithelial cell. Not all tissues and organs in the body are capable of undergoing regeneration following impairment or death. The following parenchymatous tissues of organs are not capable of undergoing regeneration: myocardium, glomerulus of kidney, central nervous system, elastic lamellae of major blood vessels, enamel of the teeth, and large defects produced in adult joint cartilage. Regeneration accompanied by some defects is possible in the following organs: skin, liver, gastrointestinal tract, and bladder. For instance, regeneration of skin restores the epidermis but not the hair follicles; sweat glands and sebaceous glands fail to regenerate. Regeneration of the stomach wall restores simple, mucus-secreting glands, but complex gastric glands fail to regenerate.

The tissues and organs capable of undergoing regeneration must possess an inherent capacity for self-renewal (periodically) under normal conditions. The tissue or organ undergoing regeneration obtains a supply of new cells by the following methods:

1. Undifferentiated cells of similar kinds are borrowed from

adjacent tissues.

2. The initial tissue and cells used in regeneration have a lower level of differentiation; thus, they are produced in a shorter period of time, and the less differentiated cells last longer.

3. In the liver the capacity for cell division is available to transitional cells, in a transitional phase of differentiation (normally these cells cannot divide).

When a less differentiated cell serves as a temporary replacement (2 above) for a highly differentiated cell, the process is known as metaplasia. It frequently requires weeks rather than days for the regeneration of highly differentiated cells and tissues. Thus, it may be necessary for the regeneration to occur by means of migration of uninjured adjacent adult cells. Squamous epithelium (adult) of the cornea of the eye can migrate over a corneal defect in six hours.

Systemic Effects of Disease

The response of living cells and tissues is always greater in extent and duration when compared to the injury or impairment present, regardless of whether death or repair of tissue ensues. For instance, the inflammatory process that precedes healing may not be localized but may include movement of both fluid and mobile cells that involves the vascular and reticuloendothelial systems. Therefore, injury provokes both a local and a systemic effect. Injury produces damage that has a tendency to spread to anatomically similar or physiologically related tissue. For instance, when a nerve is destroyed, the muscle subsequently becomes impaired. When a blood vessel is destroyed, the tissue supplied by that specific vessel succumbs. Certain distant organs to the site of injury (inflammation) have a tendency to become involved in defense. For instance, systemic reactions such as fever, leucocytosis, and acquired immunity accompany the infection of a portion of the body.

Passive and active responses of the body caused by injury or impairment show both spacial and temporal spread beyond the area of the injury and beyond the time the initial injury was produced. Extension to systemic sites is referred to as dissemination of the disease. Increasing the duration of time is referred to as prolongation of the disease. The period of time after exposure to an inanimate injury before a response is seen in the tissues is referred to as the latent period of a disease. For instance, the real extent of an electric burn is not evident in the tissues for at least a ten-day minimum period. The period of time after exposure to an infectious disease before the onset of symptoms is evident is termed the *incubation period* of the disease. Bacterial diseases have an incubation period measured in terms of days. Viral diseases have an incubation period measured in terms of weeks to months. The period of time required for the production of immunity is approximately ten to fourteen days.

The major systemic manifestations of disease are based on anatomic and physiologic interdependence. For example, anatomic interdependence would be muscle failure or paralysis following an injured nerve; organ or tissue failure following the interruption of the blood supply; and the failure of a secretory organ due to blockage of its excretory ducts. Examples of physiological interdependence are fluid and electrolyte imbalance and endocrine disturbance. When fluids accumulate in the tissues, we refer to this abnormality as edema. Edema may be due to the following etiologic factors: undernutrition, heart disease, kidney disease, and blockage of lymphatic vessels. All of these diseases are responsible for various forms of fluid imbalance leading to retention of fluids in the tissues. For instance, in chronic heart disease there may be an increased amount of blood in the lungs, liver, or spleen; this is termed *passive congestion*. As a result of massive traumas or injuries as well as burns, the damaged capillary bed retains large quantities of blood or permits leakage of fluid, thereby causing insufficient quantities of blood to be returned to the right side of the heart. The right and left ventricles fail, resulting in anoxia of all tissues. If intravenous blood (fluid) is not administered promptly, the result will be fatal. Widespread systemic impairment in the fluid and electrolyte balance occurs that is termed irreversible shock.

Endocrine glands (organs) are interrelated anatomically and physiologically. For instance, overactivity of the pituitary gland may at times be responsible for goiter (hyperthyroidism) and diabetes (hypoinsulinism). Goiter and diabetes mellitus may be influenced by adrenal secretions. The pituitary, adrenals, and thyroid glands probably alter their physiologic actions in all serious forms of diseases. The major responses due to systemic manifestations of disease are provided by the reticuloendothelial system and the endocrine organs acting with the help of the hypothalamus. The reticuloendothelial system is responsible for phagocytizing debris and foreign matter located in the lymphatic or vascular systems. This system responds to an infection in the tissues or organs by means of leucocytosis plus formation of immune bodies and lymphocytes. Leucocytosis is generally associated with fever. The pituitary and adrenal glands are related to the general adaptation syndrome (Selye). An increase in metabolic support is available to the human body under stress because of the alarm reaction that may be triggered by the release of adrenalin or ACTH from the pituitary gland.

Some cells and tissues may die and disappear. However, some tissues remain and undergo calcification with the potential to fatally obstruct a biliary or urinary passage. The replacement of cells in injured tissues may occur at a random rate until a benign or malignant neoplasm (tumor) results. Physiologic responses may become exaggerated or excessive and produce pathologic responses. All pathologic responses have their prototype in normal physiologic responses. Injury changes physiologic responses into pathologic responses. Pathology is, therefore, the result of an exaggeration of preceding physiologic responses (physiology under duress) or an exaggeration of preceding pathologic responses (pathology in excess).

References

Castiglioni, A.: *A History of Medicine.* New York, Knopf, 1941, p. 206.
MacCallum, W. G.: *Textbook of Pathology.* Philadelphia, Saunders, 1936.
Selye, H.: *Stress,* 1st ed. Montreal, Acta, 1950, pp. 5-51.
Singer, S.J. and Nicolson, G.L.: *Am J Pathol,* 65:427, 1971.
The Living Cell. Readings from *Scientific American.* San Francisco, Freeman, 1965.
Weinstein, R.S.: *N Engl J Med,* 281:86, 1969.

CHAPTER 2

CONGENITAL ANOMALIES AND HEREDITARY DISEASES

CONGENITAL ANOMALIES

CONGENITAL ANOMALIES result from hereditary defects in the germ plasma or from injuries occurring in the first three months of pregnancy. Congenital anomalies represent deficient cells available for development and maturation of the tissue or organ. One-half of 1 percent of all newborns in the United States have some type of severe congenital anomaly or malformation that is not compatible with life. Ninety percent of these newborns die within one year of birth. The incidence of serious congenital anomalies in living newborns in the United States is 1 percent. Nonfatal congenital anomalies (cataracts, deafness, defective dentition, cardiac anomalies) are acquired in the first three months of pregnancy from the following: German measles, radiation therapy or hypogonadism of the mother, incompatible blood groups between mother and child, prolonged periods of sterility (low fertility), and the elderly age of the mother (low fertility).

Congenital anomalies of the central nervous system are stated to be the most common. Most of these anomalies are incompatible with life and are present in stillborn infants. However, deformities of the extremities may be more prevalent than deformities of the central nervous system.

Heredity appears to influence the incidence of congenital anomalies since congenital anomalies are twenty-five times more common among siblings and other relatives compared to the general population. Whites have twice the number of congenital defects as blacks. When twins are born, 63 percent have some major congenital anomaly. For the most part, the major anomalies have a higher incidence in males than in females. Anencephaly is the exception, since it has a higher incidence in females.

Malformation of the central nervous system primarily results from an incomplete closure of the neural tube and its meningeal and osseous coverings. These nervous system anomalies are termed dysrhaphia or defective seam.

Hydrocephalus is a dysrhaphia characterized by dilated intracerebral ventricles containing cerebrospinal fluid. Anencephaly or arrested development of the brain is another dysrhaphia. Spina bifida or cranial bifida (failure in bony closure) with or without herniations of the meninges or neural tissue is still another dysrhaphia. Herniations may develop in the membranes of the spinal cord and are termed *meningocele* and *encephalocele*. Severe congenital anomalies incompatible with life may produce failure of closure of the neural tube, affecting the skull and spine and leaving the immature central nervous system completely exposed. The latter severe anomaly is called craniorachischisis. Less severe congenital anomalies show an open skull and immature brain, which is termed *cranioschisis*. The congenitally deformed brain is termed *anencephaly* and occurs in stillborns. Spina bifida occulta is a common asymptomatic congenital defect or dysrhaphia that requires no therapy. The spina bifida is due to the failure of fusion of spinal processes or fusion of laminae only. Spina bifida occulta occurs in 3 percent of the American adult population.

Rare forms of dysrhaphia include microcephaly, mongolism, idiocy, and cyclops. Cyclops is a failure of cleavage of the optic cup in stillborn infants.

Congenital anomalies commonly develop in the eye. An eye may be absent or small in size, and defects may be present in any optic structures. Increased pigmentation or melanosis or subnormal pigmentation (albinism) may be present. There may be congenital and hereditary strabismus, ptosis, cataracts, retinitis pigmentosa, and pathologic myopia.

Approximately 15 percent of all congenital anomalies occur in the gastrointestinal tract. A severe anomaly results from obstruction of the pylorus due to a hypertrophic muscle(s). Males are born with a large instance of pyloric stenosis. Obstruction of the intestines is approximately one-fourth as common as pyloric stenosis. Atresia is defined as an absence of a normal opening in the esophagus, stomach, anus, and bile ducts. A minor gastrointestinal congenital anomaly is Meckel's diverticulum (evagination of the ileum), which may produce symptoms similar to acute appendicitis. Megacolon, a rare congenital anomaly of the gastrointestinal tract, is the enlargement of the anatomic colon and persistence of the entire omphalomesenteric duct.

Cutaneomusculoskeletal defects occur in 11 percent of newborns in the United States. The three major defects are as follows: defects of the anterior body wall with evisceration of the heart or stomach and diaphragmatic hernias; inguinal or abnormal hernia; and harelip and cleft palate and maldevelopment of the extremities (club foot).

Inguinal hernia is the most common defect and generally affects males. Harelip and cleft palate are twice as common as congenital anomalies of the body wall, and maldevelopment of the extremities (club foot) constitutes 12 percent of anomalies.

Harelip and cleft palate have an approximate incidence of 1:1,000 to 1:2,000 or 1:3,000 live births. Thirty percent of individuals with this congenital anomaly have harelip alone, 20 percent have cleft palate, and 50 percent have both harelip and cleft palate. Other anomalies consist of defective ear cartilage and absence of one or more digits on the hand or foot.

Club foot (talipes equinovarus) has an incidence of 1:1,000 to 1:2,000 live births. It may be unilateral (43% of cases) or bilateral (57%). Club foot is frequently associated with spina bifida occulta and harelip. Club foot is probably inherited as a recessive sex-linked disease. Club foot is characterized by the following features: it is inverted, adducted, and plantar flexed; it has a small and elevated heel; and the forefoot is broad and twisted. The subject walks on the outside of the foot, causing development of bunions. Secondary pressure is referred to the bones of the club foot.

Congenital anomalies of the cardiovascular system represent 10 percent of all fatal congenital anomalies. The infants die within twelve years. Cardiovascular system congenital major anomalies consist of anomalies of the valves, narrowing of the aorta;

septal defects; transposition; overriding or stenosis of the great vessels, and patent ductus arteriosus. The patent foramen ovale is a minor congenital anomaly generally without any clinically significant findings.

Severe congenital malformations of the genitourinary system occur in approximately 0.1 percent of live births. A dysrhaphia of the urinary bladder is failure of closure of the urinary tract, termed *exstrophy of the bladder.* It occurs once in 50,000 births, and the urinary bladder drains into the surface of the abdomen. When the congenital anomaly consists of the urethra opening on the dorsal wall of the penis it is termed *epispadias;* if it opens on the ventral wall of the penis it is termed *hypospadias.* Complete absence of the bladder or a double bladder is an additional congenital anomaly. A congenital anomaly causing obstruction of the neck of the urinary bladder results in a very large or giant bladder at birth. Congenital stricture of the ureteropelvic or ureterovesical junctions is found in 5 percent of infants dying at or soon after birth. Complete absence of the urethra is incompatible with life.

Congenital anomalies of the genitourinary tract compatible with life include the following: double ureters, double pelvis, horseshoe kidney, ectopic kidney, and polycystic kidney.

Congenital anomalies develop firstly in man from arrested development or failure of proper differentiation after formation of the embryonic organ, and secondly due to an abnormal duplication of germinal tissue or an important early embryonic structure of a future organ. The majority of congenital anomalies in man are due to the first method described above. Generally, the anomaly is simply the persistence of an early phase of embryonic development of an organ that fails to reach its normal mature form. Other anomalies such as twinning, conjoined twins or monsters, and reduplication of organs are the result of the second method described above.

HEREDITARY DISEASE

Human species transmit certain characteristics from one generation to another through genes that are located in the chromatin material of the nucleus of germ cells. If the genes are abnormal or defective in some way, they have the capacity to pass on defective characteristics from one generation to another, and thus forming the basis of hereditary diseases in humans.

All body cells contain pairs of homologous chromosomes, one derived from each parent. If the chromosomes determine characteristics of the body, they are termed *dominant chromosomes;* if they fail to determine characteristics they are *recessive chromosomes.* Mendelian dominant refers to the presence of dominant chromosomes, and Mendelian recessive refers to the presence of recessive chromosomes. If both of the chromosomes determining characteristics of the body and occupying a single locus are either dominant or recessive, the chromosomes are referred to as homozygous. However, if one chromosome is dominant and one is negative occupying in a single locus, the chromosomes are referred to as heterozygous. The presence of the dominant gene means that the individual will have the dominant characteristic, regardless of whether the individual is homozygous or heterozygous. However, in hereditary diseases of man, most of the inherited diseases are determined by a dominant gene found in heterozygous individuals. If the hereditary abnormality is due to a recessive gene, the disease only becomes clinically apparent when the individual with the disease has a pair of homologous abnormal recessive genes (rare situation). The majority of individuals in a family will, therefore, be carriers of the abnormal recessive gene but will not have a clinical hereditary disease.

The following represent the four major forms of hereditary disease: Mendelian dominant traits, Mendelian recessive traits, sex-linked traits; and multiple allelomorphism. Mendelian dominant hereditary disease appears in heterozygous individuals; consecutive generations in one family are affected (one parent is affected) ; males and females have the same incidence; 50 percent of offspring are affected according to Mendel's law of heredity; normal parents do not transmit the disease; and the dominant hereditary defects are eliminated by the process of natural selection.

Examples of Mendelian dominant hereditary diseases of the central nervous system and eye include the following: Huntington's chorea, hereditary spastic paraplegia, neurofibromatosis, hereditary acoustic neurofibroma, myotonia congenita, polyneuritis, epilepsy, progressive muscular atrophy, familial periodic paralysis, tuberous sclerosis, arcus juvenilis, congenital cataract, myopia, congenital optic atrophy, angiomatosis of the retina, ectopia of the lens, congenital glaucoma, congenital ptosis, epicanthus, and retinoblastoma.

Examples of Mendelian dominant hereditary diseases of the skeletocutaneous system include the following: cleidocranial dysotosis, spina bifida, chondrodysplasia, osteogenesis imperfecta, syndactylism, brachydactylism, cervical rib, otosclerosis, Marfan's syndrome, Milroy's edema, hemorrhagic telangiectasis, urticaria, ichythyosis, keratosis palmaris and plantaris, ankylosing spondylitis, and club foot.

Examples of general Mendelian dominant hereditary diseases include the following: achlorhydria, sickle cell anemia or familial hemolytic anemia, atrophy of the adrenal with Addison's disease, goiter in cretins, and intestinal polyposis.

Mendelian recessive hereditary diseases contain the following characteristics: sporadic appearance in scattered generations of a family; affected individual has unaffected parents; appearance only in homozygous individuals; only one-fourth of a generation will have the disease; incidence is increased in the offspring when cousins marry; and survival of the recessive defect in evolution.

Mendelian recessive hereditary diseases exist and may be referred to as familial disease since they have a sporadic appearance. Mendelian recessive hereditary diseases of the central nervous system and eye include the following: Friedreich's ataxia, cerebellar ataxia, amaurotic familial idiocy, diffuse cerebral sclerosis, amytonia congenita, deaf-mutism, gargoylism, anencephaly, epilepsy, Schilder's disease (diffuse cerebral sclerosis), Wilson's disease (hepatolenticular degeneration), Mongolian idiocy, hypermetrophia, myopia, tapetoretinal degeneration, retinitis punctata albescens, choridermia, and gyrate atrophy of the retina.

Examples of Mendelian recessive hereditary diseases of the skeletocutaneous system include the following: chondromatosis, fragile bones, epidermolysis bullosa, albinism, club foot, club hand, harelip, cleft palate, torticollis, and xeroderma pigmentosum.

Examples of general Mendelian recessive hereditary diseases include the following: alkaptonuria, hypercholesteremia, angioneurotic edema, Mediterranean anemia (Cooley's anemia), celiac disease (fibrocystic disease of the pancreas), anaphylactoid purpura, Gaucher's disease, von Gierke's disease, Neimann-Pick's disease, fibrinopenia, porphyrinuria, and polymastia.

In each cell of humans, forty-seven of the forty-eight chromosomes present in the nucleus are similar in both male and female. The forty-eighth chromosome is the sex chromosome, termed Y in males and the X chromosome in females. A male receives the x chromosome from the mother and the Y chromosome from the father. A female receives an X chromosome from both mother and father. The additional genes located in the X and Y chromosomes are called sex-linked genes. Recessive defects present in the male are transmitted exclusively by females.

Sex-linked hereditary diseases have the following characteristics: Mendelian recessive; carried in the female, who does not exhibit the defect; transmitted to the male, who exhibits the anomaly because he has only one X chromosome; and theoretically possible (but rare) to have a dominant X abnormal trait or a dominant Y abnormal trait.

Examples of sex-linked hereditary diseases of the central nervous system and eye include the following: muscular dystrophy, optic atrophy (Leber's disease), color blindness, hemophilia, megalocornea, night blindness with myopia, choroideremia with blindness, extracortical aplasia, and retinitis pigmentosa.

Examples of sex-linked hereditary diseases of the skeletocutaneous system include the following: keratosis follicularis, baldness, and Heberden's nodes. An example of a general sex-linked hereditary disease is pseudohermaphroditism.

The following diseases represent examples of diseases with important hereditary predispositions: schizophrenia, organic and senile psychoses, migraine, diabetes mellitus, diabetes insipidus, mammary cancer, gastric cancer, thromboangiitis obliterans, arteriosclerosis, psoriasis, rheumatoid arthritis, osteoarthritis, gout, Heberden's nodes, hypertension, bronchiectasis, asthma, varicose veins, and hayfever.

There are three general classifications of hereditary disease based on evolution. Firstly, there are hereditary diseases that disappear, which are Mendelian dominant and incompatible with life. These hereditary diseases disappear if they are clinically manifested before mating. If the hereditary disease develops after maturity, it may persist, as in Huntington's chorea. Secondly, there are hereditary diseases that remain regardless of the principle of natural selection. These represent Mendelian recessive and sex-linked diseases that are capable of being carried and transmitted by normal people. Mendelian dominant diseases will not be eliminated by natural selection. Thirdly, new familial strains of hereditary disease occur in normal individuals from time to time due to mutation of the germ plasm.

Hereditary diseases of man might be increased in future generations as the amount of radiation being liberated is increased around the world. When experimental animals are exposed to irradiation, mutations can be produced along with new strains of hereditary diseases.

References

Bell, E.T.: *Renal Diseases,* 2nd ed. Philadelphia, Lea & Febiger, 1950.
Book, J.A.: *Hereditas, 34:*289, 1948.
Fogh-Andersen, P.: *Inheritance of Harelip, Cleft Palate.* Copenhagen, Arnold Busck, 1942.
Friendenwald, J.S., et al.: *Ophthalmic Pathology.* Philadelphia, Saunders, 1952.
Geschickter, C.F. and Copeland, M.M.: Branchogenic and other congenital cystic tumors of the neck. In Lewis, Dean (Ed.): Practice of Surgery. Hagerstown, Prior, 1955, vol. III.
Gould, S.E. (Ed.): *Pathology of Heart,* 1st ed. Springfield, Thomas, 1953.
Hicks, S.P.: *Arch Pathol, 57:*363-378, 1954.
——*Proc Soc Exp Biol Med, 75:*485-489, 1950.
Jelsma, F. and Ploetner, E.J.: *J Neurosurg, 10:*19, 1953.
Levine, A.: *Clinical Heart Disease,* 4th ed. Philadelphia, Saunders, 1951.
Murphy, D.P.: *Congenital Malformations,* Philadelphia, Lippincott, 1947.
Potter, E.L.: *Pathology of the Fetus and the Newborn.* Chicago, Year Bk Med, 1952.
Rolnick, H.C.: Anomalies and injuries of the bladder. *The Practice of Urology,* Philadelphia, Lippincott, 1949, vol. I.
Rolnick, H.C.: *The Practice of Urology.* Philadelphia, Lippincott, 1949, vol. I, 558.
Stockard, C.R.: *Am J Anat. 28:*115, 1921.
Wallace, H.M., et al.: *Pediatrics, 12:*526, 1953.

CHAPTER 3

PATHOLOGY OF CELL INJURY

VISIBLE AS well as invisible agents of injury are present in the pathologic aspect of injury. The results of the injury to tissues are generally seen in pathology, i.e. damage to tissue, defense of the tissue, and healing of the affected area in contrast to the etiologic agent causing the injury. In a small number of pathologic processes, histopathologic examination may reveal the presence of fungi, spirochetes, bacilli, or cocci as the result of histochemical staining reagents and techniques. Inanimate substances, i.e. sutures, silica, dust, asbestos fibers, and other foreign bodies may be recognized by histopathologic examination and the use of polarized light. Clinicopathologic conferences relating clinical history, physical examination, and clinical laboratory results are all vital to the differential diagnosis because the agents of disease disappear rapidly from the tissues.

There are single determinant causes of disease and death, i.e. overwhelming physical force, extreme heat or cold, potent poisons, and the rapid deprivation of oxygen and fluids all produce fatality. All of the influences predisposing to and prior to the development of the immediate cause or causes of disease are referred to as remote, distant, or preparatory etiologic factors of disease. For instance, burns, traumatic wounds, and allergies may join with bacterial invasion of tissues to initiate an infectious disease. Therefore, various injurious agents may be additive in producing disease. For instance, starvation increases the individual's predisposition to infection by tuberculosis. Deficiencies of various minerals weaken bone tissue, and a fracture results. In other words, more than one noxious agent may operate in order to produce a disease. Added insults will increasingly impair a single organ or tissue.

A series of injuries to an organ may produce a single lesion or disease by adding to the initial (original) degree of impairment. In this situation, the additional injury or injuries cause an exacerbation of the primary or original impairment.

Psychosomatic factors are one of the most common contributing factors in disease. The following are examples of diseases with structural alterations that may be influenced by emotional stress: peptic ulcer in the stomach or duodenum, irritable colon or mucous colitis, palpitation and cardiac arrythmias, exacerbations in rheumatoid arthritis, chronic skin diseases (eczema), and asthma. The greatly increasing use of tranquilizers, psychoanalysis, and hypnosis demonstrates the importance of the psychomatic component of human diseases.

SCOPE OF INJURY

Agents of injury to the body are nonselective or selective in nature in accordance with the local site of the damage produced. The nonselective agents of injury may damage any living tissue in man. Examples are extremes of mechanical force and temperature, corrosive poisons and severe degrees of anoxia, metabolic deprivations, and determinant single causes of disease or death. There is no specific affinity between the agent of injury and tissue affected.

Numerous injuries, however, have an affinity for a specific tissue or particular organ. For instance, some chemical substances exhibit a specific affinity, and this property is referred to as selective toxicity. Viruses show a selective affinity for tissues and are referred to as neurotropic, dermatotropic, hepatotropic, pneumotropic, or viscerotropic viruses. The absence of specific vitamins shows a selective affinity. Lack of vitamin D causes injuries to skeletal tissues. Lack of vitamin B_1 produces harm to the peripheral nerves. Lack of vitamin B_{12} injures the blood-forming tissues of the body, and the absence of vitamin A is harmful to the eyes.

Ionizing radiation shows selective toxicity. Some organs are radiosensitive (most readily damaged). Other organs are radioresponsive (damaged by higher dosage), and still other organs are radioresistant (resist the effect of ionizing irradiation).

Rickettsial infections attack the endothelial cells of small blood vessels. Bacterial and mycotic infections damage both the parenchyma and stromal tissues.

Aging of tissues and organs in the human body is highly selective and may be considered a negative injury to the body. The aging of the human body begins with the ovarian follicles, which contain viable ova. The viable ova undergo obliteration in females forty-five to fifty years of age. However, the testicles remain viable showing very active spermatogenesis in males up to and even beyond eighty years of age. After thirty years of age, the aging process begins in the articular cartilages of the larger joints of the lower extremities as well as in the intervertebral discs and the internal elastic lamellae of the coronary and cerebral arteries and the aorta, which may split and fragment in young adults.

Diseases of man are generally described as local and systemic; thus a distinction is made in pathology between damage or injury to a single organ compared to a series of major organs in the body. Systemic diseases of man affect numerous major organs and tissues in the body. On the other hand, local diseases affect a single structure by very selective injury to the kidney, heart, or blood vessels. A local disease may cause damage to all of the structures of a single organ. An example occurs in pancarditis, whereby the heart becomes injured as a result of rheumatic fever. All tissues, i.e. the endocardium, myocardium, and pericardium, suffer damage. Another example is pyelonephritis, where damage takes place in all structures of a single kidney. It is, however, possible for an injury to occur in only one structure within one organ. An example is glomerulonephritis, where damage is present only in the glomeruli of the kidney. In syphilis, the aortic valve and the opening of the coronary arteries are selectively damaged by the disease while the myocardium and pericardium both escape injury. Syphilis, in its late stages, damages other organs while it is selective in its injury to two areas of the heart. In modern pathology, the student understands that specific disease processes may produce injury to numerous different organic systems in the human body.

In most pathologic processes, the damage caused to tissues and organs is directly proportional to the quantity and intensity of the noxious agents attacking the body. For instance, in mechanical injury or traumatic experiences, the tissue damage that results is directly proportional to the amount of force present in the trauma divided by the overall area of contact. Another example occurs in thermal damage to tissue, where the degree of the burn is directly proportional to the degree of temperature times the duration of tissue exposure. Irradiation produces damage to the tissues in proportion to the dose of irradiation. Drugs injure tissues in direct proportion to the dosage of the drug administered. In infectious diseases, the damage to tissues and organs is proportional to the quantity of pathogenic microorganisms times their virulence. In general, the less intensity exhibited by the noxious etiological agents of disease, the greater the chance that the tissue and organ damage will be of a reversible nature. However, when severe intensity is exhibited by noxious agents of disease, the tendency is to produce irreversible tissue damage with death of the tissue or organ. The exception to the latter observation in pathology occurs in hypersensitivity reactions, where a small dosage of an allergen to which the individual has been previously sensitized may provoke the most severe reaction possible, and death.

The type of injury resulting from a noxious agent is proportional to the duration of time in which the agent is active within the body. Injury may be classified by duration into the following forms: acute, chronic, and perpetual injuries. Trauma or physical violence is an example of an acute injury. A foreign body lodged in the tissues is an example of a more chronic physical injury. The injury provoked by ultraviolet light is directly proportional to the duration of exposure and to the quantity of tissue exposed. Industrial chemicals may require prolonged periods of exposure of small amounts of the chemical before signs and symptoms of injury are evident. Some poisons, on the other hand, produce acute injury and death.

Infectious diseases may be classified into acute, subacute, and chronic forms. Many infectious diseases of man are rather persistent and, therefore, chronic in nature. For example, the following represent chronic infectious diseases of man: tuberculosis, syphilis, yaws, leprosy, and malaria. Allergic diseases of man are chronic in nature. Hay fever, asthma, and rheumatoid arthritis are allergic diseases that persist for forty to fifty years or more. When a disease shows extreme chronicity, it indicates that the etiologic agent has a prolonged effect on the body. Perpetual injuries are those injuries that affect human tissues for the life of an individual. An example is silica, which causes perpetual damage to tissues. The silica, once it becomes lodged in the lung tissue, remains there for the life of the individual, and the lung tissue can never be restored to normal function. Silica causes a perpetual fibrosis of the lung. Radioactive materials that gain entrance into the human body remain active for the lifetime of the individual, causing perpetual injury. Uranium and radioactive isotopes are examples of substances causing perpetual injury to the human body. The radioactive isotopes do diminish in intensity, due to a short half-life; the duration of radiation in the tissues is perpetual and continues to exist to infinity as smaller quantities are measured and a perpetually diseased state of an organ exists for the life of the individual. Perpetual injury to tissues is the basis for understanding the pathologic processes present in cirrhosis of the liver, chronic nephritis, and in neoplasia (cancer).

Bacteria and parasites may demonstrate geographical or seasonal variation in the incidence of prevalence of the disease they produce in man. For instance, malaria occurs in the tropical countries or tropical climates; streptococcal infections are prevalent in cold climates; rheumatic diseases are more common in cold and damp climates; amebic dysentery occurs in Mexico, Central and South America; and iodine deficiency develops in landlocked areas and mountainous areas.

Seasonal influences play a role in the causation of disease. For instance, pneumonia is common in the winter and spring; typhoid and enteric fevers occur in the summer and early fall; and poliomyelitis was a disease of late summer. Allergic diseases commonly occur in late spring and late summer because pollens are present in these seasons.

References

Adrien, A.: *Selective Toxicity*. Methuen's Monograph on Biochemical Subjects. London, Methuen and New York, Wiley, 1951.

Gray, A. and Doniach, I.: *J Clin Pathol, 23*:608, 1970.

Iseri, O.A. and Gottlieb, L.S.: *Gastroenterology, 60*:102, 1971.

Long, E.R.: *A History of Pathology*. Baltimore, Williams and Wilkins, 1928, p. 63.

McNally, W.D.: *Toxicology*. Chicago, Industrial Medicine, 1937, p. 987.

Minot, A.S. and Cutler, J.T.: *Am J Physiol, 93*:674, 1930.

Reynolds, E.S. and Ree, H.J.: *Lab Invest, 25*:269, 1971.

Trump, B.F., et al.: *Proc Natl Acad Sci, 66*:433, 1970.

Wolman, M.: *Pigments in Pathology*. New York, Acad Pr, 1969.

CHAPTER 4

RETROGRADE CELLULAR ALTERATIONS AND INFILTRATIONS (CELL DEATH)

INTRODUCTION

THE INDIVIDUAL cell of the human body has been considered the unit of the pathologic process. When noxious agents cause disease in a part of the body, it is the component units (cells) that are altered. The student of pathology must realize that impairment due to alteration of the cell is the initial or primary point of all disease processes. Cellular units of the body consist of protoplasm, which has the ability to be in a solid or liquid state. Protoplasm is a gel (colloidal material), which is composed of carbohydrates, lipids, proteins, and inorganic ions. The components of the cell include the following protoplasmic structures: nucleus, nucleolus, chromosomes, mitochondria, golgi apparatus, aster and spindle fibers. The nucleus and cytoplasm of the cell are enclosed in a semipermeable membrane through which water, nutritional materials, and waste products may pass.

When alterations occur in the cell, it indicates that changes have taken place in the protoplasm as a reaction to injury. Injured or damaged nuclei condense, break up, or simply disappear. Condensation of the nucleus is referred to as pyknosis. Nuclear disruption is referred to as karyorrhexis, and nuclear dissolution is karyolysis. The cytoplasm of cells may increase its water content and form a hydrosol, an alteration in the normal gel state of cytoplasm. If the cell absorbs or imbibes a modest quantity of water, the cell is said to undergo cloudy swelling. However, if the cell imbibes an extreme quantity of water, the cell is said to have undergone hydropic degeneration. Injured cells may contain increased quantities of fat, and the cells are said to have undergone fatty change or fatty metamorphosis. Cells may succumb to injury and become liquid in nature; these cells are said to have undergone liquefaction necrosis. When cells die, their protoplasm may be transformed from a colloidal substance into a solid gel; these cells are said to have undergone coagulation necrosis. The cell outlines are destroyed during liquefaction and coagulation necrosis.

Retrograde cellular alterations are, therefore, forms of protoplasmic damage, i.e. degeneration and necrosis. Degeneration refers to reversible forms of protoplasmic alterations. Necrosis refers to irreversible forms of protoplasmic change. Atrophy is the gross decrease in the size of an organ due to a decrease in either the number or the size of cells. Atrophy is not caused by primary or direct impairment of cells but is rather a secondary impairment caused by many factors that all interfere with nourishment of the organ.

The retrograde reversible forms of alteration are, of course, less serious in nature than the irreversible forms that produce secondary impairments. Therefore, cloudy swelling and hydropic degeneration are simply phases of reversible retrograde alterations, whereas liquefaction and coagulation necrosis are irreversible retrograde alterations. Prior to either the reversible or irreversible retrograde alteration, there is an early phase known as the chemical lesion, i.e. an invisible chemical change in the injured cell not recognizable by gross or microscopic examination. An example are sperm cells irradiated with small doses of irradiation, which show no microscopic changes, yet monstrosities are produced by the fertilized ovum.

Alterations in the structure of cells undergoing retrograde cellular alterations mean that functional impairment has taken place. Therefore, all forms of response of cells to injury actually begin with a decrease of or the loss of a vital physiologic process, and the very initial chemical degree of depletion is generally not visible by gross or microscopic examination. Cells of tissues and organs are surrounded by body fluids supplied by the blood. Damage to cellular units, therefore, also encompasses corresponding secondary alterations in the distribution of tissue fluids and blood. For instance, the color, size, and consistency of an organ are due to the proportions of parenchyma (cellular), stroma (cellular), and blood and tissue fluids (interstitial). Any alterations in the proportion of the latter four constituents may produce gross changes in the organ, which are characteristic of the disease upon gross examination by the pathologist. Alterations in the distribution of blood in the organs generally mean that secondary impairment or defense has taken place. An example is hemorrhage in an organ following alterations in the blood vessels. Hemorrhage is followed by hyperemia (congestion), a situation whereby an excess of blood accumulates in an organ, generally as a secondary effect of inflammation or heart failure. Edema refers to an abnormal increase in the quantity of interstitial fluid in the tissue or organ. Edema is generally secondary to nutritional deficiencies or circulatory alterations. The edema fluid present during infectious diseases contains leukocytes in the inflammatory exudate.

REVERSIBLE FORMS OF RETROGRADE CELLULAR ALTERATIONS IN THE PARENCHYMATOUS TISSUES
Cloudy Swelling (Albuminous Degeneration)

Cloudy swelling or albuminous degeneration is the most common reversible retrograde alteration characterized by retention of water in injured cells. There is an alteration in the normal colloidal gel of the cytoplasm in which the solid particles are clumped together, becoming visible upon microscopic examination. Microscopically, the cytoplasm of cells with cloudy swelling have a swollen, ground-glass appearance with clumps of particles. The organs affected by cloudy swelling have the following gross appearance; pale, swollen, and opaque, with a parboiled appearance. The kidney, liver, and pancreas show cloudy swelling following an infection with high fever or in patients who succumb to heat stroke or poisoning. Cloudy swelling affects the mitochondria of the cell and may readily be separated from the cytoplasm by centrifugation.

If intracellular edema is advanced, the cells become distended by fluid, and the cytoplasm becomes empty in microscopic sections. This situation is termed *hydropic degeneration of cells*. It is a reversible form of retrograde change, and the cells remain viable and have the capacity to recover to their physiologic state.

Fatty Change (Fatty Metamorphosis)

Fatty change or fatty metamorphosis is a reversible retrograde alteration, i.e. a stage of impairment that follows cloudy swelling or hydropic degeneration. Fatty change is generally found in the liver and results from a deficiency of lipotropic substances in the protein portion of the diet. The lipid is not capable of converting fats to phospholipids prior to transporting the lipids to other tissues and organs. The deficiency involves the following lipotropic substances: cystine, choline, and methionine, which provide sulfur and methyl groups to organs and tissues. Fatty change of the liver results from the inability to metabolize excessive fat when sulfur and methyl groups are exhausted due to a high fat diet, following poisoning, or during starvation.

What fat is visible in the cells of an organ that normally metabolizes the fat, the situation is called fatty metamorphosis, fatty phanerosis, or fatty change. When fat is visible between mesenchymal cells, as occurs in obesity, the situation is termed fatty deposition. When the fat is deposited in fibers in the stroma of organs or in muscle, it is referred to as fatty infiltration because it is not normally observed in these latter sites. An example is fat in the scarred heart muscle of the aged.

Reversible Vascular Alterations—Vasodystonia

Early secondary alterations occur in the endothelium of blood vessels adjacent to an area of primary injury in living tissues. Vasodystonia means a reversible form of alteration of the endothelium, causing impairment of the blood vessels. The endothelium or lining cells bulge or undergo spiking as they project into the lumen of the blood vessel. Spiking of endothelium leads to increased vessel permeability. The endothelial linings lose their normally repellent characteristics for thrombocytes, leukocytes, and erythrocytes, and endothelial stickiness ensues. In capillaries and venules the reversible vasodystonia initiates inflammation accompanied by transient vasoconstriction, then vasodilatation, intraluminal bulging of endothelium, and increased permeability of vessels. The endothelial alteration leads to passage of plasma and to emigration of leukocytes from the blood. The increased stickiness of the vascular endothelial cells with a loss of its normally repellent characteristic toward the platelets is the initial step in the alterations responsible for intravascular clotting (thrombosis).

Vasodystonia is due to vascular alteration and damage caused by injurious agents. It is well established that capillary endothelial cells are altered as a result of immediate damage caused by the injury and that the endothelial damage directly increases the permeability of the vessel wall. Vasodystonia generally is followed by inflammation and is a secondary impairment because the damage in the adjacent tissues causes the release of histamine and other substances, and axone reflexes are active upon the vessel wall. The formation of antibodies in infectious diseases may sensitize the endothelial cells of capillaries so that, if the proper antigen makes contact with the tissues a second time, these small capillaries become blocked due to thrombosis plus necrosis of the endothelial cells. The formation of thrombi and necrosis of endothelium is known as the Arthus phenomenon.

Impairment of the vascular system either following direct injury to capillaries and arterioles or by secondary impairment universally occurs if tissue is damaged that contains a blood supply. The blood supply is the major connection between the tissue responses to an injury and the local protective reactions that develop against the impairment, such as inflammation, thrombosis, and resolution.

REVERSIBLE ALTERATIONS IN CONNECTIVE TISSUES
Mucinous Degeneration

Connective tissue has been described in courses in histology or microscopic anatomy as a continuous matrix that varies greatly in its consistency. Connective tissues range from the limpid Wharton's jelly of the umbilical cord to the hardness of bone, in which there is incorporated an interlacing fabric of various kinds of fibers. The continuous matrix (connective tissue) is present in the spaces between organs and major vessels and supplies the capsule that surrounds the organs' major structures plus their supporting stroma. The fibers that make up collagen, reticulin, or elastica are composed of precipitated scleroproteins embedded in a form of mucin, i.e. a matrix of mucopolysaccharides. During pathologic processes, alterations may develop in connective tissues of organs and tissues affecting both the mucopolysaccharide ground substance and the fibrillary scleroproteins. The ground substance of connective tissue is hydrophilic, thus retaining water and absorbing electrolytes. Water is absorbed by connective tissues by hydration. The wetting of connective tissues, which have the greatest mass of collagen fibers in the body, is the first process used in the tanning industry when preparing leather for hardening by various tanning agents. The wetting process in connective tissues occurs in the following stages:

1. swelling or plumping whereby the fibrils remain intact (reversible);

2. swelling and absorption of water or salt-swelling in which the fibers are divided into fibrils and a loose fibrous texture is present (partially reversible); and

3. collagen fibers are completely dissolved and replaced by gelatin (irreversible).

In pathology, if the connective tissue becomes loose and edematous, it is termed *myxomatous change, myxedema,* or *mucoid degeneration.* These conditions are compared with the Wharton's jelly of the umbilical cord. Various pathologic conditions may produce reversible wetting or hydration of connective tissue. Reversible wetting of connective tissue accompanied by depolymerization of the polysaccharide matrix occurs in hyperimmune states, i.e. rheumatoid arthristis and hypothyroidism. Hydration of connective tissue in thyroid deficiency is myxedema. A severe but reversible change in the ground substance of connective tissues is present when vitamin C deficiency or scurvy develops. Ascorbic acid (vitamin C) is required for the production of matrix and fibrils by the fibroblasts. Deficient ascorbic acid results in resorption of the matrix of bone, cartilage, and endothelium. The condition is reversible by the administration of vitamin C.

In pathologic processes accompanied by hyperparathyroidism there is depolymerization of matrix with an increase in the quantity of serum glycoproteins. Calcium and phosphorus are released as the mineral-binding capacity of the matrix is decreased, resulting in deposits of calcium and phosphorus in different organs. The mineral deposits of calcium and phosphorus are termed *metastatic calcifications*. The calcifications, however, are reversible if the hyperparathyroid condition is reversed. In hypersensitivity states that accompany the collagen diseases, i.e. acute rheumatic fever, rheumatoid arthritis, disseminated lupus erythematosus and polyarteritis, the matrix of connective and vascular tissues is altered, causing permeability and leakage from blood vessels, with edema developed in the stroma. Early edematous changes in hypersensitivity states are reversible; however, if the hypersensitivity persists, irreversible alterations ensue such as fibrinoid degeneration and rheumatoid nodules. The latter two situations subsequently become the seat of dystrophic calcification as calcareous deposits develop in the degenerations.

The hydration of the ground substance of connective tissue is a reversible pathologic process called mucinolysis. The hydration or wetting of connective tissue by mucinolysis splits the reticulin and collagen fibers that function in the transmission of tension through the connective tissue. The liberated fibroblasts, now free of stress, lie in a fluid matrix that permits their proliferation and de-differentiation into histiocytes and macrophages. The alteration in the connective tissues may stimulate resolution and fibroblastic repair of the injured tissue.

Mucoid Degeneration of Epithelial Structures

Inflamed or irritated epithelium lining the respiratory or gastrointestinal tract causes these membranes to secrete greatly increased quantities of mucin, which is stored in the lumen of these structures. This situation is termed *mucoid degeneration;* however, it represents a form of hyperfunction or a defensive process. Mucin may be produced and liberated in great excesses in some glandular tissues, which become the site of a neoplasm. The malignant cell of the neoplasm breaks up and discharges mucin into the supporting stroma. The neoplasm is said to have undergone a gelatinous change in its character.

LEUKOCYTIC IMPAIRMENT OR ALTERATION

Leukocytes are altered when they rid the tissues and organs of noxious particles by means of phagocytosis. Some leukocytes undergo liquefaction necrosis upon attacking and phagocytizing virulent forms of microorganisms. Other viable leukocytes filled with phagocytized but undigested microorganisms are carried in the lymphatic vessels to regional lymph nodes. In the lymph nodes, other phagocytes cannibalize the circulating phagocytes with their microorganisms; some may be vital, some may be dead. The circulating phagocytes, therefore, carry the microorganisms away from the infected tissue and spread these living or dead agents to the regional lymph nodes. If macrophages attack a large foreign substance in the tissues, they must initially fuse together, forming a giant cell composed of one mass of cytoplasm with multiple nuclei. The fused giant cells are viable and mobile, and the process by which each cell is formed is irreversible, i.e. they cannot revert to separate macrophages.

NECROSIS

If injured tissues die prior to the death of the individual, their cells deteriorate, dissolve, or slough off. The irreversible destruction of tissues and organs is called necrosis and refers to both the gross and microscopic appearance of the tissue. Gangrene means massive necrosis or death of a part en masse. If the necrotic tissue becomes desiccated and shrunken into a dry, dead substance, it is termed *dry gangrene*. If the necrotic tissue undergoes putrefaction by invasion of the dead tissue by saprophytic organisms, causing partial liquefaction necrosis, the situation is termed *wet gangrene*. If ischemic tissue in an organ dies and the necrotic tissue remains as a firm and swollen region, it is termed *infarction*. If a rather large portion of the liver dies, it is transformed into a soft, yellow red material. If the latter process proceeds rapidly it is called acute yellow atrophy of the liver. When this same process occurs slowly it is called acute red atrophy of the liver. *Atrophy* is generally used here to indicate a shrinkage of the tissue or organ due to deficient nourishment. In the hepatic situation, the pathologic process is that of massive necrosis rather than atrophy.

Microscopic findings are present during necrosis and in intracellular lesions. Pyknosis means the condensation of the nucleus in a dying cell. Karyorrhexis means the breaking up of the nucleus of a cell. Karyolysis means the cell has gradually faded out. If a virus enters and injures a cell, the cytoplasm swells; this is termed *ballooning*. When liquefaction necrosis occurs in the cytoplasm of cells, this is termed *reticulosis*. The viral bodies and the precipitated cytoplasmic material in infected cells are termed *inclusion bodies*. When epithelial cells are injured in the liver and kidney, droplets of precipitated protein accumulate in the cell protoplasm prior to development of coagulation necrosis. Precipitated protein in the cytoplasm is an irreversible change termed *hyalin droplet degeneration*.

When cells, tissues, or organs die, the alterations that ensue are related to the presence or absence of enzyme systems in the necrotic tissue. For instance, if some of the enzyme systems survive, the necrotic tissue may be digested and liquefied by these enzyme systems, resulting in liquefaction necrosis. When, however, the enzyme systems are completely destroyed, the necrotic tissue produces a coagulation necrosis. Examples of liquefaction necrosis are a blister following a superficial burn, purulent exudate in an abscess, and peptic ulcers caused by the digestion of the mucosa of the stomach or duodenum. Examples of coagulation necrosis are eschar of deep burns, infarcts, and diphtheritic membranes where fibrin and dead cells are overlying a superficial ulceration.

Coagulation necrosis may be followed by the splitting up of lipids within the necrotic tissue. The latter results in a coagulum containing abundant fats and having the gross appearance of cheese. This form of necrosis is called caseation necrosis and is present in tuberculosis and syphilis. Caseation necrosis is primarily a special form of coagulation necrosis. The caseation necrosis generally develops in inflamed tissues or organs where dense collections of histiocytes or macrophages are present and the mass is avascular.

Enzyme systems present within dead cells or following their alteration by another enzyme system must attack the dead elements of the injured tissue in order to produce necrosis of tissue.

Enzyme systems (heterolytic) arising from other tissues migrate to the site of dead elements of the injured tissue by way of the circulating fluids or from the leukocytes that migrate into the injured tissue. The presence of the leukocytes in the injured tissue predisposes this tissue to dissolution.

Fat necrosis is irreversible death of cells in fatty tissue. The lipid constituent of fatty tissue is split by lipase into free fatty acids and glycerol. Fat necrosis occurs in the greater or lesser peritoneal cavities due to pancreatic diseases, which permit lipase in the pancreatic juice to pass into the adjacent structures and split up the fatty tissue.

Pathologic calcification occurs when dead tissues in the body become the site of deposition of calcium salts. Calcium salts are normally in solution as complex phosphate-carbonate salts, are readily precipitated in injured and necrotic tissues. The precipitated calcium salts are fixed in the decomposed tissues by some obscure mechanism. Examples of pathologic calcifications are calcification of the arteries and calcification of scarred tubercles in tuberculosis. Another entirely different type of pathologic calcification is termed *dystrophic calcification,* which is associated with alterations in the parathyroid glands. If hyperfunctioning parathyroid glands are present, the blood serum contains supersaturated calcium salts, and these calcium salts may be deposited in the normal epithelium of the stomach and kidney. Such hyperfunctioning of the parathyroid glands may be the result of an adenoma. Secondary hyperplasia of the parathyroid glands may follow the development of rickets, whereby the normal absorption of calcium through the gastrointestinal tract is altered. Metastatic calcification may form following the administration of excessive amounts of vitamin D in children. The excessive vitamin D increases calcium absorption in the gastrointestinal tract and increases secretion of phosphorus in the urine. Metastatic calcification produces kidney stones; it develops in the mucosa of the stomach, in the thyroid gland, and in the lungs. In these organs there is development of a local alkaline tissue following the excretion of acid, and thus, the excess calcium salts precipitate in the alkaline tissue residue.

Putrefaction is another type of liquefaction necrosis. *Clostridium welchii, Clostridium septicum,* and *Clostridium aedema-*

tiens infect and putrefy the necrotic tissue, forming liquefaction of cells and gas. The formation of gas and liquefaction of cells in necrosis is termed *gas gangrene*.

Hyaline necrosis or hyalinization is another irreversible alteration (necrosis) that develops in mesenchymal tissues. It may form as droplets of precipitated protein in epithelial cells. Hyalinization may develop in collagen fibers. When present, the collagen takes a bright pink stain with eosin, and the gross feature is a glassy appearance to affected tissues or organs. Hyalinization develops in old scar tissue, in the basement membrane of respiratory epithelial cells during chronic inflammation, and in nonvital glomeruli of the kidney. During typhoid fever, the muscle fibrils have a glassy appearance termed *Zenker's hyalinization*. Thrombi may have a glassy appearance in small blood vessels and thus are referred to as hyaline thrombi.

Amyloid is a special form of hyaline, i.e. it turns black when stained with iodine and covered with sulfuric acid. Amyloid also stains differentially with Congo red or cresyl violet. Amyloid affects the collagen fibers of the liver, spleen, and kidney and is termed *secondary amyloidosis*. The secondary form of amyloid develops after a very long-standing suppurative pathologic process such as tuberculosis, bronchiectasis, and chronic osteomyelitis. During amyloidosis, precipitated material composed of a complex of polysaccharides of globulin is secreted by macrophages in the presence of immune bodies. The early formation of amyloid takes place within the histiocytes or macrophages. Any pathologic process capable of elevating the globulin or protein component of tissue fluids above the normal levels predisposes to development of amyloidosis. The amyloid is, therefore, a special product liberated by dying macrophages or histiocytes and is consistent with the retrograde cellular alterations and infiltrations. Multiple myeloma is an example of a disease that elevates the globulin or protein content of tissue fluids and thus predisposes to amyloidosis.

Hyaline necrosis (hyalinization) and amyloidosis are due to an irreversible alteration in the ground substance of connective tissues. It is entirely possible that the high globulin composition in the matrix of the connective tissue, associated with a vitamin C deficiency, may be responsible for the amyloid alteration, i.e. a severe disturbance of local metabolism of protein.

Primary amyloidosis is a rare infiltration of amyloid in the skin, heart, bones, tongue, larynx, and joints. Primary amyloidosis is of obscure etiology. The liver may be infiltrated with amyloid and has a pale, hard, and enlarged appearance, i.e. a lardaceous or amyloid liver. Infiltration of the spleen with amyloid results in a glistening, translucent spleen. Deposits of amyloid may occur in the region of the malpighian bodies of the spleen, and this situation is described as sago spleen. When the kidneys contain amyloid infiltrations they become pale, firm, and enlarged. The renal infiltrations of amyloid occur within the vascular loops or in Bowman's capsule about the glomeruli.

Fibrinoid necrosis is an irreversible retrograde alteration of obscure etiology. Fibrinoid necrosis consists of a coagulum affecting the ground substance and collagen fibers of the connective tissue in the hypersensitivity conditions, i.e. acute rheumatic fever, rheumatoid arthritis, and collagen diseases.

Somatic death is the death of an individual as the result of the failure of several vital organ systems (cardiovascular, respiratory, central nervous system). Somatic death is to be distinguished from cell death, which does not kill the individual. The majority of injured cells and tissues causing impairment of function are irreversible alterations, but they are not fatal to the individual. The body's defensive mechanism is capable of removing the dead tissue, and the area is replaced with scar tissue (repair) or by regenerated parenchyma (regeneration). Somatic death, however, occurs promptly when the vital organ systems cease to function. Loss of body heat occurs soon after death. Rigidity of the voluntary muscles (rigor mortis) occurs within twelve hours following death and disappears in three to four days. Signs of somatic death are important in the event of medical emergencies happening in the hospital or medical office. Failure of respiration in a patient during a medical emergency can be determined by holding a mirror in front of the nose to look for condensation of moisture, or by a wisp of cotton to detect air currents. Cessation of the heart beat can be detected by using a stethoscope placed over the precordium.

PATHOLOGIC PIGMENTATIONS

The normal color of organs and tissues together with their size and consistency is a cardinal morphological feature used by the pathologist in judging the presence of pathologic processes. If the blood supply to an organ is increased, the color becomes redder or darker. However, when there is a diminished blood supply, the organ becomes pale, shrunken, and is described as ischemic. If the quantity of interstitial fluid in any organ becomes increased, it develops a pale, swollen, and limpid appearance.

Abnormal pigmentations in tissues and organs have been given an important connotation in pathology. The most vital pigmentations in pathology are produced by the following endogenous pigments in the human body: melanin, hemoglobin, lipochrome, and myoglobin.

Metals produce pigmentation in the tissues. Silver compounds that are used in pharmacology and therapeutics may be deposited in the corium of the human skin. The latter clinical pigmentation is termed *argyria*. The pigmentation of argyria consists of a slate gray color in the skin, which becomes intensified and darkened following exposure to ultraviolet sunlight. Compounds containing mercury may be applied topically to the skin, or mercury salts may be introduced by tatooing in the skin, producing localized areas of a gray color due to the presence of mercury. Ingestion of lead or bismuth is responsible for production of a black line in the gingiva, which is caused by deposition of lead or bismuth sulfide in the submucosal tissue. Rarely, gold salts used in the treatment of arthritis may produce chrysiasis, a slate gray color in the skin and mucous membranes due to deposits of gold. Radioactive gold has been used for the treatment of cancerous implants in serous cavities.

Carotinemia is a condition of the skin whereby it is stained a yellow color caused by an excess of carotinoid pigments. The excessive carotinoid pigments come from foods (carrots, which are rich in provitamin A) or are due to the improper transformation of carotene to vitamin A in the liver. During advanced pituitary diseases, e.g. in Simmond's disease or pituitary cachexia, there is a defect in the conversion of carotene to vitamin A in the liver. In castrated individuals there is also an improper conversion of carotene to vitamin A in the liver.

Anthracosis is caused by inhaled dust if it contains carbon. Black deposits of carbon occur in the lungs and mediastinal lymph nodes. Siderosis produces a rusty red color in the lungs and mediastinal lymph nodes if iron dust is inhaled. Carbon and iron dust pigments are generally harmless and do not induce pathology. However, if the inhaled dust contains silica dust, which is found in hard coal mines, pathological processes will take place in the lungs and mediastinal lymph nodes.

Dirt is the most common exogenous pigment in man. Dirt may accumulate in rough portions of the skin when soap and water cannot be used daily.

The two most vital abnormal endogenous pigmentations in man are melanin and hemoglobin. Increased deposition of melanin pigment occurs in the skin during the following diseases: Addison's disease, neurofibromatosis, malignant melanoma, benign melanoma, and hemochromatosis. The skin of the Negro and Indian races (Eastern and Western) normally has increased melanin compared to the Caucasian.

Blood pigments arise when red blood cells disintegrate. The nonglobulin part of the hemoglobin is broken down into hemosiderin and hematoidin. Hemosiderin, a polymer of ferric hydroxide, stains deep blue when treated with potassium ferrous cyanide and hydrochloric acid. This reaction is termed *Perl's reaction*. Hemosiderin may appear in macrophages in twenty-four to thirty-six hours following a hemorrhage in experimental animals. In man, hemosiderin may appear on the third day following hemorrhage. Hemosiderin forms golden brown (unstained) granules, free or within phagocytes. Hemosiderin is present in the lungs during chronic congestive heart failure and also in the liver during hemosiderosis and hemochromatosis after repeated hemolysis of red blood cells. Hemosiderin may also be located in areas of old hemorrhages.

Hematoidin is a brownish pigment excreted in the bile as bilirubin. It is iron free and is the vital pigment involved in jaundice. Hematoidin is produced by reticuloendothelial cells from destroyed red blood cells. Hematoidin is removed from the bile circulation by hepatic cells and excreted by the bile ducts to the intestines, where it is converted into urobilinogen by the action of bacteria. Half of the urobilinogen is resorbed and used to form additional hemoglobin. The other half of the urobilinogen is oxidized to form urobilin and is excreted as a brown pigment in the feces. A minor quantity of urobilin is excreted by way of the kidneys. When the flow of bile from the liver is obstructed, the individual develops jaundice because of excessive accumulation of bilirubin. The stools become white or clay colored, a sign of the absence of urobilin.

Porphyrins are iron-free tetrapyrrols related to the heme part of hemoglobin. Porphyrins are fluorescent under ultraviolet light and emit a pink red fluorescence. The most important porphyrin compound (three series of porphyrin compounds occur in nature) is a decomposition product in heme, which is excreted during a variety of adult anemias and is also present in porphyria in large quantities within the tissues.

Lipochromes are pigments related to the coloring material in egg yolks and butter. Lipochromes are located (normally) in the cortex of the adrenal gland, corpus luteum, seminal vesicles, and interstitial cells of Leydig, and the ganglion cells of the nervous system and neurohypophysis. Lipochromes are present in aging heart muscle and neoplasms, producing a yellow leaf color. Lipochromes represent lipids containing colored hydrocarbons.

Myoglobin is an iron-free pigment derived from muscle and appears as casts in the kidney when a muscle is crushed or severely traumatized. Myoglobin is a heme pigment that is related to bilirubin or hematoidin.

References

Best, C.H. and Ridout, J.H.: *Am J Physiol, 122:*67, 1938.

Ellinger, F.: Functional biology of ionizing radiations. In Gehrens, C.F., et al.: *Atomic Medicine.* Baltimore, Williams and Wilkins, 1953, p. 86.

Florey, Sir H.: *Lectures on General Pathology.* Philadelphia, Saunders, 1954.

Gansler, H. and Rouiller, C.: *Schweiz Z Allerg Pathol, 19:*217, 1956.

Gustarson, K.H.: *The Chemistry and Reactivity of Collagen.* New York, Acad Pr, 1956.

Jeghers, H. and Edwards, E.A.: Pigmentation of the skin. In MacBryde, Cyrill Mitchell (Ed.): *Signs and Symptoms, Applied Pathologic Physiology and Clinical Interpretation,* 2nd ed. Philadelphia, Lippincott, 1947.
Pearse, A.G.E.: *Histochemistry.* Boston, Little, 1954.
Rich, A.R.: *Johns Hopkins Med J, 35:*415, 1924.
Robb-Smith, A.H.T.: *Lectures on the Scientific Basis of Medicine.* London, The Athlone Press, 1954, vol. II, 1952-53.
Seyeri, C.: *J Biophysics Biochem Cytol, 2:*293, 1956.
Teilum, G.: *Am J Pathol, 32:*945, 1956.
Feld, J.J., et al.: *Proc Soc Exp Biol Med, 48:*229, 1941.

CHAPTER 5

DISSEMINATION OF DISEASE AND SECONDARY IMPAIRMENTS

THERE IS A tendency for the initial damage to tissues and organs during various pathologic processes to spread or disseminate within the human body. There is also a tendency for primary disease states to be prolonged into chronic diseases in man. The initial disease may be classified as a focal form of disease when the injury due to the noxious agent remains sharply localized to a part of an organ. The initial disease may be classified as a diffuse form of disease when the entire organ or its complete surface is injured by the noxious agent. For example, an abscess is a focal suppurative process, whereas a generalized urinary bladder infection is a diffuse infectious disease. However, so long as the focal or diffuse form of disease is confined to one organ, the situation is termed a *local pathologic process*. When several organs in the body are involved by the pathologic process the disease is termed *regional*, and when numerous organs are involved the disease is systemic in nature. In skeletal diseases, we utilize the terms *monostotic bone disease* when a single bone is involved and *polyostotic* when several bones are affected. Diffuse skeletal disease means widespread involvement of the entire skeletal system. When the disease is brief it is termed *acute;* when it is prolonged for several months, it is termed *subacute;* and when it is prolonged for years the disease is termed *chronic* in nature.

Spread of disease within the body is termed *dissemination*. The injurious agent spreads throughout the body during dissemination of a disease. For instance, during a pyogenic infection there is an initial focal abscess. However, the abscess may rupture into a major blood vessel, producing a bacteremia with subsequent development of multiple abscesses throughout the body. During a period of months or years, the abscesses may become widespread in distribution and chronic in nature. Chronic forms of tuberculosis, syphilis, and leprosy spread widely and are, therefore, examples of dissemination of disease. These diseases spread damage from a primary local lesion to other regions of the body, causing a loss of function in the other organs affected. Secondary impairment is a common factor in dissemination. For instance, the prostate gland undergoes enlargement due to testicular aging and imbalance of internal secretion in the male sex glands. The enlarged prostate gland obstructs the urinary flow from the bladder. The urinary bladder dilates along with dilatation of the ureters and renal pelvis, leading to renal insufficiency accompanied by uremia and death. The process may require ten or more years and is called prostatism, a form of secondary impairment.

Dissemination or spread of disease occurs when the noxious agent penetrates into an adjacent region or is transported to the distant organs and tissues. Penetration or extension of the injurious agent simply means that the agent passes into the adjacent tissues. Dissemination and metastasis means that the more distant organs and tissues are injured by the noxious agents.

In infectious diseases, the injurious microorganisms directly spread through the tissue spaces or normal anatomic structures present in an organ or tissue. Infectious agents spread in muscle along the fascial planes. Infectious agents in the urinary tract spread by either ascending or descending from the urinary bladder to the ureters to the renal pelvis. Pulmonary infections spread along the bronchi or by way of the pleural fluid to the surrounding tissues. When fluid is present in the serous cavities of the peritoneum, pericardium, and meninges, the infectious agents may extend from one portion of the cavity to another with relative ease.

Dissemination or metastasis to distant organs takes place by way of the lymphatics or blood stream or by combination of the two routes. Infectious diseases may disseminate by way of an anatomic structure and the lymph nodes draining this structure.

The local lesion produced in the anatomic structure plus the involved lymph nodes together are referred to as the primary complex.

Inanimate and animate forms of disease spread along predictable pathways. For instance, various poisons have an affinity for a specific organ. Heavy metals and organic solvents injure tissue at the site of ingestion, plus produce secondary impairment in the organ that is responsible for the metabolism or detoxification of the chemical, plus damage the organ responsible for excretion of the drug and its metabolic products. When soluble mercury salts are ingested as a poison, ulceration takes place in the oral mucosa, damage occurs to the liver since it is the organ where detoxification occurs, and secondary impairment proceeds to involve the bowel and kidney as organs responsible for excretion of the mercury salts. Ionizing radiations appear to pass through the body in a straight line, with the damage caused by these penetrating rays varying inversely as the square of the distance from its source.

Animate damage resulting from bacteria on animal parasites has a rather complex path of dissemination. The portal of entry is the initial site of injury, and extention subsequently occurs to the regional lymph nodes, i.e. through the primary complex. From the primary complex, dissemination occurs to distant or remote organs, i.e. to the liver, kidneys, or brain. This is referred to as secondary or tertiary stages of complete dissemination. Late involvement of distant or remote organs generally takes place by way of the blood stream. However, variations are not uncommon. For instance, abscesses may rupture and penetrate tissues that, under normal circumstances, impose an obstacle to the spread of the infectious agent. In the abdomen, the portal circulation may be utilized to transport microorganisms to the liver, where the infectious agents are filtered out and dissemination is prevented for a prolonged period of time. Leukocytes that ingest the infectious agent may be unable to destroy it. The migration of the leukocytes throughout the reticuloendothelial tissues of the body may aid in the dissemination of the infectious disease.

When major damage takes place in one organ, there is often a secondary response or secondary impairment to the primary injury by a related anatomical structure not in contact with the injurious agent. Spread or damage from the primary site occurs to a second organ or organs, causing the loss of physiologic or anatomic support from the remote organs because of mutual interdependence. For example, injury to the ganglion cells in the central nervous system may cause degeneration or necrosis in the axones of the peripheral nerve. The secondary impairment in the peripheral nerve causes an interruption in the innervation of the muscle supplied, and flaccid paralysis ensues. Another example occurs in poliomyelitis when the virus injures the motor cells in the anterior horn of the spinal cord, i.e. secondary impairment.

Obstructions may develop to the discharge of products from many secretory and excretory organs. For instance, salivary secretion may be obstructed by a stone in Stensen's duct of the parotid gland. Urinary excretion from the kidney may be obstructed by a stone or a stricture in the ureter or by compression of the ureter by a neoplasm or mass outside. Fecal material may be blocked through the bowel by adhesions or neoplasms, producing intestinal obstruction. Bile ducts may become blocked by gall stones or from pressure exerted by a neoplasm or enlarged lymph nodes, resulting in jaundice or biliary cirrhosis.

The normal passage of blood from the heart to great vessels occurs by way of the cardiac orifice, which is protected by valves preventing the return of blood into the heart chambers. Stenosis or incompetent valves may produce dilatation of the chambers of the heart, causing failure of cardiac function. All of the examples of obstruction are examples of anatomic secondary impairment.

Atrophy means an acquired shrinkage in the size of an organ due to a decrease in the number or size of its cells. Atrophy indicates that normal size was present before the shrinkage occurred. Atrophy results from inadequate nourishment of the organ caused by the following: impairment of blood supply due to narrowing of vessels; disuse atrophy occurs through loss of motor supply, immobilization, contractures; pressure atrophy results from compression of fluid or blood supply; senile atrophy occurs following decreased metabolism; starvation atrophy occurs following generalized metabolic depression; and endocrine atrophy results from decreased function of endocrine organs. (Hypoplasia should be distinguished from atrophy). Hypoplasia results from arrested development. Aplasia results from early arrest, and agenesis means complete congenital absence.

Secondary impairment is based on the principle of dependence of organs on their nerve and blood supply as well as upon anatomical pathways for transporting fluid to or from secretory or execretory organs. The more subtle secondary impairments involve the interdependence of endocrine and vital organs. For instance, when the function of the pituitary gland is impaired in the young individual, he suffers from decreased function of the thyroid, and the pituitary and gonads remain in an infantile stage of development. This condition is hypophyseal dwarfism. The secondary impairments are referred to as endocrine atrophy.

The major forms of secondary injury or secondary impairment are directly related to the interrelationships of the numerous vital organs, i.e. the bone marrow, heart, lungs, kidneys, and the liver. The number of related organs that are undermined or weakened in function by secondary impairment is directly proportional to the normal physiologic load of the organ that is initially altered or injured. For example, the heart has the function of supplying both oxygen and nourishment to all organs throughout the body through a delicate network called the vascular tree. Acute heart failure during shock or gradual heart failure in chronic congestive failure results in damage to all organs. If death takes place due to shock, all organs show a state of local areas of infarction or pre-infarction caused by the presence of a progressive hypoxia. In congestive heart failure the urine outflow from the kidneys is impaired; the uptake of oxygen by the lungs is diminished; the liver is engorged, and the cells surrounding the central vein die from anoxia; the cerebral function is depressed due to congestion; the cerebral spinal fluid pressure is increased due to delayed absorption; the secretion in the digestive tract is impaired; and the anoxia of the bone marrow stimulates an increased formation of red blood cells. Diseases of the kidney with impaired renal function cause waste products to accumulate in the blood, and the toxic affects of uremia cause depression of the cerebral and cardiac functions. Severe impairment of the lungs increases the load upon the right side of the heart, causing right heart enlargement and an increase in the number of red blood cells in the circulation. Liver impairment alters the detoxification function of the liver and places an excessive load on the kidney, resulting in the hepatorenal syndrome.

CIRCULATORY SECONDARY IMPAIRMENT

Secondary impairment of the circulatory system indicates that an excess of blood or tissue fluid occurs in various organs, which is a common occurrence in various pathologic processes. Edema is defined as an abnormal accumulation of fluid in the tissues. Fluid accumulates in the tissues due to slowing or obstruction of the circulation (blood vessels and lymph vessels). Increase in venous pressure with congestive failure or mechanical obstruction is referred to as hydrostatic edema. Because hydrostatic edema is so frequent during heart disease, it is designed as cardiac edema. The edema of congestive heart failure is produced by a number of factors, i.e. retention of sodium chloride produced by decreased filtration in the kidneys, which suffer from a decreased blood flow, and increased venous pressure in congested veins.

When a large quantity of fluid develops in the pleura due to hydrostatic edema, the situation is referred to as hydrothorax or pleural effusion. Ascites means the accumulation of fluid in the peritoneal cavity. Hydropericardium refers to the accumulation of fluid in the pericardial sac. Hydroarthrosis means the accumulation of fluid in joint cavities. Dependent edema is defined as the accumulation of fluid in the dependent portions of the body caused by congestive heart failure. Anasarca means widespread edema. Lymphedema refers to the blockage of lymphatics with an abnormal accumulation of fluid within the tissues drained by lymphatics. Nephritic edema is nutritional edema, which results from a diminished osmotic pressure of the plasma caused by a decreased concentration of albumin in the plasma.

The capillary wall is directly damaged in various forms of anoxia, chemical poisoning, and in inflammation caused by infections of chemicals. The fluid present in the tissues is termed *inflammatory edema*. Milroy's edema represents a rare, inherited edema. Myxedema results from hydration of the subcutaneous connective tissues plus lowered thyroid function.

Congestion (passive hyperemia) is the presence of increased

blood in organs as a result of circulatory stasis. Congestion commonly occurs during cardiac disease and is always accompanied by some degree of edema. Active hyperemia in an organ or part means that the normal arterial tone has been altered, and there is an increase in the amount of arterial blood that enters the local capillary bed.

Dead tissues are incapable of defending themselves; however, dead and dying tissues can stimulate reactions of secondary impairment, which are defensive and healing reactions on the part of the adjacent mesenchymal structures, reticuloendothelial system, and endocrine organs. Secondary impairment can be suffered by all tissues and organs and represents the response to an injury. The injury is always outside the tissue affected even when the injury is inherited or arises due to a congenital defect. Secondary impairment follows primary impairment and is responsible for defense; healing is always endogenous in nature.

The organ or tissue initially injured has the tendency to drag down a second organ, and the second organ drags down the third organ, etc. In transmitting impairment to other tissues and organs that are part of the mesenchymal defensive elements, the body utilizes endogenous alarming substances that are internal agents, i.e. histamine and H substances released by dying cells, acetyl choline released by axone reflexes, and thromboplastin from injured tissues. The histamine and H substances initiate inflammation, and the other substances initiate coagulation.

The body utilizes only four components for its defense and healing: the vascular endothelium, the circulating and potentially mobile cells from the reticuloendothelial system, the constituents of loose connective tissue, and the immature reserve cells of parenchymatous organs, which undergo self-renewal. The cellular elements available for defense and healing are, therefore, labile, mobile, readily replaceable, shielded, in excess, and periodically at rest.

Reference

Altschule, M.D.: *Physiology in Diseases of the Heart and Lungs.* Cambridge. Harvard U Pr, 1950.

CHAPTER 6

DISTURBANCES OF BODY WATER AND ELECTROLYTES AND OF CIRCULATION OF BLOOD

DISTURBANCES OF BODY WATER AND ELECTROLYTES

THE HUMAN BODY CONTAINS a division of body mass into the extracellular fluid, and solids in homeostasis. The compartments of fluid (water) of the body include the extracellular fluid composed of the blood plasma (4% by weight) and the interstitial fluid (11% by weight) and the intracellular fluid (45% by weight). The total of body water is 60 percent by weight, and solids make up 40 percent by weight.

The fluids (water) or the extracellular and intracellular fluid that make up the human body are surrounded externally by the skin and internally the lining of the gastrointestinal tract, bronchi, hepatic ducts, and pancreatic ducts. The intracellular body fluid is maintained in a hypertonic condition in relation to the extracellular fluid.

Water and electrolyte balance, acid-base balance, and intake from and output to the outside environment occur by way of the gastrointestinal tract and other surface areas (skin, lungs, etc.). The movement of body fluids between the body compartments depends upon the osmotic pressure produced principally by proteins, which vary in their concentration between the extracellular and intracellular fluids. During disease, intravenous fluids are administered to the body. However, in general, fluid, electrolytes, protein, and other materials enter the cells of the body by passing through the lining of the gastrointestinal tract into the blood plasma, then into the interstitial fluid compartment, and finally into the cell by passing through the cell membrane. When fluid is lost from the cell, it passes through a reverse route (cell membrane to interstitial fluid, to blood plasma, to urine, and to skin and lungs.) Some fluids are lost through the feces. During diarrhea, the loss of fluids and electrolytes through the fecal matter can be considerable.

Thirst is defined as a mechanism partially controlled by osmoreceptors in the blood vessels and in part by emotional factors.

Regulation of fluid and electrolyte balance, once the fluids and electrolytes pass across the intestinal mucosa, is dependent upon the function of the kidney. The loss of fluid and electrolytes by way of the kidney is dependent upon the acid-base balance plus the excretion of waste products and quantities of normal constituents of blood plasma. The level above which a normal substance or waste product is excreted through the urine is termed the *renal threshold* for the particular substance.

The endocrine glands have a prominent and vital role to play in the regulation of water and electrolyte metabolism. The effects produced by the endocrine glands are mediated by the central nervous system through the hypothalamic factors, whose role is to release pituitary trophic hormones and, by acting upon the hypothalamic nuclei, to produce the antidiuretic hormone. The most important hormones for regulation of the kidney are the antidiuretic hormone, aldosterone, and the third factor.

The antidiuretic hormone is produced in the hypothalamus and is excreted from the posterior pituitary gland. It is transported from the hypothalamus within axons down the stalk of the pituitary into the posterior lobe of the pituitary gland. The antidiuretic hormone acts upon the distal renal tubules. Aldosterone acts upon the proximal convoluted tubules of the kidney and conserves both water and salt. Angiotensin is the most important stimulus to the secretion of aldosterone from the adrenal glomerulosa cells. The third factor also influences sodium and water in the renal tubules. The third factor affects urine volume and content and thus water and electrolyte balance. The third factor produces a diuresis of sodium, which also carries some water.

Normal water and electrolyte metabolism is altered by pathologic processes, e.g. by diarrhea where an abnormal loss of both water and electrolytes occurs from the gastrointestinal tract. Increased loss of water occurs during hyperventilation. Both water and electrolytes are lost during sweating.

Acid-base disturbances develop in metabolic and respiratory pathologic processes. For instance, metabolic acidosis may develop in diabetes mellitus, renal failure where retention of phosphates and acids occurs, and occasionally in severe diarrhea. Respiratory acidosis is associated with chronic pulmonary pathologic processes (severe emphysema) where there is a change in the normal gaseous exchange in the lungs. Respiratory acidosis may also be associated with chronic asthma or bronchitis. The individual with acidosis has a flushed skin and demonstrates air hunger. Acidosis causes a reduction in the carbon dioxide combining power of the blood and excretion of a more acid urine with ammonia ions replacing sodium ions in the urine. Metabolic acidosis develops in wasting and starvation and intestinal obstruction where there is a loss of sodium due to diarrhea.

Metabolic alkalosis is associated with individuals who lose gastric juices containing chlorides due to vomiting. Respiratory alkalosis is associated with hyperventilation, high fevers, and lesions of the central nervous system. During alkalosis, the carbon dioxide combining power of the blood is elevated while the serum chloride is lowered, and there is loss of potassium. To keep the sodium there must be loss of potassium (potassium has a reciprocal relationship to sodium).

Loss of water and electrolytes in disease may be classified as the following forms of depletion: water, salt, and mixed salt and water due to external loss, and as mixed salt and water due to internal loss of water and electrolytes.

External loss of water in disease is caused by the following: failure of intake during nausea or coma; inability to swallow; provoked vomiting and sweating; major psychoses; weakness; esophageal stricture; and diabetes insipidus. The fluid shift consists of loss of fluid in all body compartments (extracellular and intracellular). Clinical features include hemoconcentration, oliguria, and elevated serum sodium.

External loss of salt in disease is caused by the following: salt-losing nephritis; low salt regime in cardiac disease; mercurial diuretics; lavage of the gastrointestinal tract; and excessive sweating. The fluid shift consists of extracellular loss of fluid. The clinical features are hemoconcentration, low blood pressure, polyuria, reduced serum sodium, and azotemia.

External loss of mixed salt and water in disease is caused by diarrhea and vomiting, intestinal obstruction, draining fistulae, and diabetic acidosis. There is a loss of fluid in all compartments, and more rapid shrinkage of plasma volume.

External loss of mixed salt and water in disease is caused by adrenal cortical hypofunction (Addison's disease). The fluid shift consists of a fall in plasma and extracellular volume, and a relative increase in intracellular volume. The clinical features include hemoconcentration, low blood pressure, oliguria, marked loss of weight and weakness, nitrogen retention, and loss of sodium in the urine.

Internal loss of mixed salt and water in disease is caused by burns and crush injuries in eight to forty-eight hours, peritonitis, and massive thrombophlebitis. The fluid shift consists chiefly of loss of plasma volume; however, other fluid compartments also suffer. The clinical features include hemoconcentration, oliguria, and salt retention in the body due to adrenal stimulation. Sodium and potassium are lost through leakage in injured tissues, increased production of antidiuretic hormone, and shock with hypotension.

DISTURBANCES OF CIRCULATION OF BLOOD
Edema

Edema is defined as the presence of an excessive quantity of fluid in any tissue or part of the body, i.e. within the interstitial spaces of the body. However, edema generally means excess fluid within individual cells (cloudy swelling or hydropic degeneration). Edema has also come to mean body-wide accumulations of fluid, which are located not only within the interstitial tissues but also in body cavities. One should think of accumulations of fluid in the interstitial spaces as true edema, which has a consistency similar to that of the normal interstitial fluid. At times, there is massive accumulation of interstitial fluid during heart failure, in which situation the edema is called anasarca (dropsy). Edema fluids are named according to the type and locations.

A transudate is defined as a fluid with a low concentration of protein. The protein concentration of the transudate is less than 4 percent, and the specific gravity is less than 1.012. The transudate is a clear fluid, or it may appear as a pale yellow fluid that has the consistency of the normal interstitial fluid of the body. The transudate fluid accumulates between individual cells and in the interstitial spaces of connective tissues. It may also accumulate in the different body cavities (peritoneum and pleura) where the fluid accumulates in a fashion similar to fluid accumulations in the interstitial spaces of the body. Transudate fluid, because of its low quantity of protein, rarely clots and is freely transported when pressure is applied by external forces or by an adjacent organ. Transudates are subject to gravity and gradually move toward the lower extremities when the individual is walking. In the bedridden patient, the transudate accumulates in the most dependent anatomical portion of the body, generally in the buttocks. The latter accumulation of transudate is called dependent edema. Dependent edema pits on pressure from the finger and is referred to as pitting edema. Once the pressure of the finger is removed, the fluid returns to the original area.

Exudate is a second type of edema and is defined as a fluid rich in protein. The protein concentration is greater than 4 percent, and the specific gravity is above 1.018. The protein component of the exudate is present as fibrinogen or fibrin fibers (polymerized fibrinogen). The exudate is less mobile with less pitting upon pressure because of the presence of the fibrin fibers, which form a network in the interstitial spaces. Exudates are primarily present following localized injuries to tissues and are considered a part of tissue response along with the localized inflammatory reaction. The exudate is present as a localized fluid. Areas of the body containing exudates are generally painful, and the exudate is filled with large numbers of polymorphonuclear leukocytes as well as other elements of acute inflammation.

Types of Exudates (Effusions)

Effusion is defined as an abnormal fluid present in the interstitial space or body cavities. It is synonymous with edema. Serous fluid or serous effusion is synonymous with transudate when present in excessive quantities in the interstitial fluids. Fibrinous effusion is defined as a fluid rich in protein, specifically fibrinogen or fibrin. This pathologic fluid generally accompanies inflammation and should be classified as an exudate because of the high protein concentration. Sanguinous effusion is defined as fluid containing numerous red blood cells, which color the fluid red. Grossly, this fluid appears similar to hemorrhage in the tissues. However, the sanguinous effusion has an hematocrit below 40 to 45 percent. Purulent effusion is defined as a fluid containing great numbers of polymorphonuclear leukocytes and is classified as an exudate. This exudate is associated with the acute inflammatory process. The purulent effusion appears grossly as pus, i.e. a yellow, turbid material that is very high in cells. Mixed effusion is defined as the fluid of an effusion that contains a mixture of blood, pus, cells, fibrin, etc. For instance, serosanguinous means an abundant fluid with a moderate amount of blood, fibrino-purulent means fluid containing abundant fibrin and numerous pus cells, or sanguino-purulent means a fluid containing red blood cells and pus cells.

The following special terms are used for the various types of effusions, depending upon their location in the body. *Pericardial effusion* is defined as a pathologic effusion containing more than 15 cc of serous fluid in the pericardial cavity. The pericardial cavity normally contains 5 to 15 cc of serous fluid. The pericardial effusion may be either an exudate containing fibrin (fibrinous effusion) or a transudate, in which case it is termed *hydropericardium*. If the effusion has blood as a component, it is termed *hemopericardium*. When the hemopericardium exerts pressure on the heart, the situation is termed *pericardial tamponade*. Purulent effusions also occur within the pericardium.

Disturbances of Body Water and Electrolytes 59

Pleural effusion is defined as a pathologic effusion when it is present in excess of 10 cc in each pleural cavity. Each pleural cavity normally contains 5 to 10 cc of serous fluid. Hydrothorax refers to a serous effusion; hemothorax refers to a sanguinous effusion, and pyothorax or empyema refers to a purulent effusion in the pleural cavity. Empyema may also indicate a chronic process in addition to a purulent process.

Peritoneal effusion is defined as pathologic serous fluid in excess of 25 cc within the peritoneal cavity. The peritoneal cavity normally contains from 10 to 25 cc of serous fluid. Ascites is defined as a peritoneal effusion. Ascites may consist of either serous, sanguinous, or purulent effusions, or of a mixture of the three. Anasarca (dropsy) is defined as massive edema of the body. It is a generalized, dependent type of edema and should be classified as a transudate. Anasarca is associated with cardiac failure, renal failure, and lymphatic obstruction. Pulmonary edema is the replacement of the air-filled alveolar spaces of the lungs with fluid. The edema of the lung is a transudate caused by congestive heart failure. In severe right heart failure, the individual will have pulmonary edema plus fluid in the pleural cavities. If left heart failure occurs, pulmonary congestion and edema appear early, and the pulmonary edema may be present without peripheral interstitial edema of the legs. Advanced pulmonary edema will cause difficult breathing and rapid respiration with rales in the chest as the fluid is mixed with air.

Transudates, therefore, have a tendency to be generalized whereas exudates tend to remain localized. Transudates generally result from the accumulation of excessive fluid in the body. The excess fluid passes or exudes from vessels into the interstitial spaces. Transudates, on the other hand, are always the result following failure of the kidneys to excrete sufficient quantities of fluid. Transudates are common due to heart failure where the renal arterial pressure is reduced and the venous outflow is deficient.

In portal hypertension, the blood cannot pass through the enlarged collateral veins into the circulation. The dilated collateral veins occur predominantly in the esophagus leading to esophageal varices, around the rectum leading to hemorrhoids, and in the wall of the abdomen. A varix is defined as a pathologically dilated vein. Cardiac edema is defined as the accumulation of a thin fluid, which has a low concentration of protein. It is, therefore, classified as a transudate that occurs in various sites in the body as a result of partial heart failure. Heart failure is defined as a pathologic condition in which the muscular force of the heart is insufficient to pump the blood through the systemic circulation and meet the needs of the body, which are dependent upon the activity of the individual. The heart has a great reserve, which is called upon for brief periods of time by increasing the heart rate and cardiac output as well as by cardiac hypertrophy. In a compensated individual with heart disease, the heart is capable of meeting the needs of the body. Such individuals subsequently reach the limits of compensation, and decompensation ensues, i.e. heart failure results.

Heart failure has been classified as acute or chronic. Acute heart failure is due to the following:

1. Death of a large part of the heart (large infarction) or cardiac arrhythmia or total stoppage of the heart;

2. Massive blockage of the blood flow through the lungs due to the presence of emboli; and

3. Massive trauma associated with massive hemorrhage and shock.

Chronic heart failure may be present for years, and there is a blockage and filling up of the veins on the right side of the heart. When filling up of the veins is caused by a backing up of blood, congestion develops and the pathologic condition is termed *chronic congestive heart failure*. The heart generally shows a mixture of both right and left heart failure. Backward heart failure is defined as the inability of the heart to pump the entire load of blood that is presented to it. This results in the damming back of blood into the vessels located in the lungs and peripheral venous system. Backward heart failure is accompanied by an elevated venous pressure, edema, and congestion. Forward heart failure is defined as an inadequate arterial blood pressure, which is incapable of pumping adequate quantities of blood required for normal nutrition and for the removal of waste products from the tissues. Forward and backward heart failure occur together because the cardiovascular system is a closed system.

Renal edema (nephrotic edema) is defined as a transudate or edema that occurs following renal failure caused by intrinsic renal disease. Renal edema is due to failure to properly handle sodium and water and to the lowering of the plasma protein osmotic pressure due to loss of albumin from the diseased kidney. Renal edema is a transudate with a very low concentration of protein. Edema (transudate) is evident around the eyelids (periorbital edema), but gravity does not pull the transudate to the lower portions of the body as one sees during cardiac edema.

Lymphedema is caused by congenital obstructive situations, inflammation of the lymphatics, parasitic, obstructive type of infections, metastatic neoplasms, and surgical intervention. The edema develops following obstruction of the lymphatics and failure of the lymphatic drainage. Lymphedema is a transudate generally localized to one drainage area for the lymphatics. For instance, one or both legs may be involved by lymphedema. Elephantiasis is lymphedema of both legs caused by a parasitic obstructive infection. Lymphedema appears grossly as boggy edema with some pitting. Postural edema is edema dependent upon both the venous and lymphatic return to the heart, muscle activity, and valves in the venous system. Varicose veins develop because of the loss of normal valve activity in the veins, which in turn diminishes the efficiency of muscular action. Postural edema occurs in individuals who stand for prolonged periods of time. Postural edema may be complicated by the presence of varicose veins. Venous edema is the accumulation of fluid in the tissues when there is venous obstruction to the flow from a region of the body. Hypoproteinemic edema is defined as a generalized condition in which the edema undergoes pitting and accumulates in the dependent parts of the body. Renal edema may be associated with hypoproteinemia caused by the loss of protein by way of the pathologic kidney. Inflammatory edema is an exudate containing a high concentration of protein (fibrin) plus numerous polymorphonuclear leukocytes. It is a localized edema due to increased capillary permeability to fluids and cells. Allergic edema is a peculiar variety of inflammatory edema. It is caused by a hypersensitivity response of the body to a foreign antigenic substance(s), i.e. allergens. Inflammatory cells plus numerous eosinophiles are present in the inflammatory edema. Angioneurotic edema is a widespread variety of allergic edema. Angioneurotic edema may affect the larynx, vocal cords, tongue, and lips. Obstruction and suffocation are complications of angioneurotic edema of the larynx and vocal cords.

The main causes of edema are increased permeability of the capillary and/or wall of the venule, a decrease in the colloidal osmotic pressure of the plasma protein, an increased hydrostatic pressure of the capillary and venous blood, lymphatic obstruction, decreased extravascular tissue pressure, and pathologic retention of sodium and water.

The increased permeability of capillary walls is the result of injury to the capillaries following local alterations such as inflammation, burns, blunt force, or hypoxia. A decrease in the colloidal osmotic pressure of plasma proteins accompanies liver disease with decreased production of albumin or in renal disease where there is excessive loss of plasma proteins because of the damaged kidneys. The increased hydrostatic pressure of the blood is due to deficient venous drainage in a local area caused by trauma, neoplasm exerting pressure, or heart failure, which produces general stagnation of venous blood and increased venous hydrostatic pressure. Lymphatic obstruction results from neoplasms (tumors) or infections. A rarely decreased extravascular tissue pressure occurs in the cachectic patient. Retention of sodium and water is caused by stimulation of aldosterone by the adrenal cortex or by decreased detoxification of the aldosterone hormone by the liver. One or a combination of the six main causes of edema may be operating in the production of any specific case.

Normally, not all of the fluid that passes out of capillaries into the interstitial spaces is returned to the capillaries. Fifteen or twenty percent of the fluid passes into the lymphatics from its interstitial location. The normal exchange of fluid between the interstitial spaces and the plasma is adversely affected by alterations in the following: osmotic pressure of the blood, osmotic pressure of the tissues, hydrostatic pressure of the blood, hydrostatic pressure of the tissue, and by damage to blood vessel walls. Edema of the generalized type within the interstitial tissues (subcutaneous and tissue located between musculature) is generally not harmful to the body. However, if edema develops in the brain (very limited expansion possible), the result could prove to be fatal. The latter edema of the brain is termed *cerebral edema*. On the other hand, pulmonary edema may also prove to be fatal since it may encompass so large an area that physiological air exchange is not possible.

Dehydration

Dehydration of the tissues of the body is defined as a reduction in the body fluid volume due to an output that exceeds the intake of fluid. Primary dehydration is defined as the loss of body water without any electrolytes. Secondary dehydration is defined as the loss of water plus electrolytes, i.e. generally sodium. The loss of body fluid volume takes place through the skin, lungs gastrointestinal tract, kidneys, and draining sinuses. Dehydration causes disappearance of the subcutaneous tissues of the body. The internal tissues appear dry and sticky. The body is capable of conserving water so that the interstitial spaces containing fluid are the first area to be reduced. Secondly, the cells of the body lose water, and lastly, water is lost from the blood vascular system. When the dehydration of the body is severe and there is a large reduction in the vascular blood volume, the result is the development of shock.

Hyperemia and Congestion

Hyperemia refers to active hyperemia, which is defined as an intentional relaxation of the arteriolar muscle that permits the quantity of blood entering an area of the body to increase substantially. Active hyperemia is a physiological process under the body's control. The venous outflow from an area of active hyperemia is also increased so that there is no stagnation of blood in the affected tissue. More blood enters the area with active hyperemia, more nutrients are available to the cells, and more blood leaves the area. Hyperemic blood has a high concentration of oxygen and a red color, and is high in nutrients and low in waste materials. Examples of active hyperemia are the inflammatory response of blood vessels to a local injury or the dilatation of the blood supply to the skin when the body loses heat.

Congestion is passive hyperemia, which is defined as a localized pathologic area of the vascular bed that has accumulated an abnormal quantity of blood. Passive hyperemia is generally the result of an obstruction reducing the outflow of blood plus a contribution from obstruction of the lymphatic flow. During congestion, there is stagnation of blood in the affected area. Thus, the blood remains for abnormally long periods within the blood vessels and contains a low concentration of oxygen and blue color, is low in nutrient materials, and is high in waste products. The inflow of blood to the congested area is normal until pressure increases within the congested tissue, at which time the inflow of blood decreases from the normal. Passive hyperemia results from thrombosis of a vein or from heart failure, in which case the blood pools in the entire venous system. The cause of passive hyperemia may be due to a temporary, semipermanent or permanent pathologic process, and the congestion may remain for an extended period of time. Passive hyperemia or congestion is, therefore, a pathologic entity. Chronic passive congestion is defined as a long-standing congestion.

Ischemia is defined as a localized reduction of the normal arterial blood supply to a part of the body. It is caused by an arterial venous, or capillary lesion, which produces an obstruction in the outflow of blood (congestion). The congestion subsequently prevents sufficient arterial blood from flowing into the affected area.

Hypoxia is defined as less than the normal quantity of oxygen in an individual. The individual has an abnormal quantity of blue (reduced) hemoglobin, and the color of the skin is bluish due to cyanosis. Hypoxia is also defined as the lack of oxygen to a body part in addition to the total individual.

Anoxia is defined as a complex lack of oxygen in a tissue

within the body. When the quantity of oxygen drops below the minimal level required for survival of the tissue, the result is degeneration and necrosis. Rupture of blood vessels and hemorrhage may follow necrosis of the anoxic tissue. Ischemic areas are accompanied by anoxia or hypoxia. At death, the entire body undergoes anoxia.

Anemia is defined as the reduction below physiologic limits of the hemoglobin-red blood cell mass accompanied by decreased delivery of oxygen to the tissues. During anemia, the circulating blood is unable to supply an adequate level of oxygen to the tissues for normal physiologic processes. Anemia may be caused by a reduction in the total number of red blood cells circulating in the blood. The hematocrit or percentage of blood cells in the blood drops below the normal (40 to 45%) during anemia. If the hematocrit is less than 37 percent, a definitive diagnosis of anemia is established. Females have a tendency to have a lower hematocrit than males because of menstruation. Anemia may develop in which a normal quantity of red blood cells is present when the body is unable to manufacture a normal type of hemoglobin or to produce a sufficient quantity of hemoglobin for the red blood cells. The red blood cells then cannot carrry sufficient oxygen. Anemia is also caused by chemicals that interfere with the hemoglobin-oxygen carrying mechanism. For instance, carbon monoxide saturation of the hemoglobin is responsible for the inability of the hemoglobin to bind oxygen.

Hypoxemia and anoxemia are related to the reduced quantity of oxygen present in the blood. Hypoxemia is caused by anemia, suffocation, and poisoning with carbon monoxide. Hypoxemia causes hypoxia of tissues and eventual necrosis.

Increased circulation of blood to a tissue or area of the body may occur in the following situations:

1. Well-oxygenated blood;
2. Poorly oxygenated blood with normal red cell mass;
3. Nonoxygenated blood in a part of the body;
4. Each red blood cell contains a normal amount of oxygen, but has a marked reduction in the total number of red blood cells;

5. Poorly oxygenated blood, which is also deficient in red blood cells; and

6. Well-oxygenated blood with an adequate number of red blood cells but deficient in nutrients, and rarely, with an excessive accumulation of waste products.

Decreased circulation of blood to a tissue or area of the body may occur in the following situations:

1. Partial ischemia due to heart failure, shock, partial occlusion of blood vessels in arteriosclerosis;

2. Complete ischemia due to thrombosis and arteriosclerosis with anoxia leading to necrosis; and

3. Due to congestion associated with low nutrients, low oxygen, and increased waste products.

Physiological volume of circulating blood to an area per unit of time may be associated with the following:

1. Poorly oxygenated blood;
2. Low number of red blood cells;
3. Absence of oxygen;
4. Deficiency in nutrients;
5. Excess nutrients (increased glucose in diabetes mellitus);
6. Excess waste products (urea in azotemia).

Hemorrhage

Hemorrhage is the escape of whole blood, i.e. red blood cells and plasma, from the blood vessels following a break in the blood vessel wall. Hemorrhage may accumulate in the tissues, in body cavities, or on the surface of the body following a wound. Red blood cells may escape rather slowly through the blood vessel wall without a clear break in the vessel wall. When only red blood cells (no plasma) pass (escape) through the vessel wall, the process is termed *diapedesis* rather than hemorrhage. A damaged capillary wall will frequently permit the escape of only plasma (no red blood cells). The latter situation is known as a serous or serofibrinous effusion rather than hemorrhage. True hemorrhage is reserved only for situations whereby whole blood escapes from blood vessels. Hemorrhages are given specific names primarily dependent upon the location. Petechiae are very small hemorrhages, which are usually multiple in nature. Petechiae are common on the skin and serous membranes of body cavities. Ecchymoses are large hemorrhages, which are common in the skin and form the rainbow-colored lesion called a bruise. The ecchymosis under the skin contains red blood cell hemoglobin, which gradually decomposes over a period of days. Decomposition products of hemoglobin are biliverdin, hematoidin (bilirubin), and hemosiderin. A bruise (ecchymosis) differs from an abrasion, which refers to a break in the skin. Hematoma is an accumulation of blood into a swelling and is due to an internal hemorrhage into the tissues. The blood becomes localized in the tissues and is palpable. Purpura is defined as multiple hemorrhages. Purpura is associated with the absence of platelets, and the resulting hemorrhages are quite variable in size, i.e. some are small, others are large hemorrhages. Leukemia causes the development of purpura. Purpura is similar to the hemorrhagic diathesis. Hemorrhagic diathesis is defined as a hemorrhagic tendency accompanied by large or small multiple hemorrhages and is generally due to diseases of the bone marrow, i.e. destruction of platelets caused by toxins or by leukemia. Hemorrhagic diathesis is a clinical feature of poor clotting caused by the absence of some clotting factor. Exsanguination is defined as massive hemorrhage resulting in shock and death. Hemorrhage may occur into a large cavity (pleural or peritoneal cavities), retroperitoneally, or externally from a wound.

Hemorrhage that occurs into the gut is referred to according to its location. For instance, if the hemorrhage is located in the stomach, it is termed *gastric hemorrhage.* Esophageal hemorrhage results from esophageal varices. Gastric hemorrhage and duodenal hemorrhage result following chronic ulceration. Hemorrhages in the colon are caused most often by carcinoma, whereas rectal hemorrhages result from hemorrhoids. If a moderate sized gastrointestinal hemorrhage is present high in the gastrointestinal tract, the blood will become partially digested as it moves through the gastrointestinal tract. Following defecation, the feces will appear as dark black, greasy, and foul smelling. This description of a stool is termed *melena,* which is due to partial digestion of blood as it passes through the gut along with the feces.

Massive gastrointestinal hemorrhage may also produce vomiting of blood if the hemorrhage is located in the esophagus, stomach, or upper portion of the small intestines. The vomiting of blood is termed *hematemesis*. Massive gastrointestinal hemorrhage may produce diarrhea of fresh blood or the passage of partially decomposed blood (melena). Massive blood loss into the gastrointestinal tract may overload the system of disposal of hemoglobin pigments following the breakdown of hemoglobin and produce jaundice. The yellow discoloration of the skin during jaundice is caused by the presence of breakdown products of hemoglobin, primarily bilirubin or hematoidin.

Epistaxis is hemorrhage from the nose, or a nosebleed. Pulmonary hemorrhage occurs within the lung, generally into alveolae and bronchi. Hemoptysis is defined as the coughing up of blood from the lung into the mouth. Aspiration is defined in pathology as the raising of stomach contents (which frequently contain blood) by muscle activity, through the esophagus into the pharynx and then sucked into the lungs.

Hemothorax or sanguinous pleural exudate may be mixed with pleural fluid, i.e. a transudate or exudate, and thus contains variable amounts of blood. The mixed pleural exudates are termed *serosanginous, sanguino-purulent,* and *fibrinosanguinous effusions*. Hemopericardium is defined as blood in the pericardial cavity, which may create pressure upon the heart, producing cardiac tamponade. Mixture of blood and transudate or blood and exudate may exist in the pericardial cavity comparable to mixtures described in the pleura.

Hemoperitonium is defined as pure blood in the peritoneal cavity. However, mixtures of blood and a transudate or exudate may also occur in the peritoneal cavity. Hematuria is hemorrhage into or arising from the urinary tract. The urine is, therefore, stained with blood during hematuria. Menorrhagia or metrorrhagia is defined as excessive hemorrhage arising from the vagina. Normal bleeding from the vagina with ovulation cycles is termed *menstruation*. Cerebral hemorrhage is bleeding into the substance of the brain. Hemorrhage may begin within the substance of the brain and rupture into the subarachnoid space or into the ventricles of the brain. Subarachnoid hemorrhage is defined as hemorrhage located around the brain in the region between the arachnoid membrane and the brain surface. Subdural hemorrhage is the presence of hemorrhage located between the dura and arachnoid. It is most commonly of traumatic etiology. Cerebral vascular accident is a defect in the function of the brain produced as the result of vascular disease. It includes the following hemorrhages: cerebral hemorrhages; subarachnoid hemorrhages; subdural hemorrhages, or thrombosis of a cerebral vessel without the presence of hemorrhage. Cerebral vascular accident is a term used when no specific diagnosis has been achieved or when insufficient findings are present and a definitive diagnosis cannot be made.

Hemostasis is defined as the control of hemorrhage. Hemarthrosis refers to the presence of a hemorrhage into a joint. Hemorrhagic shock is a process in the body that occurs whenever there is a sufficient quantity of blood lost from the blood vascular system. If the blood loss is rapid, the less the quantity of hemorrhage necessary to produce shock.

Arteriosclerosis

Hardening of the arteries, i.e. arteriosclerosis, is defined as all of the degenerative changes in the arterial wall that produce a thickening or proliferative artery wall. Arteriosclerosis is classified into the following forms: intimal arteriosclerosis, medial arteriosclerosis and arteriolar sclerosis.

The most common form of arteriosclerosis is intimal arteriosclerosis. It occurs in all adults and frequently may produce occlusion of the lumen of the artery and an infarction due to death of the tissue. Intimal arteriosclerosis is responsible for heart attacks. The etiology of intimal arteriosclerosis is currently obscure. Initially, there is a marked deposition of lipids in the intima of blood vessels, immediately beneath the endothelial lining cells. If the intimal lesion has a high lipid content, it is called atherosclerosis. It may eventually be proven that damage must occur to the intimal wall and that the lipids accumulate in the area of damage. It may likewise eventually be proven that the amount of circulating lipids or the size of the particles of circulating lipids is abnormal in arteriosclerosis. The lipid deposited in arteriosclerosis is cholesterol. As the intimal lesion advances, there is fibrosis in the intima and subsequently intimal calcification, which produces a greater interference with the normal flow of blood.

Medial arteriosclerosis is Mönckeberg's medial sclerosis. This form of arteriosclerosis occurs during senility as the tissues undergo senile changes. Mönckeberg's medial sclerosis is due to deposition of calcium salts in the media of larger arteries. It rarely causes interference with circulation; however, it produces a stiff aorta and stiff arteries, which cause an increased systolic blood pressure. This medial sclerosis produces so-called "pipe-stem" arteries which, although they are stiff, continue to have an adequate sized lumen.

Arteriolar sclerosis is defined as another form of arteriosclerosis, that involves primarily the arterioles and only infrequently the smallest arteries. The lesion is different from intimal and medial arteriosclerosis; therefore, it should be considered separate from arteriosclerosis.

Arteriosclerosis thus refers to intimal arteriosclerosis with considerable atheroma. Intimal arteriosclerosis is the most frequent and most vital form of arteriosclerosis. All adults possess some degree of arteriosclerosis, with more than 50 percent of the U.S. population dying of this disease and its complications. Arteriosclerosis may occur as intimal fatty streaks, which are present at birth but which gradually progress, primarily in males, to produce widespread arteriosclerosis of the cardiovascular system. The fatty deposits progress to include atheroma, fibrosis, and calcification. The final phase of this arteriosclerosis is the development of thrombosis of the lumen followed by infarction in the heart or brain, with fatal results. During arteriosclerosis, the kidney and leg may be severely but not fatally damaged.

The pathogenesis of intimal arteriosclerosis is as follows. Only the intima and subintimal areas of the artery are involved, causing an impingement on the lumen. The intima is normally composed of a layer of endothelial cells, a thin basement membrane, and an irregular layer of elastic fibers termed the *internal elastic lamina* (outside the intimal basement membrane). There are a few collagen fibers, but no cells, between the elastica and media of the normal artery. As intimal arteriosclerosis forms, the endothelial cells of the intima plus the basement membrane become separated from the elastic lamina and the smooth muscle cells of the media by means of the accumulation of mononuclear cells and lipid. The streaks and plaques seen in arteriosclerosis are composed of mononuclear cells and lipids. The arteriosclerotic lesion is, therefore, an artificial zone or layer that splits the intima as it enlarges in size. It may eventually be proven that an ulceration or erosion of the endothelial surface occurs first during the formation of the arteriosclerotic plaque. The first step may perhaps be loss of endothelial cells with the formation of a fibrin clot over the denuded area. Secondly, cells may accumulate over the internal elastic lamina in the area of the clot. Thirdly, organization of the clot into a scar (plaque) occurs plus re-endothelialization of this scar, followed by new endothelial cells that proliferate over the plaque from several directions. However, the lesion produced results as a plaque that consists of mononuclear cells, lipid, and later, fibroblasts, collagen, and calcium salts. The lesion (plaque) is located between the endothelial cells and their basement membrane on the lumen side and the internal elastic lamina that rests on smooth cells external to the plaques.

The origin of the mononuclear cells that migrate to the plaque is obscure. These cells may represent modified smooth muscle cells that migrate toward the lumen from the smooth muscle layer of the blood vessel. On the other hand, these cells may represent interstitial mononuclear cells (histiocytes or fibroblasts) that have migrated through the smooth muscle. It is also possible that they are mononuclear cells from the blood, which accumulate in the area. The lipids that become mobilized in the early atheromatous plaque are generally, a mixture of lipids, i.e. consist of free fatty acids, neutral fats, and cholesterol similar to the plasma lipids. In the more advanced arteriosclerotic plaque the primary lipid is cholesterol, which is associated with lipoproteins. Research may eventually reveal that the lipoprotein profile of the plasma is related to the formation of arteriosclerosis. This observation has not been verified.

Intimal arteriosclerotic lesions are of greater severity in males than females and occur in individuals from thirty-five to fifty years of age. In the female, however, significant intimal arteriosclerotic lesions appear in the sixth and seventh decades of life compared to forty-five years of age in males. If the female lives to advanced age, she will develop just as severe arteriosclerotic lesions as the male.

Intimal arteriosclerotic lesions generally affect the aorta and its major branches. The intimal lesion is composed of lipid, lipoprotein, fibrosis, and finally, calcification. Lesions of arteriosclerosis of the medium sized artery contain less deposition of lipid and more fibrosis when compared to large arteries. For instance, the secondary and tertiary branches of the arcuate and interlobar arteries of the kidney contain less lipid deposition than large arteries.

Upon gross examination, the initial phase of intimal arteriosclerosis appears as yellow, slightly raised fatty streaks present in the intimal lining of the blood vessel. When the fatty streaks are small, they are seen only by microscopic study after staining the intima with a fat stain. Intimal fatty streaks have been reported in children three or four years of age and with greater frequency in the teens and second decade of life. The intimal fatty streaks are believed to be reversible following the lowering of dietary fats and during malnutrition. Histopathologic examination reveals the presence of lipid, primarily as cholesterol-containing lipoproteins similar to their concentration in the plasma. The cholesterol-lipoproteins appear as droplets with cells producing foam cells located just inside the elastica (between the elastica and endothelial basement membrane.) The foam cells are believed to be smooth muscle cells or macrophages. One theory concludes that lipid is imbibed by pinocytosis, and another theory concludes that lipid is formed *in situ* by abnormal mononuclear cells. Macrophages and smooth muscle cells migrate from the media to the subintima of the vessel wall. The foam cells aggregate to form small elevated plaques or elongated streaks in the intima.

As the arteriosclerosis advances and the patient ages, minute streaks produce atheromatous plaques. The atheromatous plaque process is accelerated with hypertension. The atheromatous plaques also have free lipid in the form of globules present within cells caused by the rupture of foam cells accompanied by some inflammation, some hemorrhage, and some fibrosis. In the advanced stage of arteriosclerosis, hemorrhages occur to the wall of the blood vessel in the region of the arteriosclerotic plaque. The hemorrhage may be highly significant in final occulsion of the vessel lumen. With continued progression of the lesion, the arteriosclerotic plaque produces an elevation of the endothelium, and ulcerations may occur. The atheromatous ulcer may be associated with thrombosis, i.e. the blood blot occurs in the lumen of the vessels during life, located over the ulcer. A scar is formed following organization of the thrombus, and the endothelium grows over the organized tissue. When patients attain sixty to seventy years of age, the plaques develop a more fibrous and less atheromatous nature, with calcium salt deposition in the interstitial areas. At this stage of progression, the yellow atheroma becomes pearly grey when viewed grossly. When the atheromatous plaque completely surrounds the circumference of the vessel or assumes a very large size, it ulcerates and thromboses, or hemorrhage occurs into the plaque from one of the many vessels proliferating into the plaque as it becomes organized. Thus, the chances of complete thrombosis of the lumen of the vessel wall is very high. Complete thrombosis of the lumen of the vessel always causes tissue death. Severe arteriosclerosis with marked reduction in the lumen of the artery may cause tissue death, particularly if systemic shock is present.

In the greatly advanced arteriosclerotic plaques, the lipid becomes higher in free cholesterol and lower in phospholipids. One theory (unsubstantiated) states that, as the plaque forms and later becomes fibrotic and subsequently calcified, the nutrition of the plaques becomes inadequate and poor nutrition causes death of the foam cells that release lipids into the interstitial tissue spaces.

A mural thrombus is defined as any type of thrombus that extends from the wall of a blood vessel or from the wall of the heart into the lumen. Mural thrombi cause partial occlusion of the lumen of one of the chambers of the heart or the lumen of the aorta. The mural thrombi occur most commonly in the auricles of fibrillating hearts, in the ventricles of very dilated hearts, and in abdominal aortas affected by severe arteriosclerosis.

During the progression of intimal arteriosclerosis, the media of the blood vessel affected appears relatively uninvolved. However, in the late stage of intimal arteriosclerosis, the plaques may become large and hard and press upon the media of the blood vessel with the result that local muscle atrophy occurs with infiltration of both the media and adventitia by chronic inflammatory cells. When the media of the affected blood vessel becomes weakened, the patient may be predisposed to the development of the arteriosclerotic aneurysm. The aneurysm is a pathologic process causing the ballooning out of a blood vessel. Saccular aneurysms are round or globoid in shape and affect only a short portion of the vessel. Fusiform aneurysms have a fusiform shape and involves a longer segment of the vessel with the dilatation of the vessel wall becoming most severe in the central part of the aneurysm. Aneurysms are the result of damage to the media of the blood vessel because the media represents the main tissue of the vessel wall. The media also controls the pressure of the blood. Aneurysms primarily create eddy currents and produce stagnant blood in the pathologically enlarged lumen; secondarily, the stagnant blood is responsible for the formation of thrombi in the aneurysm. Dissecting aneurysm has a communication between the lumen of the vessel or a rupture of a large vasa vasorum with splitting of the layers of the blood vessel wall by dissection of blood. The dissecting aneurysm is generally several millimeters or one centimeter in thickness; however, the aneurysm may extend for long distances along the vessel wall. Complications of the dissecting aneurysm are rupture into the surrounding tissues and fatal hemorrhages.

The etiology of intimal arteriosclerosis is highly obscure in spite of the tremendous number of reports and theories in the literature. However, the following facts represent a summary of our present knowledge:

1. Intimal arteriosclerosis occurs in all humans. It increases with age in local intensity and scope of distribution. It must be of multiple etiologies and is an aging phenomenon.

2. Intimal arteriosclerosis is focal in nature; therefore, it is not caused by a universal pathologic process of the vascular system. The focal disease is more severe in nature in the larger sized arteries and in the aorta. Arteriosclerosis of the aorta is generally more severe in nature if located in the abdominal compared to the thoracic portion of the aorta. The reason is obscure, but in man, there is increased pressure of the blood in the abdominal aorta and this portion is more fixed. Hypertension appears to increase the severity of arteriosclerosis in the abdominal aorta and elsewhere.

3. Intimal arteriosclerosis is affected by heredity. For example, the Japanese and African Bantu have a lower incidence of arteriosclerosis than persons living in the United States. The cause is obscure and perhaps is related in some manner to the diet.

4. Intimal arteriosclerosis is increased if systemic diastolic hypertension is present. Arteriosclerosis is generally absent in the pulmonary arteries unless systemic diastolic hypertension and pulmonary hypertension are present.

5. Intimal arteriosclerosis is increased in areas of blood vessels that are under stress. For instance arteriosclerosis is increased at bifurcations and where the blood vessel is not free to expand and contract (posterior portion of the aorta where it rests against the spinal cord). The hemodynamic theory of origin of arteriosclerosis is that stress occurs by the lowering of the lateral pressure of the blood at the hemodynamic stress points.

6. Intimal arteriosclerosis occurs more frequently in males and females who have passed the menopause. Females prior to the menopause do have arteriosclerosis, but it is less severe and uncomplicated until after age fifty-five.

7. Dietary habits are related to intimal arteriosclerosis. The

obese patient with normal clinical laboratory findings has more arteriosclerosis than the nonobese patient. If the obese patients have hyperlipemia and hypercholesterolemia in addition to obesity, they are more likely to develop severe intimal arteriosclerosis. Other factors appear to be important in intimal arteriosclerosis, but the elevated lipids appear to play a dominant role. Therefore, unsaturated (vegetable) fats have been recommended to replace the saturated fats; however, this fact has not been substantiated.

8. The use of tobacco increases the severity of intimal arteriosclerosis.

9. That intramural hemorrhages may be related to the etiology of intimal arteriosclerosis is without proof. The status of new vessels in the arteriosclerotic plaque and the blood platelets may play some role. The newly formed blood vessels are more delicate and more readily ruptured, producing hemorrhages.

10. Thrombosis, however, is important in the development of complications from intimal arteriosclerosis. Fibrinolysins may be involved and activated when thrombosis develops. Thrombi formed in blood vessels may last for hours to one or two days, causing infarction; however, they can be lysed by the fibrinolysins. This situation occurs in the human heart.

11. It is possible that the type of circulating lipids and lipoproteins is important in arteriosclerosis. Lipoproteins, not lipids, in the plasma or ateriosclerotic plaque may be proven to be a most vital factor in development and prognosis of intimal arteriosclerosis.

12. Environmental influences (urban living) and socioeconomic status have not been proven to be etiologic factors since they are complicated by diet, exercise, and other factors.

13. Intimal arteriosclerosis is increased in individuals with a sedentary occupation or environment. Sudden exercise or exertion has no proven relationship to intimal arteriosclerosis regardless of the coronaries reported while straining at stool.

14. The veins of humans show no lesions similar to intimal arteriosclerosis. However, veins are affected by phlebosclerosis or a fibrotic thickening of vessel walls.

Arteriosclerosis should be considered as the result of many and various types of traumas. It is the result of many different types of injuries that occur with aging, following by repair of the damage. It is affected by the lipids present in the body, which are in turn controlled by both diet and heredity. Lipids may accumulate in the damaged wall of the vessel, and the lipids cause secondary damage, etc.

Arteriolar Sclerosis

Arteriolar sclerosis is defined as a subdivision of the general area of arteriosclerosis. It is, however, a separate entity, which affects the smallest arteries and arterioles. There are three types of arteriolar sclerosis: hyalin arteriolar sclerosis, hyperplastic arteriolar sclerosis, and necrotizing arteriolitis.

Hyaline arteriolar sclerosis results from a gradual deposition of the granular glycoprotein present beneath the elastic lamina (external to the elastic lamina) in arterioles of larger caliber. Histopathologically, this material present appears bright red and is a glossy and structureless mass called hyalin. The hyalin has a very fine granularity and contains ferritin granules. Arteriolar sclerosis is related to slowly progressive diastolic essential hypertension. There is a direct association between hyalin arteriolar sclerosis and hypertension. Hyalin arteriolar sclerosis is rarely seen, outside of the spleen, except in hypertensives and diabetics. Within the spleen, hyaline arteriolar sclerosis probably develops and progresses with aging. The deposition of hyaline interferes, in time, with the normal flow of blood when the size of the vessel lumen is decreased. The etiology of the hyalin is obscure. Perhaps it is diffusion of normal or abnormal plasma proteins. No evidence is available to prove that the hyalin represents an antigen-antibody complex as seen in lupus erythymatosis and glomerulonephritis. Hyalin may contain gamma globulins and fibrin.

Hyperplastic arteriolar sclerosis is a proliferative type of lesion in which layers of cells develop in the intima between the endothelial basement membrane and the smooth muscle or elastica. The proliferating cells in the intima may be either mesenchymal cells or migrated smooth muscle cells similar to the origin of cells in intimal arteriosclerosis. There is a reduplication and/or degeneration of the internal elastic lamina in hyperplastic arteriolar sclerosis. The many layers of proliferating cells and the reduplication of the internal elastic lamina appear to be separated by clear spaces (perhaps artifact or edema). Because of the microscopic appearance of this hyperplastic lesion, it has been called onion-skin arterioles. Hyperplastic arteriolar sclerosis is primarily associated with rapid, progressive, and severe hypertension.

Necrotizing arteriolitis (fibrinoid change or fibrinoid necrosis) is another type of lesion involving arterioles. It is generally considered as acute degeneration, necrosis, and inflammatory response often superimposed on fibrinoid necrosis or change. Necrotizing arteriolitis consists of (1) edema; (2) deposition of eosinophilic granular material and fibrin deposited in vessel wall; (3) necrosis; and (4) thrombosis of arterioles. Necrotizing arteriolitis is associated with individuals having long-standing hypertension and hyalin arteriolar sclerosis or in young individuals who develop severe hypertension and hyperplastic arteriolar sclerosis. If the hypertension and vascular alterations are rapid or increase in severity, the condition is called malignant or accelerated hypertension. Arterioles show fibrinoid necrosis, and the necrosis is generally present with thrombosis or rupture and complete interruption of the blood flow. Necrotizing arteriolitis is common in the kidney and produces malignant nephrosclerosis and uremia.

Hypertension (High Blood Pressure)

High blood pressure is a common disease with obscure cause(s). It is more common in females than males by two to one. During the heart beat or systole, the most important element is the force of the heart and the elasticity of the aorta. Between the heart beats or diastole, the blood pressure (diastolic blood pressure) is primarily dependent upon the size of the arterioles. Normally the systolic blood pressure is 100 to 150 mmHg and the diastolic blood pressure is 70 to 90 mmHg. The systolic blood pressure must always be higher than the diastolic blood pressure.

Hypertension may be classified into diastolic or systolic hypertension. Diastolic hypertension is the most frequent form and is prominent in middle age. It begins as an intermittent spasm of the arteriole wall, producing intermittent elevations of the diastolic blood pressure. The systolic blood pressure is elevated secondarily. Spasm eventually becomes permanent, and the arterioles become involved with arteriolar sclerosis. Diastolic hypertension appears concurrently and simultaneously with arteriolar sclerosis. Diastolic hypertension is generally associated with the severe form of arteriosclerosis. It has not been proven that the hypertension is the cause of arteriosclerosis. Hypertension appears only to accelerate the continued progression of a preexisting arteriosclerosis. Over 90 percent of instances of diastolic hypertension have no definitive or apparent cause and are, therefore, termed *idiopathic* or *essential hypertension*. Essential hypertension is commonly associated with individuals under stress and in individuals with labile emotional patterns. A blood pressure of 150/90 mmHg is indicative of diastolic hypertension. In 5 to 10 percent of individuals with diastolic hypertension, the disease is considered to be due to renal or endocrine disease.

Systolic hypertension is an aging disease probably caused by the loss of elasticity of the aorta due to the presence of Mönckeberg's medial arteriosclerosis or calcification of the media and the degeneration of the elastica. This form of hypertension has a typical blood pressure of 200/80 mmHg and rarely causes complications.

The following three observations illustrate the interrelationships between hypertension and arteriosclerosis:

1. Intimal arteriosclerosis causes vascular occlusion with infarction;

2. Arteriolar spasm and/or sclerosis causes diastolic hypertension above 90 mmHg; and

3. Medial arteriosclerosis (Mönckeberg's sclerosis) causes systolic hypertension with systolic blood pressure of 180 to 200 mmHg. The diastolic pressure is 80 to 90 mmHg (normal).

Blood Volume and Shock

Blood volume is defined as the plasma and red and white blood cells and represents all material or elements circulating in the arteries, veins, and capillaries of the body. The blood volume is approximately 5 percent of the total mass of the human body, or about 3600 to 6000 cc. The blood volume tends to be constant primarily at the expense of the interstitial fluid and secondarily at the expense of the cellular fluid. When disease or injury occurs the normal blood volume may be decreased below a critical level, i.e. less than 75 percent of normal volume, wherein shock results.

Shock is a situation of the body whereby there is inefficient circulation of blood caused by the following:

1. An imbalance between the size of the vascular bed and the blood volume, and

2. An inability on the part of the heart to produce enough force to drive the blood in a normal fashion.

Shock occurs if the blood pressure drops below 90/60 mmHg (only general rule with exception for small females). In order to diagnose shock, one must observe the following clinical signs and symptoms: lethargy, confusion or coma, weak and rapid pulse, oliguria, cold and clammy extremities, and pallor. The normal renal function, is reduced, and urine outflow is low or completely absent.

There are three types of shock, i.e. hypovolemic, cardiogenic, and low-resistance. Hypovolemic shock is caused by injury, hemorrhage, burns, salt and water depletion. The blood volume may be low in red blood cells and low in plasma. Peripheral resistance is high, cardiac output is diminished, and venous pressure is normal or low.

Cardiogenic shock is caused by myocardial infarction, heart failure, pulmonary embolism, and cardiac tamponade. The blood volume is high or normal. The peripheral resistance is high with arterioles contracted. Cardiac output is greatly diminished and venous pressure is increased.

Low-resistance shock is caused by gram-negative septicemia with endotoxins, toxins, acidosis, adrenal insufficiency, drugs, electrolyte imbalance, and neurogenic reflex. The blood volume is normal, peripheral resistance is low with dilated arterioles, cardiac output is diminished, and venous pressure is low.

Differentiation of shock into primary and secondary forms is obsolete and should be abandoned. Primary shock has in the past referred to an acute reaction to stress. It is the immediate reaction due to neurogenic stimuli, which results in vascular relaxation and the pooling of blood in capillaries. There is a fall in blood pressure and failure of the right heart to fill, leading to asystole or stoppage of the heart for a few seconds. The brain becomes hypoxic, and temporary unconsciousness occurs. The latter is known as fainting (syncope). Recovery is generally prompt as the body defensive mechanisms come into play. Today, we do not use the term *primary shock,* and the term *shock,* therefore, refers to secondary shock.

Reduction in Blood Volume

The causes of reduction in blood volume are hemorrhage, burn shock, massive infection, massive trauma (crush syndrome), severe dehydration, and Addison's disease (adrenal cortical insufficiency). Internal or external hemorrhage leads to hemorrhagic shock, a form of hypovolemic shock. The concentration of the blood and the hematocrit remains normal for the first six to eight hours following hemorrhage. After this period, the blood will be diluted by the movement of water passing into the vascular compartment. The plasma begins to regenerate in one to two days, and the red blood cells regenerate after three to seven days. Complete restoration of blood requires three to four weeks following extensive loss. The more rapid the loss of blood, the less loss of the blood required to cause shock.

Burn shock is caused by partial destruction of the blood by the heat present at the time of the burn with the loss of a few red blood cells. However, burns predominantly produce leakage of plasma from the damaged capillaries. Hemoconcentration of the blood is normal, and the hematocrit is elevated in burn shock.

Massive infection is capable of causing shock. Shock results primarily by a direct action of bacterial endotoxins or toxins on capillaries, which causes paralysis of arteriole, muscle with arteriole, and capillary dilatation and/or leakage of plasma. There may be some role played by the central nervous system action in causing the vascular paralysis. Gram-negative microorganisms are primarily the etiologic agent.

Massive trauma (crush syndrome) produces reduction in

blood volume and causes shock. The following mechanisms appear to be responsible for the shock:
1. toxic products released from the damaged tissue (these play a major role);
2. hemorrhage;
3. direct physical capillary damage from the injury; and
4. occasional hypoxia.

Surgical procedures cause trauma; extensive procedures, particularly extensive handling of the gut, may cause surgical or traumatic shock.

Severe dehydration may result in the loss of blood volume. Addison's disease (adrenal cortical insufficiency) may result in loss of salt and water with a decrease in blood volume, causing a direct effect on the heart and great vessels, and causing shock. Shock is the most common cause of death in Addison's disease.

An increase in the size of the vascular bed in man may be due to hypoxia, toxins or poisons, infections, massive trauma, brain lesions, and neurogenic factors. The increase in the size of the vascular bed is rarely responsible for shock by itself.

Cardiac shock is generally due to myocardial infarction caused by the occlusion of a coronary artery. The efficacy of the heart becomes reduced from normal so that the available force is less than required to pump the blood.

Irreversible shock occurs when the general breakdown in body metabolism has advanced to the point where restoration of the normal human circulation is not possible. If the circulation is restored, however, the tissues have undergone such damage that shock recurs in a few hours and the patient succumbs. Shock leads to hypoxia, hypoxia leads to more shock, etc., until death occurs. Metabolic alterations are capable of causing similar situations that contribute to promoting shock.

The pathology of shock encompasses a generalized parenchymatous degeneration, focal zones of necrosis of tissues, capillary and venous dilatation and congestion, petechiae, and edema. The terminal pathologic events include pulmonary edema. As the blood pressure falls, the kidney goes into either oliguria (partial reduction in the flow of urine) or anuria (complete cessation of the flow of urine. If shock should be prolonged for more than a few hours, extensive degeneration of the renal tubules (acute tubular necrosis) is the result. Since the distal nephron is generally most severely damaged during shock, this situation has been termed *lower nephron nephrosis*. Fatty infiltration of the liver and heart occurs during shock, indicating cellular damage due to poor circulation of blood. The adrenals also show stress reactions, and acute gastrointestinal ulcerations (acute stress ulcers) may develop during the shock state. On rare occasions, a large area of the gastrointestinal tract will show hemorrhagic necrosis during shock.

Blood Clotting

The human body has a mechanism for stopping hemorrhages. When the blood vessel is severed, there is an immediate spasm of the muscle in the vessel wall near the severed end or cut, which stops or slows the blood flow. When the severed blood vessel is very small, the severed end may be filled with platelets, i.e. a platelet thrombus develops. The absence of blood platelets is responsible for many small hemorrhage (petechiae). When a larger vessel is severed, the mechanism for stopping the hemorrhage is formation of a fibrin blood clot formed primarily of fibrin, blood platelets, and other blood elements within the lumen of a blood vessel or in the heart of a living person.

The normal circulating blood stream contains the following elements:

1. Fibrinogen, a liquid protein formed in the liver;

2. Platelets, small portions of cells called megakaryocytes, which grow in the bone marrow. On rupture, platelets release thromboplastin;

3. Prothrombin, a complex chemical (alpha 2 globulin) made in the liver from vitamin K;

4. Calcium;

5. Thromboplastin, a chemical not actually present in the plasma but formed in various ways. It is formed from broken down platelets, from lacerated tissues, or from a combination of red blood cells and plasma; and

6. Antienzymes such as fibrinolysins and antithrombin-globulin, which interfere with blood clotting. Hemophilia is a congenital bleeding disease and, therefore, should be classified here.

When an injury occurs to tissues of the body, the following takes place:

1. Prothrombin in the presence of thromboplastin and other factors produces thrombin; and
2. Liquid fibrinogen in the presence of thrombin plus plasma calcium produces solid fibrin.

The solid fibrin clot forms outside of a blood vessel, i.e. in the tissues. A thrombus forms inside the blood vessel and seals off the severed portion of the blood vessel. The blood clot in the area of tissue damage also acts as a framework upon which the repair process begins. It should be remembered that the clotting mechanism is balanced by a fibrinolysin mechanism of the body, the function of which is to dissolve the blood clot.

Hemorrhagic diseases are present when the blood clotting mechanism in man fails because of a deficiency of the required materials. For instance, the liver manufactures the fibrinogen and the prothrombin. Only rarely is the fibrinogen deficient. However, in severe liver diseases associated with jaundice, the prothrombin is generally decreased, producing multiple bleeding areas termed *hemorrhagic diathesis*. Prothrombin may be measured by the time it requires a standard mixture of blood to clot. The latter is termed the *prothrombin time* and is reported as a percent of the normal. A prothrombin time below 25 percent means we may expect bleeding. Platelets are manufactured by the bone marrow. Platelets are the main, but not only, source of thromboplastin. They act to terminate small hemorrhages by means of formation of platelet thrombi. Thus, when there is a destructive process in the bone marrow caused by leukemia, chemicals, etc., small hemorrhages invariably follow and are termed *thrombocytopenic purpura*. The platelets normally have a reading of 150,000 to 250,000 per cubic millimeter. A platelet value below 30,000 indicates hemorrhage is present.

Thrombosis

Thrombosis is defined as the formation of a solid mass derived from the constituents of the blood within a blood vessel or the heart cavities during life. This is a defensive and useful process intended to protect the individual from the loss of blood from the vascular system. However, thrombosis may occur in occasional situations where it is unneeded, and the result is a harmful accident.

The most common causes of thrombosis are damage to the blood vessel wall, interference with the blood flow leading to stasis, abnormalities of the clotting mechanism, and hyperconcentration of the blood.

Damages to the blood vessel wall are due to arteriosclerosis (may partially block blood flow), trauma to vessel, inflammation around an underlying cardiac infarct, infection (subacute bacterial endocarditis), polyarteritis nodosa (immunologic or allergic disease), hypoxia, frostbite or burn, and necrotizing arteriolitis (fibrinoid necrosis with malignant hypertension).

Interference with the blood flow leading to stasis is caused by heart failure; immobilization (in legs of bedridden patients); varicose veins; blockage of vessel by atheroma, neoplasm, etc.; eddy currents; and arteriosclerosis. Abnormalities of the clotting mechanism are due to the variations in inhibitors or to abnormal substances. Increased clotting may be seen in patients with neoplasms (carcinoma of the pancreas). Hyperconcentration of blood results following dehydration or polycythemia, i.e. a disease where the red blood cell mass is markedly increased.

When the thrombus forms in the heart chambers and aorta, it tends to occur as a plaquelike substance, which covers only one part of the circumference of the chamber or aorta. It is, therefore, referred to as a mural thrombus. The mural thrombus may form upon a diseased heart valve. The latter thrombus hangs into the lumen of the heart chamber and is termed a *vegetation.* If the initial thrombus forms in the medium or small vessels, it begins in a vessel with blood flowing normally. A small clot forms in this vessel, then propagates around the wall of the blood vessel to circumscribe the lumen. The clot then begins to build up alternating layers of platelets and white blood cells mixed with fibrin to give a layered effect (laminated effect), which gradually causes occlusion of the vessel lumen. The central portion of the lumen of blood vessels is the last area of the vessel to be occluded. Alternating layers of blood platelets and blood cells and fibrin are visible grossly and microscopically and are called the lines of Zahn.

The thrombus, being an antemortem blood clot, must be differentiated from the postmortem clot (clot formed within vessels after death), clots that form within the tissues or outside the body after hemorrhages, and emboli.

Grossly, examination of a thrombus reveals a firm, mottled pink, gray, and yellow mass. Microscopically, the thrombus contains lines of platelets alternating with layers of fibrin containing white blood cells and some red blood cells. Beginning organization may be seen microscopically (small blood vessels, white and red blood cells) at the periphery of the thrombus. When the mechanism of thrombosis is complete, the blood clots rapidly in adjacent vessels above and below the thrombus. Clotting may proceed for some distance from the initial site of occlusion and is termed *propagation of the thrombus.*

The postmortem clot has a uniform dark red color like currant jelly. If clotting is rapid it appears as a partially red, dependent part. If clotting is slow it appears as a partial, pale, grayish yellow part. The slow clotting allows time for the red blood cells to settle out and form a chicken-fat clot. The postmortem clot is moist, elastic, and retracts from the wall so that it may not completely fill the lumen of the blood vessel. Clot retraction prevents the postmortem clot from filling the lumen of the blood vessel.

Venous thrombosis due to stasis in a vein is termed *phlebothrombosis.* If the venous thrombosis is due to an infection of the vessel wall, its condition is termed *thrombophlebitis.* Clots caused by phlebothrombosis are frequently located in the leg veins or in the pelvic veins, and are not strongly united to the vessel wall. Therefore, they tend to break off readily, and emboli result.

Embolism and Thromboembolism

Embolus is defined as any foreign substance freely circulating in the blood stream during life. A thrombus, which is composed of constitutents of the blood, is a foreign substance and should be considered an embolus once it moves from its site of origin. Thrombi are considered the most common form of emboli. The following types of emboli occur in man: thrombi, fat, bone marrow, neoplastic cells, air, gases, amniotic fluid, and atheromatous material. Some emboli are infected by invasion of microorganism and are termed *septic emboli*. Emboli may develop in the arteries, capillaries, veins, or lymphatics of man.

Thromboembolism is defined as the process of thrombosis, which is followed by the breaking off of a portion of the thrombus, which is then carried in the circulation to a distant site where it occludes another vessel. The embolus lodges in another vessel of smaller diameter, and subsequently, a secondary thrombosis develops around the lodged embolus. Thrombi produce emboli; however, the embolus does not assume the shape of the blood vessel in which it becomes lodged. Emboli may be coiled structures or are crammed into a blood vessel of smaller caliber. Emboli may arise from older thrombi and, therefore, have a pink color and firm consistency. After the embolus has lodged in a distant vessel, it is common for an additional or new thrombus to form around the embolus. This fresh thrombus is darker red in color and has a more gelatinous consistency when compared to the lodged embolus. If the embolus is large, the patient frequently succumbs. If the patient does not die immediately, there is formation of a secondary thrombosis directly around the embolus plus necrosis (infarction) of the tissue or organ supplied by the occluded vessel. When the embolus is not fatal, the secondary thrombosis around the embolus propagates so that it fills the entire lumen of the vessel. The older embolus will be more pink in color, more firm in consistency, and appear coiled. The recent (secondary) thrombosis is more red in color and gelatinous in consistency. Thrombi remaining at their site of origin can cause complete occlusion of vessels.

Thromboembolism commonly occurs in the deep veins of the

leg and as embolization in the lungs. Thrombi also form in the veins of the pelvic periprostatic plexus from which emboli travel to the lungs. Auricular fibrillation (a rhythm disturbance in the auricle of the right side of the heart) may result in the formation of a thrombus within the auricle. The latter thrombus breaks off and may be transported to the lungs. If a thrombus (mural) is present on a valve of the right side of the heart, it may break off and also be transported to the lung. The venous and right heart thrombi are all stopped by the capillary plexus of the lungs. A thrombus may also develop in the left auricle or on a valve on the left side of the heart. A mural thrombus of the left side of the heart may produce secondary emboli, which are transported to the distal arteries.

Infarction

Infarction is defined as a form of tissue necrosis during life. The cells of a tissue die during infarction, while the individual lives on. The necrosis of tissue has the capacity to stimulate a reaction to the dead cells, and this bodily reaction differentiates necrosis from simple postmortem changes. Infarction is one form out of many forms of tissue necrosis; it is necrosis of tissue caused by the loss of an adequate blood supply. Infarction is an ischemic type of tissue necrosis, ischemia being defined as the lack of an adequate blood supply. Infarction is commonly (not universally) the result of the sudden occlusion of a vessel, which produces ischemic necrosis, i.e. coagulation necrosis in a tissue without an adequate collateral circulation. Infarctions, however, are not always associated with the sudden occlusion of a vessel. Some instances of infarction do not produce coagulation necrosis, but in its place liquefaction necrosis is evident as in infarction in the brain. Venous occlusion may represent the etiology of an infarct in certain tissues and regions of the body. Collateral circulation may be present in an area, but inadequate due to occlusion of the collateral vessels. A temporary partial loss of the blood supply to the brain may result in infarction. However, an extended partial loss of the blood supply or a short, one-hour loss of all of the blood supply to a muscle or tendon generally does not result in infarction. In summary, the more highly differentiated the tissue, the more sensitive is the tissue to development of an infarct from reduction of the blood supply.

Microscopically, the central zone of the infarct shows coagulation necrosis or liquefaction necrosis with a fading out of cell and tissue outlines. An acute inflammatory reaction occurs surrounding the outline of the coagulation necrosis (infarct). Polymorphonuclear leukocytes occur initially, and subsequently, repair is present with fibrosis, large mononuclear cells, and new blood vessels. In small infarcts the dead cellular debris may be removed by phagocytosis, and scar tissue results. In larger infarcts it may be incapable of being removed; thus, a mass of hyalinized necrotic tissue occurs in the center of the infarct, surrounded by a band of scar tissue at the periphery of the infarct. Some infarcts that undergo liquefaction necrosis (brain) produce cystic spaces in the affected tissue.

The causes of infarction are arteriosclerosis with or without thrombosis, periarteritis or thrombophlebitis with thrombosis, thromboembolism, torsion of the intestine or testicle with blockage of the blood supply. Infarction may occur in a tissue, but the pathologist fails to find an occluded vessel. This type of infarction is the result of a temporary ischemia occurring in a highly susceptible tissue (brain) or is due to a thrombus that has subsequently been removed by fibrinolysins.

Cerebral infarcts are principally the result of arteriosclerotic thrombosis. These infarcts appear as pale yellow in color, unless complicated by secondary hemorrhage, and consist of liquefaction necrosis and cystic spaces. Pulmonary infarcts assume a wedge shape because the arteries fan out in their distribution to the tissues. Pulmonary infarction results from arterial emboli from the leg or from prostatic veins. The normal lung has a double blood supply. Therefore, pulmonary infarcts are rare in this organ. When they do develop, they appear as red, somewhat raised areas of necrosis containing abundant blood and are, therefore, called hemorrhagic infarcts. The presence of blood occurs because of the double blood supply. Other organs with a double or collateral blood supply also produce hemorrhagic infarcts. Thrombosis of the mesenteric artery produces infarction in the small intestines and a portion of the colon. The thrombosis is caused by embolization of the mesenteric artery, i.e. an arterial embolus, and is accompanied by abundant hemorrhage. However, less hemorrhage is present in the arterial embolization compared to a mesenteric venous occlusion plus infarction, where massive hemorrhage is present. Infarction of the liver, spleen, and kidney results in anemic coagulation necrosis. The renal infarct develops as a rectangular-shaped infarct in the cortex of the kidney because of its blood supply and distribution.

Arteritis

Arteritis is defined as acute inflammation of an arterial wall, including the aorta. Arteritis is caused by bacteria and viruses. Arteritis is accompanied by a great concentration and mobilization of polymorphonuclear leukocytes and antibodies; therefore, infectious arteritis is only rarely a primary arteritis. Arteritis develops when large numbers of microorganisms are lodged in an artery and constitute a portion of an embolus in an infected heart valve. The infected heart valve is called bacterial endocarditis. Thus the infected embolus is the cause of the arteritis. Arteritis may undermine and weaken the wall of an artery or the aorta producing the aneurysm. When an aneurysm is caused by infection, generally from the infected emboli, it is known as a mycotic aneurysm. Mycotic aneurysm has no relationship to the fungi but is bacterial or viral in origin.

Polyarteritis nodosa is a form of arteritis whereby an acute immunological disease is present in the arterial wall. Acute inflammation is present throughout all coats of the vessel wall. Polyarteritis nodosa is generally accompanied by an associated thrombosis and secondary infarct in the area supplied by the altered vessel.

Arteries frequently traverse areas of inflammation in the tissues and organs of the body. For example, pneumonia may produce a secondary type of arteritis in the arteries passing through the pulmonary tissues. This secondary type of arteritis is less commonly accompanied by thrombosis, but when thrombosis does occur with secondary arteritis, the infarction that results in regions close to the original infection is termed *septic infarct*.

Venous Disorders

Phlebosclerosis is defined as the scarring of the wall of the vein and is similar to arteriosclerosis in arteries. Phlebosclerosis is only rarely of a severe, occlusive nature and primarily consists of a minimal increase in the fibrous tissue of the wall of the affected vein. The scarring of the wall of a vein is commonly associated with increased venous pressure and generally a stagnant venous blood flow. Therefore, phlebosclerosis is common in regions containing varicose veins, and these areas are also likely to reveal thrombosis.

Varicose veins develop in veins when the valves that direct the blood flow to the heart are incompetent. The normally present valves may be congenitally missing, or the veins may begin to stretch as aging occurs, allowing the valve to develop incompetencies. Individuals who stand on their feet for long periods of time tend to develop varicose veins in the lower extremities. However, varicose veins also may develop in the esophagus (esophageal varices) and in the rectum (hemorrhoids). Thrombosis commonly develops in varicose veins because of the stagnant venous flow.

Thrombophlebitis is defined as a combination of phlebitis and thrombosis. It may develop in any region of the body when an infected vessel is present. Primary thrombophlebitis occurs more commonly in the legs. The thrombus has a tendency to be attached to the vessel wall because of the inflammation and is less commonly set free to embolize distant vessels.

Phlebothrombosis is defined as a combination of dilated veins, stagnant blood flow, plus phlebosclerosis and thrombosis. Only a minor inflammation reaction ensues, and the thrombi are thus not sufficiently attached to the vessel wall. Thrombi are, therefore, the most common cause of thromboembolism from veins.

References

Balis, J.U., et al.: *Exp Mol Pathol, 3*:511, 1964.
Berger, S.: *Can Med Assoc J, 102*:1271, 1970.

Bernstein, A.: *Acta Chir Scand, 62*:124, 1927.
Bland, J.H.: *Clinical Metabolism of Body Water and Electrolytes*, Philadelphia, Saunders, 1963.
Burnell, J.M. and Schribner, B.H.: *JAMA, 164*:959, 1957.
Byrne, J.J.: *N Engl J Med, 275*:543, 1966.
Catt, K.J., et al.: *Lancet*, 6 March 1971, p. 459.
Chien, S. and Gregersen, M.I.: In Mountcastle, V.B. (Ed.): *Medical Physiology*. St. Louis, Mosby, p. 262-283.
Chobanian: *J Clin Invest, 47*:595, 1968.
Christy, J.H.: *Am Heart J, 81*:694, 1971.
Daoud, A., et al.: *Exp Mol Pathol, 3*:475, 1964.
Deykin, D.: *N Engl J Med, 283*:636, 1970.
Deykin, D.: *Calif Med, 112*:31, 1970.
Edelman, I.S. and Leibman, J.: *Am J Med, 27*:256, 1959.
Edelman, I.S., et al.: Body composition: studies in the human being by the dilution principle. *Science, 115*:447, 1952.
Elton, N.W., et al.: *Am J Clin Pathol, 39*:252, 1963.
Finberg, L., et al.: *JAMA, 184*:187, 1963.
Fox, C.L. and Nahas, G.G.: *Body Fluid Replacement in the Surgical Patient*. New York, Grune, 1970.
Franklin, K.J.: *A Monograph on Veins*. Springfield, Thomas, 1937, p. 410.
French, J.E.: In *International Review of Experimental Pathology*, New York, Acad Pr, 1966, vol.V, 253.
Friedman, M., et al.: *Am J Clin Pathol, 45*:238, 1966.
Friedman, M.: *Adv Cardiol, 4*:20, 1970.
Gauer, O.H., et al.: *Annu Rev Physiol, 32*:547, 1970.
Geer, J.C.: *Am J Pathol, 47*:241, 1965.
Geer, J.C., et al.: *Am J Pathol, 38*:263, 1961.
Goldzieher, J.W.: *Fed Proc, 29*:1220, 1970.
Haddy, F.J.: *Ann Intern Med, 73*:809, 1970.
Homans, J.: *N Engl J Med, 250*:148, 1954.
Hume, M., et al.: *Venous Thrombosis and Pulmonary Embolism*. Cambridge, Harvard Pr, 1970.
Inman, W.H.W.: *Br Med Bull, 26*:248, 1970.
MacFarlane, R.G.: Blood coagulation in theory and practice. In *Lectures on the Scientific Basis of Medicine*. London, The Athlone Press, 1953, vol.I, pp. 244-266, 1951-52.
Maxwell, M.H. and Kleeman, C.R.: *Clinical Disorders of Fluid and Electrolyte Metabolism*. New York, McGraw, 1972.
Moore, F.D.: *N Engl Med J, 273*:567, 1965.
Mudge, G.H. and Vislocky, L.: *J Clin Invest, 28*:482, 1949.
Nahas, G.G (Ed): *Ann NY Acad Sci, 133*:1-274, 1966.

Naide, M.: *JAMA, 148*:1202, 1952.
Parker, F. and Odland, G.F.: *Am J Pathol, 48*:197, 1966.
Pitts, R.F.: *Physiology of the Kidney and Body Fluids: An Introductory Text,* 3rd ed. Chicago, Year Bk Med, 1974.
Sherry, S., et al.: *Thrombosis.* Washington, D.C., Natural Academy of Sciences, 1969.
Shoemaker, W.C.: *Surg Gynecol Obstet, 132*:411, 1971.
Simpson, K.: *Lancet, 239*:744, 1940.
Singer, R.B. and Hastings, A.B.: *Medicine (Baltimore), 27*:223, 1948.
Smith, F.C.: *Am J Surg, 40*:131, 1926.
Spaet, T.H. and Gaynor, E.: *Ad Cardiol, 4*:47, 1970.
Spiro, D., et al.: *Am J Pathol, 47*:19, 1965.
Statland, H.: *Fluid and Electrolytes in Practice,* 2nd ed. Philadelphia, Lippincott, 1957.
Singer, R.B. and Hastings, A.B.: *Medicine (Baltimore), 27*:223, 1948.
Stengle, J.M.: *Blood, 35*:867, 1970.
Stormorken, H. and Owren, P.A.: *Semin Hematol, 8*:29, 1971.
Straus, R., et al.: *Am J Clin Pathol, 41*:352, 1964.
Symposium on Atherosclerosis. *Am J Med, 46*:657, 684, 691, 735, 741, May, 1969.
Symposium on Hypertension. *Circ Res,* Suppl. 1, May, 1969.
Tedeschi, L.G., et al.: *Hum Pathol, 2*:165, 1971.
Texon, M., et al.: *JAMA, 194*:1226, 1965.
Ward, P.A.: *Am J Pathol, 54*:121, 1969.
Warren, S. and LeCompte, P.M.: *The Pathology of Diabetes Mellitus,* 3rd ed. Philadelphia, Lea & Febiger, 1952, p. 130.
Webber, A.J. and Johnson, S.A.: *Am J Pathol, 60*:19, 1970.
Weisberg, H.F.: *Water Electrolyte, and Acid-Base Balance,* 2nd ed. Baltimore, Williams and Wilkins, 1962.
Winters, R.W.: *The Body Fluids in Pediatrics.* Boston, Little, 1973.
Wooley, C.F.: *Arch Intern Med, 125*:126, 1970.
Wright, H.: *J Pathol, 54*:461, 1942.
Wynn, V.: *Clin Sci, 14*:669, 1955.

CHAPTER 7

INFLAMMATION

INFLAMMATION IS DEFINED as a vascular response of the body when any tissue is injured and is an example of physiology under duress. The injury to the tissue may result from physical, chemical, or thermal factors or from infectious microorganisms. Inflammation cannot take place in nonvascular tissues, i.e. joint cartilage and the lens of the eye. Inflammatory responses occur in the tissues from the following injuries: sunburn, insect sting or bites, boil or furuncle, and hives of hypersensitive subjects. Inflammation should be viewed as an extraluminal vascular defense mechanism, which is supported by adjacent tissues. During the inflammatory response, there develops a concentration of leukocytes and plasma cells outside the vessel wall in the local injured or damaged area.

In inflammation increased fluid and cells escape from the capillaries. There is reduction of the venous return, with the excessive fluid passing into the lymphatics.

The inflammatory or vascular response to an injury consists of the following phases:

1. A vasokinetic phase whereby small blood vessels constrict, then undergo dilatation accompanied by increased hydrostatic pressure and increased permeability;

2. A fluid phase characterized by extravasation of plasma due to increased intravascular pressure and permeability with formation of inflammatory edema; and

3. A leukocytic phase characterized by emigration of white blood cells with formation of a cellular exudate.

The three phases of the inflammatory response are generally initiated within thirty minutes after the tissue is injured; however, if the injury is chemical or electrical burns, it may require several hours for these responses to occur.

An immediate response occurs in the affected area in instances of pyogenic inflammation (abscess caused by staphylococci). The local vessels undergo a temporary vasoconstriction, followed by rapid dilatation of the small arteries and capillaries. Capillary permeability increases, and plasma plus red blood cells passes through the vessel wall. The plasma is extravasated, and the red blood cells pass through the vessel wall by a process termed *diapedesis*. Initially, the circulation of blood is accelerated because of the capillary dilatation. However, the current of blood is slowed since the loss of plasma produced a greater viscosity, which is associated with an irritated endothelium, whose cells bulge into the lumen of the vessel to slow the circulation. The leukocytes present in the slowed circulation move from the center of the lumen to the periphery, where they come in contact with the irritated endothelium and subsequently pass through the vessel wall by ameboid motion. When the leukocytes adhere and line up along the endothelial wall of the vessel, the process is referred to as margination. When the leukocytes migrate by ameboid movement through the vessel wall, the process is referred to as emigration. When the leukocytes are present in the tissue and migrate toward microorganisms or particulate matter and debris, the process is referred to as chemotaxis. The vasokinetic phase of inflammation encompasses vasoconstriction, vasodilatation, and increased permeability of vessel walls. The immediate local inflammatory response takes from thirty minutes to twelve hours. When the injury is caused by bacterial infection, the first four hours of the inflammatory response constitute the most important aspect of this response. The immediate local response of inflammation serves the following functions:

1. The extravasated fluid helps to dilute any toxins in the tissues;

2. The leukocytic exudate phagocytizes the microorganisms, foreign particles and debris, and portions of other leukocytes destroyed during phagocytosis; and

3. The plasma contains opsonins, complement, and properdin, which represent bacteriostatic substances in the serum. All of the above have the capacity to neutralize the injurious substance or invading microorganisms and are further supported in neutralization by enzymes liberated by the dead and dying leukocytes. Fibrin is precipitated in the later stages of the inflammatory exudate and forms a coagulum with local defensive properties. The localization or protective function of fibrin is absent during the early (immediate) phase of the inflammatory response.

Lymphorrhagia (dilatation of lymphatics) occurs when the inflammatory edema compresses the veins, but dilates the lymphatics in the injured area. This early inflammatory response is the defense of tissue by dispersion of the injury to the reticuloendothelial system through the lymphatics. Within minutes after injury and the inflammatory response, there is a dilatation of lymphatics and increased permeability of these vessels. This results in increased return of tissue fluids (edema) by way of the dilated lymphatics and a reduced return by way of the venous system. Lymphorrhagia, therefore, is a rerouting of the inflammatory edema by way of the regional lymph nodes. Thus, the regional lymph nodes may show enlargement (lymphadenopathy), which is common during infections or hypersensitivity reactions. From the lymph nodes the inflammatory edema passes through lymphatics to the blood stream and subsequently to the liver, bone marrow, and spleen, i.e. into the reticuloendothelial system of the body. Leukocytes in the area of inflammation phagocytize the invading microorganisms entering the lymphatics to the lymph nodes to the blood stream to the liver, spleen, and bone marrow. In this way the living microorganisms are exposed to the reticuloendothelial system of the body. The spreading of the infectious microorganisms to the body's systemic defense by dispersion in addition to the localized defense is vital in streptococcal and other virulent infections. The virulent microorganisms are delayed in the lymph nodes and can be phagocytized at this point. The microorganisms that pass through the lymph nodes are phagocytized and disappear in the spleen, liver, and lymph nodes, i.e. by the systemic defensive mechanism present in the reticuloendothelial system of the body. Defense by dispersion of microorganisms involves the spleen, liver, and bone marrow in thirty minutes to a few hours after the inflammatory response occurs.

Resolution may occur in twenty-four hours in a minor inflammatory response to a small injury. Macrophages mobilize in the injured area in twenty-four hours and phagocytize debris, dead erythrocytes, and dead leukocytes. When a foreign material or organism (sutures, asbestos or silica, or tubercule bacilli) enters the tissues, the initial mobilization of the polymorphonuclear exudate is of short duration. It is replaced by macrophages and histiocytes in the inflammatory exudate, resulting in a granulomatous inflammation. Macrophages develop from monocytes in the blood stream and migrate to the area of damage in twelve hours. Macrophages simultaneously develop from immature tissue fibrocytes in the affected area. Macrophages have the capacity to phagocytize large particulate matter or microorganisms with a waxy capsule or larger fungi. The leukocytes do not have this capacity. Macrophages fuse together forming giant cells if larger matter or microorganism must be phagocytized. Tissues that contain giant cells plus macrophages form a granuloma or tubercle. In an abscess, granulocytes predominate. In foreign body reactions, tuberculosis and fungal infections, the histiocyte is the predominant cell in the inflammatory exudate. Plasma cells develop from reticulum cells in the area of damage. Plasma cells produce and elaborate antibodies, which aid in destroying certain infective microorganisms. The systemic response to inflammation is a delayed response involving the reticuloendothelial system, which produces the immune bodies against virulent microorganisms or foreign substances (proteins).

Inflammation is initiated with reversible alterations of the endothelial cells of vessels (vasodystonia). The vasodystonia is due to the following factors:

1. The injured and dead cells release histamine and histaminelike substances that cause dilatation of capillaries and venules and increased permeability of capillary walls;

2. The blood vessel alterations are further aided by axone reflexes with peripheral sensory nerves transmitting a motor impulse

to dilate small blood vessels; and

3. The endothelial cells of the capillaries may be irritated or damaged directly by the irritant or microorganisms, causing increased capillary permeability. Adrenal cortical activity (cortisone) and the general adaptation syndrome have no influence upon the early phases of inflammation or immediate tissue responses.

Granulocytes present in the inflammatory edema demonstrate an attraction or force in the exudate to numerous infective microorganisms and noxious matter. This attraction or force is called chemotaxis. Leukocytes migrate in a direct path by chemotaxis toward microorganisms or noxious particles in the inflammatory edema.

Pyogenic inflammation refers to the mobilization and accumulation of both living and dead polymorphonuclear leukocytes around clumped or dead microorganisms. This situation produces a pyogenic exudate or abscess. The abscess consists of a central zone of dead tissue, dead leukocytes, fibrin, and infective microorganisms. Surrounding this central area of liquefaction necrosis is a peripheral zone of polymorphonuclear leukocytes. The leukocytes phagocytize the infective microorganisms and undergo liquefaction necrosis, causing the abscess to increase in size. Pressure builds up in the central liquified necrotic zone, and the abscess ruptures after pointing onto an adjacent exterior body surface. When evacuation cannot occur on the surface, the abscess extends itself along the path of least tissue resistance through the fascial planes, and secondary abscesses ensue. Macrophages and fibroblasts mobilize around the periphery of the abscess, forming a connective tissue limiting wall in the unaffected adjacent tissue.

Polymorphonuclear leukocytes and histiocytes utilize a similar process to phagocytize particulate matter and microorganisms. These cells engulf the particulate matter, and cellular enzymes cause their digestion and disappearance. Only the histiocytes contain the enzyme lipase, making it capable of phagocytizing microorganisms with lipid materials in the capsule.

Abscess formation in organs, i.e. the liver, brain, and kidneys, occurs in the stroma of these organs, and the inflammation is called interstitial inflammation. Membranes and skin contain inflammatory exudates, and these responses are called membranous inflammation. Membranous inflammation, therefore, occurs in either the serosa or mucosa of these membranes. When an abscess develops in an organ as interstitial inflammation, a pus-containing cavity is formed in the organ. Healing generally occurs by fibrosis (scar) since rather large areas of the organ may be destroyed.

The following represent examples of pyogenic infections: appendicitis, cholecystitis, diverticulitis, pyelonephritis, endocarditis, thrombophlebitis, septicemia, osteomyelitis, adenitis, serositis, arthritis, prostatic abscess, conjunctivitis, pyelitis, cystitis, cholecystitis, carbuncle, furuncle, scarlet fever, erysipelas and puerperal sepsis.

Superficial inflammatory responses are termed *mucositis* and *serositis*. Mucositis is an inflammation of the mucous membranes of the body. The mucosa contains dilated blood vessels, has a red color and puffy appearance, and drains a ropy fluid. In the common cold, the nasal mucosa drains a mucoid fluid from the surface, termed *rhinorrhea*. The initial mucoid secretion in the common cold is a catarrhal inflammation. The clear exudate becomes mixed with pus and is referred to as mucopurulent. Mucositis may develop in the mucosa of the respiratory tract and nasopharynx, conjunctival surface of the eye, gastrointestinal tract and mucosa of the gall bladder and hepatic ducts, the endocervix, endometrium, and fallopian tubes, and the lining of the male genital tract.

Serositis is defined as inflammation of the serous cavities of the body, i.e. the meninges, pleura, pericardium, peritoneum, and surfaces of the joints. The fluid present in serositis becomes mixed with mucin and blood and is termed *serosanguineous*. Serositis may develop a purulent exudate containing more fibrin and is termed *fibrinopurulent*. Fibrin is precipitated from the exudate and unites the visceral and parietal layers of a serous cavity, called the bread and butter effect. In serositis, the inflammatory exudate is within a serous cavity of the body. The fibrinopurulent inflammatory exudate, if it becomes large, tends to unite the serosal surfaces, and adhesions result. Adhesions formed in this manner become dense following organization and resolution, resulting in permanent fibrous adhesions of the serosal surfaces of serous cavities.

Mucositis and serositis produce diffuse inflamation involving large surfaces or an entire organ. Interstitial inflammation is the opposite, whereby the exudate tends to be localized. The abundant quantity of fluid present in mucositis and serositis dilutes and flushes away the various noxious materials and organisms, thereby producing only limited ulceration due to necrosis. Exceptions, however, occur in the case of diphtheria and typhoid fever. In diphtheria, a necrotic sloughed tissue is mixed with the purulent exudate on the surface of a mucous membrane. The latter exudate plus sloughed necrotic cells and fibrin is called a diphtheritic membrane, and the overall inflammation in diphtheria is called diphtheritic inflammation.

Mucositis and serositis proceed to resolution and healing (repair). Interstitial inflammation proceeds to scarring and fibrosis because necrosis is very common.

Granulomatous inflammation is defined as a local (focal) histiocytosis. Large histiocytes occur in the granulomatous exudate, developing from monocytes of the blood and enlarging their cytoplasm during phagocytosis. Histiocytes also form from immature fibroblasts and endothelial cells. In damaged connective tissue, the inflammatory edema stimulates formation of histiocytes during the inflammatory phase and also during the phase of resolution.

In the tubercle or infectious granuloma, the histiocytes are the predominant cells because the microorganisms generally contain a lipid-containing capsule. Histiocytes contain lipase and are effective in phagocytizing the organisms with the lipid capsule. Histiocytes ingest suture material, large particles, dead leukocytes, and injured erythrocytes. Macrophages may also contain immune globulins and, therefore, migrate to lesions produced by a hypersensitivity reaction.

Soluble antigen appears in the area of inflammation within

one-half hour and is only partially counteracted at the end of one week. However, in the regional lymph nodes draining the area of inflammation, the soluble antigen is completely destroyed in three or four days because of the presence of lymphocytes, which produce antibodies.

During chronic (prolonged, delayed) inflammation, lymphocytes and plasma cells become the predominant cells in the inflammatory exudate. When the microorganism causing syphilis enters the tissue and blood stream, there is no reaction on the part of the body for ten or more days, at which time acquired immunity develops. After ten days the inflammatory exudate first appears at the initial site of infection, i.e. the primary lesion develops. The primary lesion of syphilis consists of plasma cells and lymphocytes. Chronic inflammatory exudates also accompany both viral and rickettsial infections as well as allergic inflammation. Eosinophils accompany the plasma cells and lymphocytes during the allergic inflammation. The plasma cells and lymphocytes probably function by producing antibodies. The lymphocytes are associated with circulating antibody formation. The plasma cells are associated with immunity present in localized tissues.

Eosinophils are mobilized in the tissue during the inflammatory reactions due to parasites. They also mobilize in allergic inflammation, in nasal polyps during hay fever, and in bronchial secretions during asthma. The basophilic granulocytes of the blood contain heparin, and they may bring anticoagulates to aid in reabsorption of the inflammatory exudate.

Acute pyogenic exudate has also been called serogranulocytosis (edema fluid plus polymorphonuclear leukocytes). The histiocytes migrate to the site of injury within approximately ten hours phagocytize debris and dead leukocytes, resulting in resolution. Histiocyte mobilization and resolution are, therefore, the beginning of the process of healing (repair). Granulation tissue is evident when a pyogenic inflammation undergoes healing. It consists of a core of necrosis surrounded by a zone of fibroblasts, proliferating capillaries, and fibrous connective tissue. Therefore, inflammation, resolution, and repair are all present in granulation tissue.

Histiocytes mobilize within thirty-six hours when the granulocytic inflammatory exudate is incapable of resolving the foreign body and persistent microorganisms. When highly persistent foreign bodies are present, the histiocytes fuse together producing giant cells, and the granuloma is evident. The granuloma soon becomes encased by fibrous connective tissue. The dead histiocytic cells undergo hyalinization, with the development of a healed tubercle in tuberculosis or a gumma in syphilis. The granuloma becomes a scar when repair is completed.

SECONDARY DEFENSIVE RESPONSES: FEVER, LEUKOCYTOSIS, AND IMMUNITY

Infections or severe damage to tissues or organs elicit not only the local inflammatory reaction but are further supported by defensive measures from the central nervous system, the endocrine system, and the reticuloendothelial system. The secondary defensive responses are fever, leukocytosis, immunity, and the general adaptation syndrome (Selye).

Fever (Pyrexia)

Fever results from an alteration in the heat control center, which is located in the hypothalamus. The heat control center of the hypothalamus functions by balancing heat production against heat loss from the body so that a normal temperature of 98.6°F is maintained. Pyrexia (fever) is the result of direct injury to this neurogenic center or its connections. Lesions of the central nervous system may produce pyrexia. Specific drugs, sunstroke, or intracranial hemorrhage may cause a depression and interference with the heat control or heat-regulating center and produce neurogenic pyrexia. Fevers usually result following invasion of the tissues by microorganisms or by the introduction of foreign proteins. The latter is antigenic hyperpyrexia, which accompanies the majority of infectious diseases.

Increased heat production in the body through accelerated metabolism, i.e. muscle exercises, is offset by an increase in the amount of heat loss through the skin and increased sweating, with evaporation of water from the surface of the body. Sweating is, therefore, a major mechanism of regulating metabolic heat when the outside temperature is greater than the temperature within the body. In fever, the body temperature is raised by conserving body heat. This occurs by means of a chill where there is peripheral vasoconstriction and diminished secretory activity of the sweat glands, contraction of smooth muscle fibers of the skin, and drawing together of the limbs with shivering, all of which produce heat through muscular contraction. It generally takes a period of thirty to ninety minutes (prodromal period) to conserve body heat and produce an elevation in body temperature. Once the prodromal phase has past and the fever is established, the blood vessels in the skin dilate, the face is flushed, and sweating occurs with a rise or fall of temperature.

Fevers rarely exceed 106°F. The increase in the amount of heat lost during fever is counterbalanced by excessive metabolism plus increased heat production. The increased heat production may rise to as great as 50 percent above normal. The basal metabolic rate increases approximately 7 percent for every degree of temperature. The latter is accompanied by a decrease in the blood sugar and the serum phosphate without any change in the blood levels for potassium, calcium, magnesium, creatin and creatinine. When the fever is prolonged, the body survives on proteins and fats, since the carbohydrate storage in the liver and muscles becomes exhausted. When the fever is high and prolonged, a marked congestion develops in the brain and all of the visceral organs associated with petechial hemorrhage. The greatest cellular alterations occur in the liver, brain, and kidney. In instances of advanced severe hyperpyrexia, the alterations of lower nephron nephrosis develop, accompanied by pigmented casts in distal convoluted tubules.

Pulse rate increases during pyrexia by approximately ten beats per minute with each degree of increase in body temperature. Headache may accompany fever, and cerebral function is disturbed, with the patient suffering from restlessness, insomnia, and delirium.

If the body temperature should rise to 112°F, convulsions,

coma, and death occur because of the action on the brain tissue. Prolonged fever produces dehydration and wasting, and may lead to circulatory collapse.

Leukocytosis

The leukocyte count in normal individuals ranges from 4,000 to 10,000 white blood cells per cubic millimeter of blood. Sixty percent of the white blood cells are polymorphonuclear leukocytes. The circulating blood also is normally composed of 15 to 30 percent lymphocytes, 4 to 8 percent monocytes, up to 1 percent basophils, and 1 to 3 percent eosinophils. Infections are caused by pyogenic cocci (streptococci, staphylococci, pneumococci, gonococci, and meningococci). Diphtheric microorganisms produce a marked leukocytosis of 15,000 to 30,000 white blood cells per cubic millimeter. Later on, with increasing local defensive mechanisms present, there may be a relative increase in lymphocytes, monocytes, and eosinophils. During the early stages of leukocytosis, the eosinophilic count may become depressed by the general adaptation syndrome. If an overwhelming infection occurs, leukopenia develops because of toxic reactions within the bone marrow.

The increase in the white cell count during leukocytosis due to an infection arises from the following sources:

1. Mobilization of leukocytes from the sinuses of the spleen, bone marrow, and lymph nodes;

2. More rapid maturation of the adult forms from the immature (myelocytes) cells; and

3. Increased production of leukocytes due to hyperplasia of the bone marrow.

Stress phenomena (strenuous exercise, pain, burns, trauma) provoke the general adaptation syndrome (Selye) and produce a leukocytosis with an eosinopenia and lymphopenia. Severe infections similarly produce a stress phenomenon, and the leukocytosis that results is endocrine in nature.

Marked eosinophilia occurs in parasitic infections and allergic diseases. Monocytosis or lymphocytosis is present in tuberculosis, whooping cough, and glandular fever. The local tissue or primary reactions have an ability to alter the character of the leukocytosis.

Immune Reaction

Acquired immunity is a specific humoral defense or resistance, which occurs when living microorganisms and their products invade tissues and organs of the body. Acquired immunity is not universally produced. For instance, there is no acquired immunity to the common cold. The cells that produce an acquired immunity are from the reticuloendothelial system, i.e. the lymphocytes and plasma cells of the spleen and lymph nodes and the lymphoid follicles of the pharyngeal and gastrointestinal tracts. These cells produce specific immune substances or globulins, which are termed *antibodies*. The offenders, i.e. proteins, polysaccharides, perhaps lipids that provoke the immunity, are called antigens. Antigens are either rather large molecules with a molecular weight greater than 10,000, or simple organic compounds combined with proteins forming the antigenic complex. The organic compounds that combine with proteins are termed the *haptens*. Acquired immunity occurs when noxious antigens provoke the reticuloendothelial system to elaborate, circulate, or deposit antibodies in the tissues.

Circulating Antibodies

Immune responses of circulating humoral antibodies are readily demonstrable in the serum and can be measured in the clinical laboratory. The following terms and their definitions have been employed for the different immune properties of the serum antibody, although one variety of altered globulin is generally concerned. Opsonin adheres to bacteria and aids phagocytosis. Lysin destroys or lyses bacteria in the presence of complement, a normal protein component of the plasma. Agglutin produces clumping or agglutination of bacteria. Precipitin produces aggregation of soluble antigens. Antitoxin neutralizes toxins. Hemolysin is a lysin against red blood cells in the presence of complement. Hemagglutinin produces agglutination of red blood cells.

The circulating antibody is present in the blood, lymph, cerebrospinal fluid, or aqueous humor of the eye of immune individuals. During acquired immunity, the circulating antibody is present in seven to twenty days following exposure to an antigen. In individuals with natural immunity, the antibody is genetically predetermined and, therefore, is present at birth. There is a difference betwen protein and polysaccharide antigens with reference to the degree and persistence of the two antibody responses. Polysaccharides produce a maximal antibody response, which persists for some time following a single dose of antigen, and subsequent doses do not increase the antibody titer. In contrast, the antibody response to protein antigens is increased in titer and duration following a second dose given in two weeks and booster dose after twelve months.

Antigens may be denatured following treatment with formalin or other chemicals. Toxicity of the antigen is reduced without diminishing the immune provoking capacity. The lowering of the toxicity of the antigen is important in the prevention of disease through artificial inoculation. Example of its use is in the prevention of tetanus and diphtheria.

Antigen generally has its first contact with cells of the respiratory tract, gastrointestinal system, or skin. The immune responses following the latter contact develop over a period of several weeks and are protective in nature. Inoculation of antigen may result in accelerated immune responses, i.e. hypersensitivity. Hypersensitivity reactions include the following: anaphylaxis, Arthus phenonemom, Shwartzman phenomenon, and Koch's phenomenon. During these hypersensitivity reactions, the immune response is transformed to a harmful reaction by two methods. First, the antigen gains access in high concentration to diffusion membranes, i.e. vascular endothelium. Second, once the immune response has occurred, the injected substance may be in direct contact with the antibody in high concentration for a short period of time. The highly severe hypersensitivity (allergic) reactions are the result of the antigen-antibody reaction following the use of a needle and syringe during inoculation.

Antibodies that become attached to the tissues are termed *sessile antibodies*, and the organ to which the antibody is attached is termed the *shock organ*. There are heat stable and heat labile antibodies. Circulating heat stable antibodies neutralize antigens upon contact by the phenomenon of precipitation or flocculation. Heat labile antibodies occur in allergic individuals and are termed *reagins*. Reagins may be transferred to a nonsensitive individual, and he will react to a specific antigen by intracutaneous administration. The environment of man is full of antigens (bacterial, etc.) and, if given the opportunity, the human body will respond to all of them.

Immunity of the human body to some substances is a physiologic state and does not always have to be acquired following exposure to an antigen. Once an individual is exposed to specific offending agents (antigens), the individual may acquire a specific immunity. These are neutralizing antibodies. In other instances, the immune response may be irrelevant or damaging to the individual, and this process is called hypersensitivity (allergy).

References

Douglas, S.D.: *Blood, 35*:851, 1970.
Ehrich, W.C.: *Mt Sinai J Med NY, 15*:337, 1949.
Florey, Sir H. (Ed.): Inflammation. In *Lectures on General Pathology.* Philadelphia, Saunders, 1954, p. 63.
Gabbiani, G., et al.: *J Exp Med, 153*:719, 1972.
Harris, H.: *Br J Exp Pathol, 34*:276, 1953.
Harris, H.: *J Pathol, 66*:135, 1953.
Hay, E.D.: *N Engl J Med, 284*:1033, 1971.
Hersh, E.M. and Body, G.P.: *Annu Rev Med, 21*:105, 1970.
King, E.J.: Silicosis. In: *Lectures on the Scientific Basis of Medicine.* London, The Athlone Press, 1954, vol. II, 1952-53.
Lattes, R., et al.: *Am J Pathol, 29*:1, 1953.
Lichenstein, I.L., et al.: *Surg Gynecol Obstet, 130*:685, 190.
McMaster, P.D. and Hudack, S.S.: *J Exp Med, 61*:783, 1935.
McMaster, P.D.: Lymphatic participation in cutaneous phenomena, *The Harvey Lectures.* Lancaster, PA, The Science Press Printing Company, 1942, Ser. XXXVII, pp. 227-266, 1941-42.

Menkin, V.:   *Dynamics of Inflammation.*   New York, MacMillan, 1940.
Miles, A.A.:   *Lectures on the Scientific Basis of Medicine.*   London, The Athlone Press, vol.III, 1953-54.
Pillemer, L., et al.:   *Science, 120:*279, 1954.
Pullinger, B.D. and Florey, H.W.:   *J Pathol, 45:*157, 1937.
Schoefl, G.I.:   *J Exp Med, 136:*568, 1972.
Teilum, G.:   *Am J Pathol, 32:*945, 1956.
Ward, P.A.:   *Arthritis Rheum, 13:*181, 1970.
Zucker-Franklin, D.:   *Semin Hematol, 5:*109, 1968.

CHAPTER 8

RESOLUTION, ORGANIZATION, REPAIR, AND REGENERATION

RESOLUTION, ORGANIZATION, AND REPAIR

INFLAMMATION IS UNIVERSALLY PRESENT during injury to tissues. Trauma to the tissues produces an inflammatory defensive response in the first several hours following the blood clotting and thrombosis of traumatized vessels. If secondary infection does not complicate the inflammatory defensive response, prompt resolution and removal of exudate occur. This process of cleaning up the debris by histiocytic cells from the blood stream and adjacent tissues is called resolution. When the area is cleared of debris and the microorganisms are phagocytized, the adjacent fibroblasts and capillaries proliferate to form new cells and capillaries, which grow into the area of inflammation. The latter is the beginning of the process of fibrotic repair. It is possible to have resolution and fibrotic repair overlapping one another. In granulation tissue, we find inflammatory defensive response, resolution, and fibrotic repair overlapping each other.

Organization of the area of inflammation means that resolution and fibrotic repair are overlapping one another. Eventually, as healing proceeds, fibrous tissue alone is present as a replacement tissue for the injured area. The final process of fibrotic repair is the presence of a scar (cicatrix). During resolution, large quantities of the inflammatory exudate are removed from the tissues by liquefaction and phagocytosis.

The macrophage, endothelial cells, and fibrocyte or fibroblast take part in the process of fibrotic repair. The latter three tissues are all of mesenchymal origin. The histiocyte (macrophage) is mobilized first at the site of resolution. Fibroblasts then migrate into the area after the macrophages clean up the debris. Fibroblasts proliferate in the area of resolution and produce fibrils in the area. The proliferating fibroblasts are followed by endothelial cells, which proliferate and form new capillaries. Therefore, a simultaneous ingrowth of new capillaries and new fibrous connective tissue occurs during fibrotic repair. Fibroblasts may be stimulated to undergo mitosis due to anoxia, dead tissues, and the sulfhydryl radical. The presence of a gradual increase in tension in the tissue causes maturation, whereby fibers are formed in the area of repair.

If the injured tissue cannot be approximated, i.e. an open wound results, granulation tissue will proliferate and fill in the wound outline. If foreign bodies remain in the wound, they may stimulate phagocytosis and fibrosis. After the granulation tissue fills the wound, reticulin fibers and immature collagenous fibers form and mature into dense collagen fibers. The dense collagen fibers exert pressure, compressing the open capillaries in the area, and produce an avascular repair process. Fibrotic repair is not present in the central nervous system because connective tissue is minimal or absent. However, glial tissue or astrocytes are present, and their function is to perform the repair process in the nervous system. The glial tissue produced in repair of the central nervous system is a much slower process when compared to fibrotic repair in other areas of the body.

When repair occurs, the injured tissue will promptly return to its physiologic state, provided no tissue has been destroyed. The latter is defined as healing by primary intention, whereby a scar of fibrous tissue is very minimal. There is no need for fibrotic repair during healing by primary intention. Primary intention passes through the following stages: damage due to laceration of skin and blood vessels; defense by blood clotting superficially and thrombosis of vessels; resolution with histiocytic cells by phagocytosis; repair by fibroblasts and capillaries (organization); and regeneration of surface epithelial cells.

Healing by secondary intention is healing by granulation tissue. If a large wound or an infected wound is present, healing occurs by means of secondary intention. Secondary intention indicates the presence of an ingrowth of new blood vessels, proliferating connective tissue, and an inflammatory exudate, all of which produce granulation tissue. The granulation tissue develops after the third or fourth day following the occurrence of the large wound. This granulation tissue is moist to wet and occupies the entire wound or defect in the tissue. The surface may bleed easily since it contains numerous capillaries without a covering epithelium. When tension develops in the large wound, fibroblasts lay down collagen fibers, which unite the wound into one mass.

The healing of an ulceration on a mucosal or skin surface is based on the presence of three zones, i.e. the ulcer is covered with debris, precipitated fibrin, and an inflammatory exudate. This superficial zone rests upon a layer of granulation tissue composed of proliferating capillaries and fibroblasts. The latter zone rests upon a layer of dense fibrous tissue. These same three zones (necrosis with inflammatory exudate, granulation tissue with budding capillaries and fibroblasts, and fibrosis) are also present in the wall of a chronic abscess, vegetations on heart valves, and in chronic gastrointestinal ulcers. For instance, the zones of healing in a chronic peptic ulcer include the following: (1) debris and inflammatory exudate; (2) persistence of an area of necrosis; (3) granulation tissue; and (4) fibroblasts.

Healing by secondary intention is several times (weeks to months) the duration of healing by primary intention (days) and is dependent upon the following factors: size of the wound, persistence and severity of infection, type of organ involved, and overall health of the individual.

Thrombosis is a defensive response of the body. Resolution occurs in a thrombus in blood vessels of moderate size or in the chambers of the heart in approximately forty-eight to seventy-two hours after thrombosis occurs. During resolution the thrombus may be (1) completely digested, (2) reduced in size, or (3) dislodged. When the adjacent wall of the blood vessel or heart chamber has become necrotic, organization of the thrombus occurs. In approximately five to seven days, fibroblasts and new capillaries proliferate, and buds of endothelial cells arise from the intima, forming new vessels. The thrombus following organization shows recanalization by new blood vessels. Organization of thrombi located in heart valves and in veins may become calcified.

Gliosis is a type of repair by substituting glial cells for the destroyed cells of the central nervous system. The ganglion cells of the nervous system undergo necrosis, and macrophages attempt to resolve the injured or destroyed cells. In three or more weeks the glial cells proliferate, migrate, and grow into the damaged area. The astrocytes or glial cells that proliferate during nervous system repair have a prolonged life and remain in the damaged area for years. However, glial tissue and glial cells may undergo degeneration and produce psammoma bodies (grains of sand in the brain). The psammoma body arises from degenerated glial cells that have undergone calcification.

Repair of bone tissue passes through several stages. First is an organizing hematoma between the fractured ends of a bone, followed by formation of the callus. When healing begins in the periosteum, the healing is preceded by formation of cartilage; fibrosis develops before the regeneration begins.

Fibrotic repair may lead to complications, i.e. strictures, adhesions, stenoses, and contractures. Fibrotic repair and the fibrosis produced may cause constricting bands of tissue or adhesions to develop. Adhesions are defined as fibrosis that binds together into one unit normally separate tissues and organs. Strictures are disabling fibrosis that causes the obstruction of a ductal system. Stenoses are fibrosis that causes a narrowing of vital organs of the body. Contractures are fibrosis that produces limitations to normal muscle movements. Contraction of a scarred heart valve following rheumatic fever produces a deformity causing heart strain and may cause cardiac failure. The uniting of joint surfaces by adhesions in rheumatoid arthritis may cause ankylosis, and abdominal adhesions have been reported to cause intestinal obstructions.

REGENERATION

Regeneration is defined as the tissue's ability or capacity to replace lost parenchymal cells in kind following their loss through injury or physiologic wear. Most tissues have the capacity to undergo regeneration; however, there are tissues such as ganglion cells of the brain, cardiac muscle fibers, and renal glomeruli that lose this ability shortly after birth. Regeneration is, therefore, different from fibrosis or scarring. Both scarring and regeneration take place in repair or healing; however, indifferent stromal tissues bridge the defect during scarring but specialized parenchymatous cells are present in regeneration. Regeneration is restricted, whereas scarring is possible in every organ.

Organ systems, such as the bone marrow, skin, mucosa of the gastrointestinal tract and liver, undergo cyclical replacement of mature adult cells that are lost daily. Complete regeneration occurs in these tissues once a month. Circulating red blood cells are replaced every 120 days. During menstruation, two-thirds of the uterine mucosal lining is replaced every twenty-eight days. White blood cells are replaced every three to seven days. Granulocytes are replaced daily. These are all examples of physiologic regeneration.

Regenerating tissue may alter its differentiation to meet functional requirements or stress. For instance, connective tissue cells in the skeletal system can elaborate either fibroblasts, cartilage, or bone. In the ampulla of the nipple, the lining cells may form epidermal, ductal, or lobular epithelial cells. Thus, there may be a shift in regenerating cells from one route of maturation to another under physiologic as well as pathologic processes. In pathology this latter change in the pathway of maturation in regeneration of tissues is called metaplasia.

Following injury and impairment, excessive regeneration may occur in which development and maturation become superimposed upon an increase in cellular division (mitosis). The latter circumstances may lead to hyperplasia, i.e. overgrowth of a tissue due to an increase in the number of cells. On occasion, a benign neoplasm may result in place of the hyperplasia.

The normal regenerative cycle consists of the following three phases: proliferative or reproductive cycle with its cellular division; maturation or differentiation cycle with its resting cells; and the adult or functional phase with its specialized structure. The third phase of the renewal cycle may be divided into adult functioning cells and those cells that undergo death and desquamation or resorption.

Pathologic regeneration may occur as either focal or diffuse regeneration. The focal pathologic regeneration is termed *reparative hyperplasia* and is secondary to a local defect caused by damage. The tissue that replaces the local defect migrates into the local defect from the adjacent normal parenchyma. In the specialized mesenchymal structures of the body, such as tendon and synovial membranes, the migration and proliferation of immature fibroblasts appear similar to the early phase of fibrous repair. However, a different situation exists when two-thirds of the liver or a portion of respiratory mucosa or of the adrenal gland is excised. Following excision, a diffuse regeneration ensues. The remaining adult mature cells located in the adjacent normal tissue undergo de-differentiation; they expand and migrate and undergo successive mitoses. Reparative hyperplasia appears in two forms, i.e. the focal response involving migration and proliferation of adjacent reserve cells, and the atypical or diffuse response that involves de-differentiation of mature adult cells. Some of the adult cells migrate and proliferate, but the majority divide in place.

Diffuse hyperplasia occurs when an entire tissue or organ undergoes pathologic regeneration. Diffuse hyperplasia leads to abnormal enlargement of the tissue or organ and may be stimulated by an endocrine abnormality or increased blood supply due to chronic inflammation. Hyperplasia is present during inflammation and increased blood supply is present in infections provoking large lymph nodes and enlarged spleen. Selective impairment of adult functioning mature cells leads to a diffuse hyperplasia of the bone marrow and is present when red blood cell maturation is altered by the absence of vitamin B_{12} in pernicious anemia. Diffuse hyperplasia is a dysfunctional hyperplasia without a direct injury to the immature cells that precede the adult functioning cells.

The main causes of hyperplasia of cells and organs are exactly the reverse of the causes of atrophy. Atrophy is defined as a decrease in the size of an organ due to a decrease in the number or size of its cells. Atrophy is caused by pressure, diminished blood supply, and diminished nourishment, and by endocrine disturbances. On the other hand, hyperplasia is caused by decompressing the limitations of an organ when focal cellular degeneration occurs in the organ. Hyperplasia also occurs when there is an increased blood supply and nourishment to the tissue as well as by increased stimulation following endocrine alterations.

Reparative hyperplasia occurs in the following mesenchymal structures: ligaments, tendons, fascia, capsule of visceral organs, skin (derma), the synovial membranes of joints, and in bone tissue following fractures. In a fractured bone, hemorrhage, thrombosis, inflammation, and resolution follow the fracture. Reparative hyperplasia also occurs in the following epithelial membranes; respiratory epithelium, gastric mucosa, skin, and renal tubular epithelium.

Diffuse reparative epithelial hyperplasia may occur in the liver. If 70 percent of the rat liver is excised, the liver will be reconstituted in fourteen to twenty-one days to its original volume. However, an enlarged size may develop in twenty-one to twenty-eight days due to epithelial hyperplasia. Following partial hepatectomy, the stimulus to cellular division of hepatic cells is probably the result of both an increased metabolic uptake from the blood after release from compression and an increased blood supply. All of the portal blood passes through the remaining portion of the liver following partial hepatectomy. Reparative hyperplasia in the liver after hepatectomy is diffuse in nature, rather than focal, due to the tremendous increase of the blood supply to the remaining hepatic cells.

Diffuse dysfunctional hyperplasia occurs in the mesenchymal structures of the body, i.e. in mesenchymal tissues that are not associated with hematopoesis and in the connective tissues forming the stroma of organs of epithelial origin. For instance, any factor that leads to a decreased life span of adult mature erythrocytes, i.e. hemorrhage, hemolytic anemia, absence of vitamin B_{12} will stimulate hyperplasia of the erythropoietic tissues of the bone marrow. Loss of adult functioning cells or decrease in their function or maturation or shortening of their life span will induce hyperplasia.

Diffuse hyperplasia may occur in the following epithelial structures: thyroid gland, mammary gland, prostate gland, and adenohypophysis. Thyroid hyperplasia may occur by interfering with its thyroxin-producing functions, either by withholding iodine or administering propylthiouracil. Hyperplasia of the chromophobe cells of the adenohypophysis results when animals are maintained on prolonged estrogen. Mammary and prostatic hyperplasia have been produced in animals by endocrine stimulation.

An injured tissue has several sources of newly added cells in hyperplasia. The injured tissue increases its capacity for proliferation by adding to the number of cells present for mitosis by the following methods:

1. Modulation of mature cells that normally do not divide occurs in reparative hyperplasia of the liver and respiratory epithelium;

2. Migration of reserve cells from adjacent tissue;

3. Extending division to the indifferent reserve cells or withholding cells from maturation, i.e. by retention.

The concentration of increased numbers of replaceable cells at sites of tissue damage applies to pathologic regeneration plus to thrombosis, inflammation, resolution, and fibrous repair. However, the accumulation of immature types of cells for proliferation after injury is not free of the hazard of neoplasia. If the accumulation of immature dividing cells grows to an excessive proportion, a benign or malignant neoplasm becomes probable unless the excessive cells undergo necrosis by outgrowing their nutritional supply. The only real prerequisite for neoplasia is a repetition of or a persistent injurious agent acting selectively upon adult mature functioning cells.

References

Ariel, I.M.: *Radiology,* 57:561, 1951.
Boling, L.R.: *Arth Otolaryngol,* 22:689, 1935.

Brues, A.M., et al.: *Arch Pathol, 22*:658, 1936.
Cameron, G.R.: The tissue cell. In *Pathology of the Cell*. Springfield, Thomas, 1951, p. 443.
Clark, E.R. and Clark, E.L.: *Am J Anat, 64*:251, 1939; *67*:255, 1940; *66*:1, 1940; *81*:233, 1947.
Cooper, Z.K. and Schiff, A.: *Proc Soc Exp Biol Med, 39*:323, 1938.
Cronkite, E.P.: The hematology of ionizing radiation. In Behrens, Chas. F. (Ed.) : *Atomic Medicine*, 2nd ed. Baltimore, Williams and Wilkins, 1953.
Dickie, M.M. and Woolley, G.W.: *Cancer Res, 9*:372-384, 1949.
Engelstad, R.B.: *Acta Radiol Supply, 19*:1-94, 1934.
Fogg, L.C. and Cowing, R.F.: *Cancer Res, 11*:23, 1951.
Friedman, N.B. and Shields, W.: *Arch Pathol, 33*:326, 1942.
Geschickter, C.F. and Byrnes, E.W.: *Arch Pathol, 33*:334-356, 1942.
Geschickter, C.F. and Copeland, M.M.: *Tumors of Bone*, 3rd ed. Philadelphia, Lippincott, 1949, p. 265.
Goddard, J.W. and Sommers, S.C.: *Lab Invest, 3*:197, 1954.
Mason, M.L. and Allen, H.S.: *Ann Surg, 113*:424, 1941.
Maximow, A.A. and Bloom, W.: *A Textbook of Histology*, 6th ed. Philadelphia, Saunders, 1952, p. 63.
Osgood, E.E.: *Natl Cancer Inst, 18*:155, 1957.
Paul, J.H. and Freese, H.L.: *Am J Hyg, 17*:517, 1933.
Schrader, F.: *Miltosis, 2nd ed.* Irvington-on-Hudson, Columbia U Pr, 1953, p. 54.
Schafer: Paul W.: *Pathology in General Surgery*. Chicago, U of Chicago Pr, 1950, p. 335.
Smith, H.W.: *The Kidney, Structure and Function in Health and Disease*. Oxford, Oxford U Pr, 1951, p. 783.
Smith, C.H., et al.: *Blood, 10*:707, 1955.
Sutherland, A.M.: *J Pathol, 71*:403, 1953.
Turner, C.D.: *Anat Rec, 73*:145, 1939.
Van Dyke, J.H.: *Arch Pathol, 56*:613, 628, 1953.
Von Gaza, W.: *Arch f klin Chir, 121*:378, 1922.
Warren, S.: *Arch Pathol, 34*, 1942; *35*, 1943. Aug. p. 443-450; Sept. p. 562-608; Oct. 749-787; Nov. 917-931; Dec. 1070-1084; Jan. 121-138 and Feb. 304-352.
Weiss, P.: *The Principles of Development*. New York, HR&W, 1939, p. 424.
Wilhelm, D.L.J.: *J Pathol, 65*:543, 1953.
Williams, J.W.: Regeneration of the uterine mucosa after delivery, with especial reference to the placental cite. *Surg Gynecol Obstet, 22*:664, 1931.
Womack, N.A. and Cole, W.H.: *Arch Surg, 23*:466, 1931.

CHAPTER 9

DISEASES OF AGING

THE HUMAN BODY ASSUMES a progressive state of aging (negative balance) from maturity to senior ages. This contrasts significantly with a positive state of balance that exists from birth to maturity. All organs in the human body show some decline in physiologic processes from maturity to senior age. The sexes differ widely in their rate of aging (negative balance of organs), and there is a difference in the same sex in the aging of one organ compared to that of another organ.

Gonads undergo alterations in the geriatric patient. Female gonads show involutional changes during climacteric from forty-five to fifty years of age. Ovaries shrink to one-third their adult mature size. Live births never occur after fifty years of age. Aging ovaries are accompanied by the following changes: thinning of the cortex of ovary with increased fibrous tissue replacing follicular structures; cystic atretic follicles and hyalinized corpora albicans; and fibrosed mass (corpora fibrosum) representing degenerated follicles. A stromal hyperplasia occurs in the thecal cells capable of secreting very small quantities of estrogen.

Mammary epithelium undergoes atrophy, and the metaplasia occurs in the sweat glands during climacteric. Fat replaces the fibrous stroma of the mammary gland. Uterine endometrium becomes cystic with aging, and the myometrium becomes hypertrophic. The mucosa of the vulva and vagina show leukoplakia and kraurosis plus pruritis with senile vulvitis.

In the male, age fifty years, there is no similar atrophy of the testes compared to that described for the ovary. Tubular epithelium of the testes and some active spermatogenesis commonly occur after eighty years of age. The majority of males show a 25 percent reduction in spermatogenesis in adult life. Seventy-eight percent of males over eighty years of age are sexually impotent. Seventy-five percent of males between eighty and ninety years of age develop hypertrophy of the prostate gland. Cellular hypertrophy is thought to result from failure of spermatogonia or the failure of spermatocytes to undergo cell division. The cells of the prostate gland will increase in size as glycogen accumulates in the cytoplasm.

The sexual decline and impotency due to aging are related only to the gonads and have no relationship to the distribution of various diseases or to the difference in the longevity of the two sexes. An example is the fact that neither female castrates or male castrates (eunuchs) show any premature aging. The gonadal alterations in the climacteric are not dependent upon the pituitary gland and its failure to function properly.

Cardiovascular alterations occur in the geriatric patient and proceed at a pace accelerated by various chronic diseases. The major cause of death after seventy years of age is senile myocardial insufficiency where no other cause of death is present at necropsy. A great increase occurs in phosphorus, calcium, and magnesium in the media of the aorta during aging. Esters of cholesterol and sphingomyelin are both lipids that show an increase in the aorta during aging. The renal plasma flow and basal metabolic rate show a decline with aging. Thrombotic occlusion of peripheral arteries is a disabling complication of aging in males from sixty to eighty or more years of age. Intimal proliferation may narrow or occlude the lumen of blood vessels. This process is increased in rate and in severity by hypertension. Retinal arteries and retinal veins show varicosities. The majority of the aging process in the geriatric patient begins with degeneration in the mesenchymal tissues of the body, particularly the blood vessels of the heart, brain, retina, and kidneys. Arteriosclerosis is correlated with aging. Systemic arteries that transport the higher blood pressure suffer more than the pulmonary circulation (lower blood pressure).

Changes in the skeletal mesenchyme occur in the geriatric

patient. The knee and hip joint cartilage undergo aging after the age of thiry years, becoming friable and frayed in a progressive fashion. Osteoarthritis is believed to begin in 97 to 100 percent of individuals over sixty-five years of age. Osteoporosis develops in the spinal column, leading to midthoracic kyphosis in about 50 percent of males and females after sixty years of age. Individuals over sixty-five years of age have degenerative joint disease and show some radiographic evidence of osteoporosis.

Intervertebral cartilages undergo regressive alterations from maturity (30 years of age) to sixty years of age. The intervertebral cartilage are penetrated by connective tissue and small blood vessels with necrosis, calcification, lacerations, and hemorrhages occurring with aging. Aging of these cartilages may be complicated by rupture and herniation of the nucleous polyposus, generally within the lumbar region. The nucleous polyposus has a fluid consistency and is present in the center of the intervertebral disc, where it is under great internal pressure. The fluid content of the nucleous polyposus decreases with age. The intervertebral disc becomes dry and fissured and shows a marked reduction in its water content as aging proceeds. The elasticity of the lung is also diminished during the aging process as is the configuration of the thoracic cage.

Skin undergoes aging in geriatric patients. The skin is loose, pigmented, and has an increased amount of keratotic areas on the exposed parts of the body. Skin generally demonstrates the following alterations during aging: the epidermal ridges and depressions are lost, and the epidermis decreases in thickness in some areas and increases in others (atrophy and hyperplasia); there is a decrease in the number of hair follicles, sebaceous and sweat glands; there is occasional hypertrophy of one hair in the nose, ears, and eyebrows; and there are zones of hypermineralization and demineralization found by microincineration. Aging of the skin results in changes that are localized, patchy, and irregular.

The lens (epithelial tissue) of the eye is the site for development of cataracts during aging (65 to 81 years of age). Cataracts are more common in females than males over sixty-five years of age.

Gastrointestinal tract changes occur during aging in geriatric patients. Diverticulosis increases with each decade of life. Aging is accompanied by the following gastrointestinal disease: diverticulitis, gall bladder disease with gall stones, peptic ulcer, achlorhydria. Increase in the alkalinity of the gastrointestinal tract during the aging process is associated with rather poor absorption of calcium and iron.

The following diseases may be considered diseases of the geriatric patient or of old age: carcinoma, diabetes mellitus, cirrhosis of the liver, emphysema, infections (pneumonia and tuberculosis, bronchitis, influenza), hypertension, right-sided heart failure, arteriosclerosis, osteoarthritis, and hypoproteinemia or malnutrition. Geriatric diseases are, therefore, precipitated by aging, and in turn, the geriatric diseases cause acceleration of the aging process. For instance, diabetes mellitus, progeria, irradiation, and xeroderma pigmentosum accelerate the aging process.

Mental and cerebral changes accompany aging and are primarily due to sclerosis of the cerebral vessels. However, both economic and social status of geriatric patients is highly conducive to mental illness. The senile brain is decreased in weight and size with an increase in the amount of cerebral spinal fluid. There is disappearance of neurons, and gliosis is present along with deposition of calcium salts and protein-lipid combination pigment.

The vitality and repair processes characteristic of young individuals are progressively decreased or lost during aging. Aging brings along with it the numerous geriatric diseases, i.e. metabolic diseases which are reversible. It is well established that the endocrine or metabolic disease termed *diabetes mellitus* actually is capable of accentuating every aspect of aging. For instance, all of the various forms of atherosclerosis develop ten years earlier and are much more prevalent in individuals with diabetes mellitus. Cancer has a higher incidence in diabetics than in nondiabetics. The disease termed *progeria* is an example of an endocrine disease that imitates the aging process. The patient with progeria dies at twenty-five years of age from coronary disease and shows all of the senility alterations accompanying the geriatric patient.

Ionizing radiation emanating from small but repeated exposures to radiologists, etc., is a form of aging. Following repeated exposures, the elastic tissue undergoes degeneration, and collagen fibers undergo hyalinization and an increase in quantity.

Malnutrition appears to be more prevalent in advancing ages and is accompanied by hypoproteinemia or hypoalbuminemia. Diarrhea is common in the aged individual, and there is some modification in normal intestinal absorption in the aged. There is a decrease in the amount of body water after sixty-five years of age. The loss occurs from the intracellular water component of the body, and cells shrink in volume. The shrinkage produces a relative increase in the extracellular water. The cells of the aged also lose sodium along with the water loss. The aged obese individual does not tolerate well an acute water and electrolyte depletion because the reserve of water is less than in the nonobese individual. The lung becomes rigid and emphysematous during aging. There is an interference with the elimination of carbon dioxide by the lungs of aging patients, particularly the aged with very early respiratory acidosis. The aging lung shows a reduction of vital capacity and increased residual air. The quantity of carbon dioxide expired in aging patients is approximately one-half that of individuals in middle life. The pulmonary physiology of aging patients limits their physical performance because there is a reduced capacity to transport oxygen from the lungs to the tissues of the body. Oxygen uptake by the tissues proceeds at a slower rate in the aging subject, and increased quantities of lactic acid remain in the tissues during exercise.

References

Albright, J.F., et al.: *Exp Gerontol, 4:*267, 1969.
Bell, E.T.: *Arch Pathol, 49:*469, 1950.
Buck, R.C.: *Arch Pathol, 51:*319, 1951.
Greech, O., et al.: *Geriatrics, 11:*284, 1956.
Dodds, E.C.: Research on aging. In *Lectures on the Scientific Basis of Medicine.* London, The Athlone Press, 1953, vol.I, 1951-52.

Folsome, C. E., et al.: *JAMA, 161*:1447, 1956.
Goldstein, S.: *N Engl J Med, 285*:1120, 1971.
Harman, D.: *J Am Geriatr Soc, 17*:721, 1969.
Harman, J.W.: *Am J Pathol, 22*:712, 1950.
Health and Demography, U.S. Dept. of Health, Education and Welfare, Public Health Service, Bureau of State Services, National Office of Vital Statistics, Oct. 1956, from material prepared by Halbert L. Dunn, Chief, National Office of Vital Statistics.
Heckel, N.J.: Diseases of the bladder, the prostate and the urethra. In Steiglitz, Edward J. (Ed.): *Geriatric Medicine,* 3rd ed. Philadelphia, Lippincott, 1954, pp. 603-620.
Hertig, A. and Mansell, H.: Female genitalia in pathology. In Anderson, W.A.D.: *Pathology,* 3rd ed. St. Louis, Mosby, 1957.
Liu, R.K. and Walford, R.L.: *Exp Gerontol, 5*:241, 1970.
Monroe, R.T.: A clinical and pathological study of 7941 individuals over 61 years of age. In *Diseases of Old Age.* Cambridge, Harvard U Pr, 1951.
Moore, R.A.: *J Urol, 50*:680, 1943.
———Symposium on endocrinology of neoplastic diseases. *Surgery, 16*:152, 1944.
Parker, R.T., et al.: *Geriatrics, 11*:235, 1956.
Poos, E.E.: *Geriatrics, 11*:83, 1956.
Smith, F.C.: *Am J Surg, 40*:131, 1926.
Sniffen, R.C., et al.: *Arch Pathol, 51*:293, 1951.
———*Arch Pathol, 50*:295, 1950.
Sommers, S.C.: *Lab Invest, 4*:166, 1955.
Sommers, S.C.: *Am J Pathol, 32*:185, 1956.
Sommers, S.C. and Lombard, O.M.: *Arch Pathol, 56*:462, 1953.
Stanton, E.F.: *Am J Obstet Gynecol, 71*:270, 1956.
von Hahn, H.P.: *Gerontologia, 10*:174, 1964/65.
Walford, R.L.: *The Immunologic Theory of Aging.* Copenhagen, Ejner Munksgaard, 1969.
Wright, I.S. and McDevitt, E.: *Ann Intern Med, 41*:682, 1954.

CHAPTER 10

ACUTE INFECTIOUS DISEASES

PRINCIPLES OF INFECTIOUS DISEASES VERSUS INFLAMMATION

DEFINITION OF INFECTION. Infections are inflammations resulting from injury to tissues by living parasite organisms.

FACTORS RELATED TO ORGANISMS. The lesion that develops in infectious diseases depends upon pathogenicity, virulence, mode of growth, products produced, adaptability, protective capsules, motility, tissue specificity, and the number of organisms in the tissues.

FACTORS RELATED TO THE TISSUES. Bacterial proteins are necrotoxins, which are capable of destroying the tissues of the host. Exotoxins are secreted by the organisms. Endotoxins are liberated after death of the organisms. The spreading factor converts the hyaluronic acid gel of the tissues into a liquid. An edema-producing factor is present in tissues. A fibrinolysin factor hastens the breakdown of fibrin in the exudate. Coagulase acts locally in tissues producing coagulation of plasma and fibrin-formation. Leukocidin is present in infected tissues and is a poisonous compound to leukocytes. Hemolysin causes hemolysis of red blood cells in infected tissues.

VIRULENCE AND ADAPTATION OF LIVING AGENTS OF DISEASE. Bacteria are living agents capable of adaptations. The virulence of an organisms is a mechanism of adaptation. A strain of organism may, through successive generations, pass on to their offspring an increase in virulence.

BACTERIAL SPECIFICITY. Some organisms grow poorly in one tissue but rapidly in another tissue.

Factors Related to the Host. The constitution, age, nutrition, endocrine status, immunity and hypersensitivity, type of tissue involved, and previous injury or disease are the main factors. In diabetes mellitus, the carbohydrate content of the tissues causes an increased susceptibility to infection. In vitamin A and vitamin C deficiencies, the tissues become more susceptible to infections. Endocrines influence the ability of tissues to resist infection. ACTH therapy acts to permit the spread of infections. Infections are common in hypoadrenalism, hypopituitarism, and hypothyroidism. Immunity influences the invasion of organisms into the tissues. Hypersensitivity is an exaggerated antigen-antibody response producing widespread necrosis in tissue. Previous injury or disease influences the type of tissue reaction resulting from living organisms.

Organisms' Influence on Tissues. When living organisms produce necrosis of epithelial cells, the resulting lesion is an ulcer. Organisms may cause necrosis and liquefaction of cells, and the resulting lesion is an abscess. When bacterial toxins produce excessive tissue necrosis with putrefaction, the result is gangrene.

Systemic Effects of Infectious Diseases. The systemic effects of infectious diseases include chills, fever, malaise, nausea, vomiting, aching joints, and loss of appetite.

Complications of Infectious Diseases. Complications are primarily due to the spread of the infection locally or systemically by way of the vascular system. The local spread of infection produces an abscess, cellulitis, sinus, and fistula. The hematogenous spread of infection produces a bacteremia, septic thrombus, septicemia, and pyemia. The diffuse spread of infection through the tissue produces a cellulitis.

Disturbances in Healing. Failure of resolution of an exudate results in a disturbance in healing. Contraction of collagenous tissue occurs during aging. Scar tissue pulls upon a joint with the development of a contracture; therefore, the extremity cannot be extended.

Incidence of Bacteremia in Infections. Following a tonsillectomy, 30 percent of individuals develops a bacteremia. Mastication produces a transient bacteremia in 55 percent of individuals. After extraction of teeth, a transient bacteremia is present in 75 percent of individuals.

ACUTE BACTERIAL DISEASES

Staphylococcus Infections

Staphylococci are hemolytic organisms producing necrotoxins, which are responsible for necrosis of epithelium, and enterotoxins, which are responsible for food poisoning. Acute inflammatory lesions due to *Staphylococcus albus* drain spontaneously, resulting in minimal necrosis. *Staphylococcus aureus* is more pathogenic than *Staphylococcus albus*. A boil or furuncle of the skin is due to *Staphylococcus aureus*. A carbuncle is a group of boils or a diffuse distribution of furuncles. Staphylococci produce felons, infected finger tips. When the staphylococcus infection occurs around the nail, the infection is termed *paronychia*. Necrotoxins produced by staphylococci affect bone tissue by provoking necrosis and osteomyelitis. Impetigo is a staphylococcus infection of the epidemis of the skin. Superficial pustules develop but break down readily, forming shallow ulcers. A staphylococcal bacteremia may result in osteomyelitis of bone tissue. Osteomyelitis due to *Staphylococcus aureus* is a chronic disease and is extremely difficult to eradicate.

Streptococcal Infections

Streptococcus pyogenes or beta-hemolytic streptococci are the most pathogenic streptococci. Alpha- and gamma-hemolytic streptococci are the least pathogenic. Streptococcal organisms cause septicemia during wound infections of the hands and face.

Phlegmon, i.e. suppurative cellulitis, is a spreading, diffuse, necrotizing, and poorly outlined inflammation due to streptococcal organisms. Erysipelas is an acute group A hemolytic streptococcal inflammation involving the extracellular portion of the dermis. Erysipelas produces sharp, well-defined borders in the affected tissues. The duration of the inflammation is from four days to two weeks. The inflammation is usually self-limited; however, septicemia is a possible complication. The Quincy sore throat and retropharyngeal abscesses are due to streptococcal infections. Ludwig's angina is a hemolytic streptococcal infection of the soft tissues of the neck, submandibular area, and floor of the mouth.

In scarlet fever, a streptococcal septicemia is caused by beta-hemolytic streptococci. Pink skin rash, high fever, sore throat, involvement of the skin and mucous membranes, and a strawberry tongue are the main symptoms. The mucous membranes and the skin frequently undergo ulceration.

Diplococcus Infections

Diplococcus pneumonia types 1, 2, and 3 are responsible for lobar pneumonia. Lobar pneumonia may be divided into red hepatization, gray hepatization and resolution. If failure of resolution occurs, carnification, abscess, or gangrene develops in the lung. When resolution takes place, the leukocytes liberate a fibrinolytic enzyme which produces a liquid exudate. Following failure of resolution the lung becomes solid, i.e. carnification is present.

NEISSERIA GONORRHEA. *Neisseria gonorrhea* is responsible for limited tissue necrosis. *Diplococcus gonococcus* provokes an acute suppurative infection of mucous membranes.

NEISSERIA MENINGITIDES. Exposure to *Neisseria meningococci* may result in epidemic meningitis. A bacteremia occurs in every case of meningococcus infection. Acute bacterial endocarditis may result from the bacteremia. A sore throat is the initial symptom; however, in twenty-four hours a septicemia is present. Multiple confluent petechial hemorrhages occur in the mucous membranes.

PSEUDOMONAS AERUGINOSA. Pseudomonas infections occur secondary to starvation, diabetes mellitus, or following successful treatment with antibiotics. Cellulitis of the maxillofacial regions may be due to *Pseudomonas aeruginosa*.

Corynebacterium diphtheriae is the only pathogenic group of *corynebacterium*. Adults acquire immunity by contracting diphtheria or by immunization. Intoxication may occur with toxemia. The organisms remain on the surface of the pharynx and nasopharynx, producing exotoxins that cause necrosis.

Hemophilus pertussis or whooping cough generally occurs in children under five years of age. A mild upper respiratory infection occurs, accompanied by coughing. Severe coughing ensues, which lasts from three to four weeks. Paroxysmal states of coughing occur every four to five hours.

Friedländer's bacillus occurs in debilitated individuals as a secondary infection, causing a diffuse lobar or patchy type of pulmonary infection.

TYPHOID FEVER. Typhoid microorganisms enter the body through food or contaminated water and enter the lower gastrointestinal tract and Peyer's patches of the colon. As the disease progresses, lymphoid proliferation occurs in the reticuloendothelial system.

PTOMAINE POISONING. Food poisoning is generally due to *Staphylococcus aureus;* however, it may be due to *Clostridium botulinum.* When the organisms and toxins are ingested they are abosrbed by the host and cause symptoms of ptomaine poisoning. Botulism is due to organisms that are capable of surviving for long periods of time. The organisms produce a potent neurotoxin.

CLOSTRIDIUM TETANI. *Clostridium tetani* grow within necrotic tissue. A true toxemia results, along with a slight local reaction. The neurotoxin of *Clostridium tetani* is a stimulatory toxin, producing clonic contraction of muscles of the jaws. The muscles of the face and mastication undergo contractures. The contractures are painful and spread rapidly to the trunk, where every muscle undergoes contraction while the patient is conscious.

CLOSTRIDIUM WELCHII. *Clostridium welchii* organisms are responsible for gas gangrene. *Clostridium welchii* grow in necrotic tissues, producing an exotoxin that causes local necrosis of tissue due to the formation of gas.

GLANDERS BACILLUS. Glanders bacillus penetrates intact skin, therefore, laboratory workers may develop glanders disease. Lymphadenopathy and septicemia develop with a generalized pustular rash.

BRUCELLOSIS. Brucellosis, also termed *undulant fever,* is a viral disease characterized by nervous exhaustion, psychoneurosis, low-grade fever, weakness, malaise, and joint pains.

References

Banatvala, J.E.: *Br J Haematol, 19:*129, 1970.
Banatvala, J.E., et al.: *Lancet, 1:*1205, 1972.
DeJongh, D.S., et al.: *Am J Clin Pathol, 49:*424, 1968.
Evans, A.S.: *N Engl Med J, 279:*1121, 1968.
Frenkel, J.K.: *Fed Proc, 28:*179, 1969.
Frenkel, J.K., et al.: *Science, 167:*893, 1970.
Gerber, P.: *Lancet, 2:*988, 1972.
Grady, G.F. and Kensch, G.T.: *N Engl J Med, 285:*831, 1971.
Hart, P.D., et al.: *J Infect Dis, 120:*169, 1969.
Hirshaut, Y., et al.: *N Engl J Med, 283:*502, 1970.
Jawetz, E., et al.: *Review of Medical Microbiology,* 9th ed., Los Altos, Lange, 1970.
Klainer, A.S. and Beisal, W.R.: *Am J Med Sci, 258:*431, 1969.
Marcial-Rojas, R.A.: *Pathology of Protozoal and Helminthic Diseases.* Baltimore, Williams and Wilkins, 1971.
Mitchel, D.N. and Rees, R.J.W.: *Lancet, 2:*81, 1969.
Novick, R.P.: *Fed Proc, 26:*29, 1967.
Spaulding, W.B. and Hennessy, J.N.: *Am J Med, 28:*504, 1960.
Spector, W.G.: *Int Rev Exp Pathol, 8:*1, 1969.
Stuart, B.M. and Pullen, R.L.: *Arch Intern Med, 78:*629, 1946.
Tamm, I. and Eggers, S.J.: *Am J Med, 38:*678, 1965.
Third International Conference on Sarcoidosis. *Acta Med Scand,* Suppl. 425, 1964.
Thompson, J.G.: *South American Med J, 38:*696, 1964.
Trauger, D.A.: *Am Rev Respir Dis, 87:*582, 1963.
Watanabe, T.: *Bacteriol Rev, 27:*87, 1963.
Winship, P.: *Am J Clin Pathol, 23:*1012, 1953.
Zimmerman, L.E. and Rappaport, H.: *Am J Pathol, 24:*1050, 1954.

CHAPTER 11

SPECIFIC GRANULOMATOUS INFLAMMATIONS

Introduction

CHRONIC GRANULOMATOUS INFLAMMATION encompasses specialized types of inflammatory responses, which are protracted processes extending for prolonged periods of time (chronic). The chronic granulomatous inflammations have specialized characteristics in common despite a different etiology. However, the basic distinguishing features of chronic granulomatous inflammation can be altered by the living agent causing the disease. The granulomatous inflammation is chronic (prolonged) in nature because the causative microorganism persists within the tissue and thus continue to influence the body's reaction to this injurious agent for a prolonged period. The causal agent of chronic granulomatous inflammations is a living microorganism (bacterium, fungus, virus) or a foreign body whose chemical composition and toxic potential play a significant role in determining the outcome of the tissue reaction.

CHRONIC INFLAMMATION

The chronic inflammatory response differs from the acute inflammatory response in the following ways: It shows a marked degree of tissue involvement plus a proliferation of mononuclear cells; it has a greater involvement of lymphocytes and marked connective tissue response; polymorphonuclear leukocytes are not abundant; tissue necrosis may accompany this response; and granulation tissue is formed followed by various degrees of scar tissue.

Chronic inflammation may cause severe damage to the anatomic structure of an organ and cause altered physiologic function by the organ. For example, severe tuberculosis and mycotic infections of the lungs or severe damage caused by post-necrotic scarring after hepatitis in the liver and extensive chronic pyelonephritis in the kidney greatly reduce the organ's normal physiology.

Obstruction of vital tissues and organs due to scarring associated with chronic inflammation has severe clinical manifestations. Contraction and distortion resulting from fibrosis (repair) accompanying peptic ulcers may lead to pyloric stenosis (hourglass constriction) of the stomach. Regional enteritis is an example of an advanced chronic inflammatory process of obscure etiology. It leads to considerable fibrosis and scarring of the wall of the intestines, resulting in intestinal stenosis and obstruction. Another example is gonorrhea accompanied by urethritis in males, which may lead to scarring and stricture of the urethra with some blockage of urinary flow.

The events leading to the development of a chronic inflammation and its consequences include the following: causal agent produces tissue necrosis; necrosis causes an acute response in the tissue; the causal agent survives, producing continued local damage; local damage causes either the viable agent to multiply and spread to a new site or local damage is responsible for antigens, which stimulate antibody production; and local damage is eventually partially healed by scarring.

GLANULOMATOUS RESPONSE AND GRANULOMA

If an individual has never been exposed to tubercle bacillus, introduction of this microorganism into the lungs results in a series of defensive mechanisms terminating in the primary focus. There is a very brief infiltration of polymorphonuclear leukocytes into the tissue, and numerous inhaled tubercle bacilli are phagocytized by mononuclear cells. The tubercle bacilli are not destroyed within the phagocyte; in contrast, they multiply quite freely and subsequently destroy the phagocyte, which causes them to be freed. An immune response is gradually developed to the antigens of the tubercle bacilli, and a cellular reaction takes place within the primary focus. The result is necrosis of cells in the center of the primary focus. The latter series of events is repeated over and over.

The inflammatory response in the tissues to the presence of tubercle bacilli has the following characteristics: lesions develop with an extensive cellular response, i.e. a proliferative (productive) response; or lesions develop where a fluid exudate is the predominant feature, i.e. an exudative response.

The early proliferative (productive) lesions are composed of central cluster of microorganisms plus necrotic cells and debris surrounded by a zone of mobilization of cells. The accumulating cells at the periphery of the lesion are mononuclear cells derived from monocytes migrating from the blood stream. In addition, macrophages make up part of the mononuclear cells. Monocytes are cells arising from bone marrow stem-cells, which are mature cells by the time they migrate from the blood stream to the site of injury. The mature monocyte has no capacity for mitosis or ability to synthesize nucleic acids. The mononuclear cells near a lesion of tuberculosis are not undergoing mitosis, but do have a long lifespan and are capable of morphologic alterations and cytoplasmic changes in response to their surroundings.

Mononuclear cells associated with lesions of tuberculosis appear to resemble the epithelial cells. This morphologic alteration in the mononuclear cells is due to the presence of tubercle bacilli. The monocytes may become organized into syncytial clusters of cells once they phagocytize the tubercle bacilli or their products. The cells in the syncytial cluster contain a variable number of nuclei located within a large cytoplasmic mass. The tuberculous lesion shows the presence of "epithelioid" mononuclear cells in a peripheral location. Some epithelioid mononuclear cells further become organized into multinucleated giant cells as the epithelioid cells coalesce. The giant cells associated with the tuberculous lesion are characterized by the presence of pseudopodia and a peripheral location for the nuclei so that they appear as a horseshoe. The multinucleated giant cells with peripheral horseshoe nuclei are termed *Langhans' giant cells*. Langhans' giant cells are also believed to be formed by nuclear replication without any cell division. As the tuberculous lesion ages, accumulations of lymphocytes develop peripherally around the developing lesion. Lymphocytes migrate to the tuberculous lesion initially from the blood stream and subsequently from the lymph nodes. The lymphocyte function is for the formation of immunoglobulin. Plasma cells may be present and are active in the synthesis of protein (immunoglobulin).

Fibroblasts subsequently appear around this chronic granulomatous lesion. The chronic granulomatous lesion of tuberculosis may undergo healing, whereby the centrally located necrotic tissue is largely removed by phagocytosis and replaced by collagenous connective tissue produced by fibroblasts. The healed lesion is low in vascularity. The tuberculous lesion is, therefore, a circumscribed nodular type of lesion consisting of a central zone of epithelioid cells, giant cells with some degree of necrosis, a peripheral accumulation of lymphocytes and plasma cells and fibrosis. The latter lesion is defined as a granuloma (tubercle). Chronic granulomatous inflammation is a prolonged inflammatory response by the body in which the granuloma is always produced. The granuloma has been termed a *tubercle* resulting from infection with *Mycobacterium tuberculosis*.

The tuberculous lesion may be self-limiting. The defensive mechanisms of the infected individual may overcome the microorganisms, cause resolution of the lesion (granuloma), and produce a fibrous nodule at this site. In still other cases, the tuberculous lesion cannot be confined or healed, and the mass of the lesion is increased by expanding peripherally in all directions. The central zone of necrosis increases in size, and in the gross state the fresh specimen has the appearance of soft cheese. Therefore, the necrosis is termed *caseous necrosis* or *caseation*. Small satellite tubercles (granulomas) may develop at the periphery of the main tubercle and are caused when bacillus-laden monocytes migrate from the main granuloma into normal adjacent tissue. The satellite tubercles subsequently coalesce with the main granuloma, increasing the mass of the granulomatous lesion.

Tubercle bacilli or infected phagocytes migrate along the lymphatic channels and eventually enter the bronchial lymph nodes at the hilum of the lung. The granulomatous inflammatory process is repeated in the lymph nodes in rapid fashion. The lymph nodes, therefore, become greatly enlarged, and their normal structures are replaced by a large mass of caseous, necrotic material containing tubercle bacilli.

Original granulomas (tubercles) are primarily microscopic lesions. However, as the initial granuloma grows, it soon becomes a greyish, round, and readily visualized structure appearing grossly as millet seeds. Thus, the numerous granulomas are called "miliary tubercles." The small initial granulomas result in the formation of a larger or "conglomerate tubercle." Conglomerate tubercles become quite large and extensive in nature, consisting primarily of caseous necrosis and debris surrounded by a peripheral zone of cells described for the typical chronic granulomatous inflammatory process.

In time, widespread dissemination of tubercle bacilli and miliary tubercles occurs to other parts of the body distant from the primary locus. Dissemination of tuberculosis occurs by the involvement of blood vessels in the chronic granulomatous inflammatory process as very large numbers of tubercle bacilli invade the blood stream. Metastatic miliary tubercles may arise at any distant site, in almost any tissue and organ, since the tubercle bacilli are seeded in any organ of the body and arrive by way of the arterial system. Miliary tuberculosis runs a rapid course, carrying the patient into a downhill course, which requires chemotherapy to save the patient.

Primary tuberculosis may be manifested at any site where the tubercle bacilli are introduced into the body. For instance, a primary focus of tuberculosis may occur in the intestinal tract, leading to mesenteric lymphadenopathy and tuberculosis peritonitis. Primary tuberculosis of the tonsil leads to involvement of the cervical lymph nodes. Destruction of the cervical lymph nodes by caseation necrosis may result in dissemination of tuberculosis into the soft tissues of the neck with development of the "cold abscess," i.e. an abscess formed by collections of caseous necrotic material with a rise in the skin temperature seen in acute pyogenic abscesses. The cold abscess spreads to adjacent tissues along the lines of least resistance, and eventually, it discharges caseous necrotic material on the surface of the skin after forming a tuberculosis sinus.

In subjects who have had a previous primary infection with tubercle bacilli, or have been vaccinated with BCG, a positive tuberculin reaction and a delayed type of immune response or hypersensitivity to tuberculosis antigens will be demonstrated. The response of the latter subjects to a subsequent infection by the tubercle baccillus will be considerably modified. The following characteristics are present in the individual's response to this subsequent infection: it is harder to acquire the tubercle bacillus infection due to some degree of immunity; therefore, there is value to the BCG prophylaxis; a very active cellular (monocyte) response occurs early; if the developing granulomatous lesion persists, they progress more slowly and occur by direct extension rather than by the rapid dissemination through the lymphatics; the more localized the primary focus the less rapidly progressive the lesion is; and widespread miliary dissemination is less common and occurs late in the disease. The delayed type of immune response to tuberculosis antigens, which occurs in an individual vaccinated with BCG, may not be productive of total immunity. However, it will modify the body's response to the tubercle bacillus and should be considered as an adjunct to the protection of humans against tuberculosis infection.

FATE OF CHRONIC GRANULOMATOUS INFLAMMATIONS

Caseation necrosis or liquefaction of the granuloma occurs in other chronic granulomatous infections in addition to tuberculosis. Cellular necrosis may occur in granulomas accompanied by softening and autolytic liquefaction, i.e. a "soft tubercle" develops. The latter type of granuloma develops in tuberculosis and in some deep mycoses. Hard tubercles refer to granulomas in which necrosis and softening do not take place or are minimal. Hard or nodular granulomatous lesions are characteristic of the chronic granulomatous disease termed sarcoidosis. The production of necrotic or liquefied material is important in granulomas when considering their potential for dissemination of the infection.

For instance, caseous material that contains numerous microorganisms may have ready access to blood vessels, and thus, dissemination occurs. A caseous mass may erode and destroy the bronchus. The necrotic material is coughed up, leaving a cavity filled with numerous pathogenic microorganisms. A focus of caseation necrosis may erode into a serous body cavity accompanied by the formation of pleural and peritoneal lesions, or the caseous focus may invade the subcutaneous tissue and form the cold abscess.

Infectious granulomas without the formation of soft tubercles do not undergo extension and follow an entirely different pattern or fate than the soft tubercles. The fate of a granuloma is dependent upon multiple factors in addition to the nature of the etiologic agent. If the body is capable of eradicating the etiologic agent, healing ensues as necrotic tissue is removed by phagocytosis and fibrosis but no blood vessels replace the necrotic material. Rather large scarring may result. Large caseous masses may be sterile; however, they present a problem to the phagocytes. The large caseous mass is generally surrounded by a capsule composed of dense, vascular, fibrous connective tissue forming a partially walled off mass. The latter lesion undergoes varying degrees of calcification (pathologic). Healing of the chronic granulomatous inflammatory response is often incomplete, accompanied by destruction of tissue and extensive fibrous scarring and impaired physiology of the involved organ.

EXAMPLES OF CHRONIC GRANULOMATOUS INFLAMMATION (DISEASE)

Granulomas present in chronic granulomatous inflammations may be classified as infectious granulomas, spirochete granulomas, other bacterial granulomas, mycotic granulomas, and noninfective granulomas.

The infectious granulomas are tuberculosis, leprosy, and other mycobacterial granulomas. Tuberculosis is tuberculous granulomatous inflammation previously described in this chapter.

Leprosy is a chronic granulomatous inflammatory disease caused by *Mycobacterium leprae*. Prolonged and very close contact are prerequisites for the establishment of this granulomatous infection in the majority of individuals. *Mycobacterium leprae* probably enters man through the skin or mucous membrane of the upper respiratory system. From the respiratory tract the infection probably spreads through the branches of the peripheral nerves.

Tuberculoid leprosy is that form of the infection in which the skin and peripheral nerves are principally involved. Tuberculoid leprosy is a slow, progressive, symmetrical process, which disseminates along the adjacent peripheral nerves. The sensory nerves are primarily infected by the *Mycobacterium leprae*. Granulomas subsequently develop in the skin and peripheral lymph nodes. Few leprae microorganisms are present in the granulomas of the skin and peripheral lymph nodes.

Lepromatous leprosy is a second form of this granulomatous disease. In this form, there is involvement of the skin and mucous membranes. The granulomas generally develop in the following parts of the body: skin, mucosa, peripheral nerves, larynx, testes, and distal portions of the hands and feet. Lepromatous leprosy progresses very rapidly. Large granulomatous lesions form, and subsequently, they fuse together to form large disfiguring cutaneous patches. The disfiguring is termed *leonine facies*. Various forms of the disease may be contained in the same infected individual.

The intradermal injection of lepromin (suspension of killed *M. leprae* from lepromatous leprosy) produces a reaction similar to the tuberculin test. Subjects who have leprosy respond in forty-eight hours with a tuberculinlike response. Four weeks following injection of lepromin, a raised, papular response occurs. The lepromatous form of leprosy represents a poor immunologic response to the antigens of the *M. leprae*.

Complications due to neurologic involvement develop late in the disease and include sensory loss, muscle wasting, considerable crippling of the hand, and blindness. Long-term leprosy is accompanied by amyloidosis and secondarily infected ulcers. The ulcers are the result of involvement of the sensory nerve fibers by *M. leprae*.

Other mycobacterial granulomas produce systemic granulomatous infections that are identical to tuberculosis, i.e. *Mycobacterium bovis,* the Battey-Ovian bacillus, and *M. kansasii.* These granulomatous infections are not identical to tuberculosis because their transmission is probably not airborne, and they demonstrate a resistance to antituberculosis drugs. They are more difficult to irradicate than tuberculosis. However, their lesions in the tissue are similar to those of the *Mycobacterium tuberculosis.*

The swimming pool granuloma is caused by *Mycobacterium balnei.* This mycobacterium is present in swimming pools, and the site of entry into the body is abraded skin. This mycobacterium produces local granulomatous nodular lesions, which become necrotic and ulcerate, resulting in elevated granulating tissue. Histopathologic findings are identical to tuberculosis; however, the lesion is localized at the site of the infection with some local extension. Treatment is satisfactory to antituberculosis drugs.

Mycobacterium ulcerans is another granuloma, but is much more destructive than the swimming pool granuloma. This mycobacterium produces rather large ulcerating granulomas, which extend throughout the full thickness of the skin and into the underlying muscle.

SPIROCHETE GRANULOMAS

Syphilis is a spirochete granuloma caused by the *Treponema pallidum.* Syphilis may be congenital or acquired. Acquired syphilitic infections are venereal in origin. Acquired syphilis is divided into three evolutional stages, i.e. primary stage, secondary stage, and the tertiary stage.

The primary stage is termed the *chancre,* a hard, painless lesion of granlomatous inflammation. The chancre readily undergoes ulceration at the initial site of inoculation of the treponema. The chancre develops in the genitals, but the following areas are also involved in venereal contact: penis, labia, cervix, anal region, lips, and mouth. Spirochetes of *Treponema pallidum* can be demonstrated in the tissue by histopathologic examination and a dark-field examination of the exudate removed from the lesion.

The chancre consists of an intense cellular response, with

plasma cells, monocytes, and small lymphocytes accumulating around the small blood vessels. The blood vessels show proliferation of the endothelial cells and a fibroblastic proliferation of the vessel wall, causing closure of the lumen and decreased flow of blood. The endarteritis obliterans of small blood vessels is a common feature of the syphilitic granuloma. The primary chancre undergoes healing in about three months, with very little scarring. No massive systemic dissemination occurs during the primary stage; however, early dissemination of microorganisms occurs from the inoculation site to the regional lymph nodes, i.e. the inguinal lymph nodes become enlarged and tender.

Secondary syphilis develops from two to twelve weeks following the appearance of the chancre. It appears as a disseminated secondary stage producing mucocutaneous eruptions, which vary tremendously in clinical morphology. Mucous patches are greyish white lesions formed in the oral cavity, pharynx, and tongue. The mucous patches undergo ulceration and are termed *snail-track ulcers*. The mucocutaneous eruption appear in the following forms: macular, maculopapular, and pustular lesions in great abundance in certain cases. Papilliform, brown-colored lesions called condylomata lata may develop in the anal-genital region.

Histopathologic findings of secondary syphilis are endarteritis obliterans, an intense plasma cell, and the presence of lymphocytic infiltration around the small blood vessels. The secondary lesion is teeming with spirochetes. Secondary syphilis is highly contagious. Condylomata lata are accompanied by severe epithelial hyperplasia and hyperkeratosis in their location in the anal-genital region. Systemic symptoms occur but are not severe. There is a generalized lymph node enlargement, recurrent fever, malaise, headache, and a patchy alopecia with a moth-eaten scalp. Eye manifestations, i.e. iritis or neuroretinitis, develop in a few patients with secondary syphilis.

Tertiary syphilis is the advanced stage of syphilis, which does not appear clinically for numerous years following the quieting of the secondary stage. Approximately two-thirds of syphilitic patients will never develop the tertiary stage.

The gumma is the primary lesion of tertiary syphilis. It is a firm, nonsuppurative, granulomatous inflammation developing anywhere in the body. The gumma consists of a central necrotic region resembling caseation necrosis, but it does not change to liquefaction necrosis as seen in tuberculosis. The caseation necrosis occurs as a focus invested with an infiltrate of small lymphocytes and plasma cells plus a limiting zone of proliferating fibroblasts. Foreign body giant cells and epithelioid cells are present. Small gumma lacking caseation necrosis may develop in many cases.

The gumma is the primary, classic lesion of tertiary syphilis. However, lymphocytes, plasma cells, fibroblastic response, and endarteritis obliterans and perivascular mobilization of cells are all significant tertiary findings. Tertiary syphilis is the disseminated form of syphilis and is important because it produces rather large lesions in the cardiovascular and central nervous system. Endarteritis obliterans of the vasa vasorum occurs in tertiary syphilis. The endarteritis leads to medial necrosis of vessels and scarring. Scarring is a characteristic of syphilitic aortitis accompanied by loss of elasticity, dilatation of the aorta, and widening and stretching of the aortic valve ring. When the valve cusps become thickened and scarred, severe degrees of aortic incompetency develop. Fibrous scarring, once extensive, causes rigidity of the aorta plus a weakening of the aortic wall. Thus, this weakened wall predisposes the aorta to formation of an aneurysm. The ostia of coronary arteries are affected by tertiary syphilis and become narrow, limiting the flow of blood to the myocardium. The final result of all cardiac alterations is aortic regurgitation with compensatory, left ventricular hypertrophy, episodes of angina, and aortic aneurysm.

Manifestations of meningovascular syphilis develop in the central nervous system. Neurosyphilis is therefore a manifestation of the tertiary stage of syphilis.

Congenital syphilis is the final form of this spirochete granuloma. Congenital syphilis produces syphilitic osteochondritis, destruction of the bridge of the nose, resulting in a saddle nose, a variety of skin rashes, snuffles, and involvement of some of the internal organs in the syphilitic granulomatous inflammation.

Proliferative, chronic periostitis is a late manifestation of congenital syphilis and produces the skeletal deformity called sabre tibia.

Skin rashes of various types develop as multiple lesions during congenital syphilis. The skin rashes consist of lymphocytes, plasma cells, and fibroblasts in a perivascular accumulation and epithelial hyperplasia.

Visceral manifestations occur in congenital syphilis but are highly variable. The liver may become fibrotic due to a pericellular fibrotic reaction. The lung may reveal a different interstitial pneumonia with marked infiltration by lymphocytes and monocytes. Alveolar spaces are decreased in size or obliterated and are termed *pneumonia alba.*

Yaws, bejel, and pinta are examples of nonvenereal spirochetoses occurring in tropical countries and having an obscure relationship to venereal syphilis. Yaws is a spirochetoses caused by *Treponema pertenue* infections, pinta is caused by *Treponema carateum,* and bejel is caused by a variant of *Treponema pallidum.* All three of these nonvenereal spirochetes are identical in morphology to *Treponema pallidum,* and all of them probably represent variants of the same microorganism. All three spirochetoses produce histopathologic lesions similar to those of the syphilitic lesion. Yaws and pinta produce a primary lesion like the chancre. Bejel produces a primary lesion (chancre) in the oral cavity, i.e. multiple ulcerations of the oral cavity. All three spirochetoses have a secondary stage consisting of mucocutaneous lesions. Yaws produces a tertiary stage and gummas develop in the skeleton and skin. Tertiary stage of pinta is accompanied by cardiovascular and nervous system manifestations.

OTHER BACTERIAL GRANULOMAS

Brucellosis, tularemia, and lymphogranuloma venereum are other important bacterial granulomas. Brucellosis (undulant fever) results from infection by three small, gram-negative bacilli, i.e. *Brucella melitensis, Brucella abortus,* and *Brucella suis.* These three parasites live on goats, cows, and pigs respectively. Contact with infected animals or drinking contaminated milk produces the infection.

Acute brucellosis is marked by undulant fever, leukopenia, and granulocytopenia. Chronic brucellosis primarily causes involvement of the liver and spleen, lymphadenopathy, and bone marrow lesions. Chronic lesions contain small, nodular granulomas composed of a central zone of necrosis surrounded by a zone of epithelioid cells, giant cells, plasma cells, and lymphocytes. The chronic lesion of brucellosis is difficult to separate from the chronic tuberculosis granuloma. The nodular granuloma of brucellosis may develop in the lung, kidney, and testes. Granulomas of brucellosis coalesce to produce extensive, necrotic zones, which subsequently undergo healing by absorption, fibrosis, and calcification. Brucella infections give a positive skin test (brucellin test), which represents a manifestation of a delayed type of immunity of brucella antigens.

Tularemia is an infection caused by the gram-negative bacillus, *Pasteurella tularensis,* which occurs as a parasite of rabbits, squirrels, opossums, mice, rats, foxes, quail, pheasants, and some varieties of snakes. The human chronic granulomatous infection occurs by handling infected animals, eating improperly cooked infected meat, by the bite of an infected tick, fly, or mosquito. One infected person does not transmit the disease to another person. The primary lesion occurs at the site of entry into the body. The disease occurs in several forms, i.e. ulceroglandular (skin and regional lymph nodes), diffuse lymphatic, and pneumonic variety. The primary lesion of the skin consists of a central zone of liquefaction necrosis plus a cellular response consisting of polymorphonuclear leukocytes, lymphocytes, and giant cells. The mixed granulomatous and suppurative lesion of tularemia develops anywhere in the body.

Lymphogranuloma venereum is a venereal disease caused by the parasite *Bedsonia*. This parasite is related to ornithosis, the agent causing psittacosis. *Bedsonia* organisms are like rickettsiae but have characteristics of bacteria, possess both RNA and DNA types of nuclei acid, multiply by binary fission, have bacterial type of cell walls, and enzyme systems supporting metabolism.

Lymphogranuloma venerum infection produces an initial

small, vesicular lesion, which undergoes necrosis and ulceration. The regional lymph nodes are enlarged and matted into one mass. The lymph nodes demonstrate a chronic granulomatous inflammatory reaction consisting of an irregular, stellate area of necrotic tissue, and a peripheral area of epithelioid cells and multinucleated giant cells. The infected lymph nodes break down, adhere to overlying tissue, and drain purulent material to the outside by way of sinuses. Late manifestations of lymphogranuloma venereum demonstrate further lymphatic dissemination plus fibrosis and strictures of the genital tract and rectum. Widespread lymphatic involvement and fibrotic repair lead to lymphatic obstruction and local elephantiasis of the labia, scrotum, and penis.

MYCOTIC (FUNGAL) GRANULOMAS

Various fungi have pathogenic properties and produce systemic and local infections with a chronic granulomatous pattern. For the most part, the pathogenic fungi are classified into two important groups, i.e. *Deuteromycetes* and *Ascomycetes*.

Parasitic fungi infect man in a number of ways. The following five general areas are involved in humans:

1. Superficial fungal infections of the mucous memberane or skin (dermatomycoses or ringworm and candidiasis);

2. Local inoculations due to contact (sporotrichosis) with limited local and lymphatic dissemination;

3. Deep-seated chronic granulomatous infections of the viscera, beginning in the lungs (histoplasmosis, coccidiodomycosis, cryptococcosis) or in the alimentary tract (actinomycosis, candidiasis), with a risk of dissemination throughout the entire body.

4. Secondary fungal infections of body cavities or cysts by opportunistic fungi;

5. Attack by fungi that are primarily saprophytic but may become very dangerous parasites if the immune mechanism is surpressed, i.e. aspergillosis, phycomycosis in patients on antitumor agents, steroid therapy or irradiation.

Tissue reactions in the human body induced by the presence of fungi depend upon the specific fungus in question. The fungi that belong to *Deuteromycetes* produce chronic granulomatous lesions similar to the tubercle of tuberculosis i.e. they form epithelioid lesions resembling the mycobacterial granulomata. The specific fungus can only be distinguished by a demonstration of the causal fungus. Therefore, caseous necrosis is present in coccidioidomycosis, histoplasmosis, and blastomycoses, but the granuloma with caseous necrosis is rare in other fungal infections. Actinomycosis produces gross suppurative lesions with prominent abscess formations.

Coccidioidomycosis is a chronic granulomatous fungal infection caused by *Coccidioides immitis* in arid areas of southwestern part of the United States, and North Mexico. Humans are infected by inhaling the arthrospores of this fungus. The primary infection is, therefore, established in the lungs.

The arthrospores form a tissue phase in the form of a capsulated spherical body (spherule). The wall of the spherule ruptures and liberates numerous minute endospores, which in turn produce more spherules.

Coccidioidomycosis produces pulmonary chronic granulomatous inflammation similar to the tubercles of pulmonary tuberculosis. The cellular reaction in the pulmonary inflammatory lesion consists of epithelioid cells, giant cells, and small lymphocytes. Caseation necrosis is present in the granuloma of coccidioidomycosis. Dissemination of the infection takes place by means of direct extension, lymphatic spread, and on occasion, by the hematogenous route. The clinical disease appears similar to tuberculosis.

Individuals in the southwestern United States who acquire the primary infection generally undergo healing of the lesion by fibrosis, and this is the usual end result of the disease. In the southwestern United States, 90 percent of a given population will acquire the primary infection, and healing occurs spontaneously. The coccidioidin skin test is a delayed type of immune response analogous to the tuberculin test, which is used to determine the incidence of this fungal infection.

This fungal infection rarely is disseminated throughout the body; however, systemic spread does occur with very serious manifestations ending in fatalities. When dissemination occurs, miliary coccidioidomycosis affects any organ. Meningitis is a complication of miliary coccidioidomycosis. Amphotericin B is effective in disseminated coccidioidomycosis.

Histoplasmosis is a chronic granulomatous inflammatory process caused by *Histoplasma capsulatum*. Spores (10-15 microns) are inhaled and give rise to a yeastlike cell, which reproduces by budding. The spores are phagocytized by macrophages, and most fungi are intracellular. The yeasts multiply within the macrophages, causing the death of macrophages and liberation of yeasts into the tissues. The macrophages are thus used for local extension of the disease by disseminating the yeast during its migrations.

The solitary pulmonary granuloma is always the primary lesion unless the individual has had heavy exposure to numerous spores through the many small, nodular lesions widely distributed throughout the lungs. The regional lymph nodes are involved and may contain caseation necrosis.

Primary histoplasmosis generally heals by fibrosis, and calcification is common. The individual becomes sensitized to the antigens of *Histoplasma capsulatum*, and a histoplasmin test is available to show significant cross-reaction with the coccidioidin test and with similar reactions induced by other fungi.

Dissemination of *Histoplasma capsulatum* is very rare concerning the great number of primary fungal infections. When widespread dissemination has occurred, secondary histoplasmosis granulomas become established through the body. For instance, the liver and kidneys are markedly involved by granulomas. Disseminated granulomas occur in the kidneys, adrenals, heart, serous cavities, and meninges. A fatal termination is usually the case.

Blastomycosis is a deep mycosis caused by infection by *Blastomyces dermatitidis*. The conidiospores are the infecting agents and are introduced by inhalation, producing disease in the host.

The initial lesion of blastomycosis consists of a primary pulmonary complex. The blastomyces organism may provoke an acute suppurative response. However, more commonly, the tissue contains epithelioid granulomas similar to tubercles, with or without caseous necrosis. The majority of lesions subside, and healing of the primary focus results.

Dissemination of blastomycosis is rare. However, if it does occur, cutaneous lesions are prominent; they appear as firm, granulomatous nodules with raised margins and ulceration. The multiple skin lesions develop when an active focus of blastomycosis is present in the lungs. The pulmonary lesions spread for a number of years throughout the circulation. The lesions of blastomycosis located in the skin show pseudoepitheliomatous hyperplasia, microabscesses containing organisms, and epithelioid granulomas with giant cells.

Dissemination of blastomycosis occurs particularly to the skeleton, kidney, and prostate, producing a systemic blastomycosis.

Chromoblastomycosis is a rare, subcutaneous mycotic granuloma caused by *Fonsecaea, Philalophora,* and *Cephalosporium.* This mycosis occurs in the skin and subcutaneous tissues of the lower extremity. The granuloma consists of pseudoepitheliomatous hyperplasia, microabscesses, and large areas of destruction of tissue. The mycosis does not undergo systemic dissemination.

Paracoccidioidomycosis or South American blastomycoses is a deep mycosis caused by infection by *Paracoccidioides brasiliensis.* This form of blastomycosis begins with a pulmonary primary granuloma, which may consist of varying degrees of caseous necrosis. Dissemination is widespread, with every organ system involved, and a marked lymphadenopathy is present. The skin contains destructive, ulcerating granulomas, with the organisms having a predilection for the mucocutaneous junctions of the lips and eyelids. South American blastomycosis extends rapidly and produces severe destruction of soft tissues. Dissemination involves the internal viscera, with destruction and mutilation of organs. This variety of blastomycosis is limited to South America, particularly Brazil.

Sporotrichosis is a superficial fungal infection in man, which is confined to the skin, subcutaneous tissues, and regional lymph nodes associated with the superficial skin lesions. Dissemination to the viscera does not take place during sporotrichosis. However, pulmonary primary lesions have been reported.

Sporotrichosis is caused by infection by *Sporotrichum schenckii*. The organism enters the human body through small abrasions present in the skin. Thus, this fungal disease is common in gardeners who have numerous minor abrasions that are easily contaminated by *Sporotrichum schenckii*, which reside on plants and bushes in the garden.

Sporotrichosis develops into an ulcerated, indolent, chronic granulomatous primary lesion at the initial site of inoculation. The infection extends from the inoculation site through the lymphatic channels to the regional lymph nodes. The primary granulomatous lesion, the infected lymphatics, and the infected regional lymph nodes are involved by a chronic, granulomatous, inflammatory process composed of epithelioid cells, tuberclelike lesions (granulomas), different degrees of caseation necrosis, and Langhans' giant cells. The tuberclelike lesions are very similar to the tubercle of tuberculosis. *Sporotrichum schenckii* organisms cannot be detected in histopathologic sections; however, they can be detected by the use of fluorescent-antibody techniques.

Although the primary pulmonary lesion of sporotrichosis has been reported, it is of rare occurrence. Pulmonary sporotrichosis is a slowly progressive, granulomatous pneumonitis with caseation necrosis. The caseous necrosis may erupt into a bronchus, leading to cavitation and severe pulmonary fibrosis.

Actinomycosis and nocardiosis represent deep mycoses caused by an infection with organisms of the order Actinomycetales. Actinomycosis is a fungal infection caused specifically by *Actinomyces israelii, Actinomyces bovis* and by other members of this genus. Nocardiosis is a fungal infection caused by *Nocardia asteroides* and *Nocardia brasiliensis*.

Actinomycosis is generally caused by infection by *Actinomyces israelii*. *A. israelii* resides in the oral cavity and tonsillar crypts as saprophytic fungi. The organisms are present in an anaerobic environment with low oxygen tension, which is quite suitable for the growth of *A. israelii*. When the fungi enter into the tissues following local trauma or tooth extraction, they are residing in an unnatural habitat.

Actinomycosis is common in the mandible (lower jaw) and

soft tissues of the neck. Actinomycoses infection infiltrates widely and undergoes formation of abscesses with multiple sinuses draining pus and *Actinomyces israelii*.

Histopathological examination of a tissue specimen from actinomycosis reveals a suppurative as opposed to a chronic granulomatous inflammatory response. The following are characteristic of actinomycosis: abscess formation, extensive tissue destruction, and yellow granules (sulfur granules) within the purulent material. The sulfur granules are visible with the unaided eye. Microscopic study of the sulfur granules reveals that they consist of a tangle of slender, branching hyphae with clublike ends arranged surrounding the periphery of the mass. This arrangement has led to the use of the term *ray fungus* to describe the organism. Sulfur granules are only present in infected tissues and cannot be grown in cultures in the laboratory.

Actinomycosis infection also produces a primary pulmonary lesion or infections in the gastrointestinal tract leading, to formation of the periappendicular abscess and subsequent peritonitis. *A. israelii* organisms enter the blood stream by radicles of the portal venous system with infection of the liver, resulting in formation of extensive, destructive liver abscesses. Widespread dissemination occurs in actinomycosis with lesions developing in distant sites, i.e. bones and visceral organs.

Nocardial infections demonstrate some similarities and some differences when compared to actinomycosis. Nocardial species tend to produce primary pulmonary infections. The tissue response of humans to nocardial infection is more variable than in actinomycosis, and in chronic nocardial infections the typical tuberculoid granuloma is present, behaving like lesions of tuberculosis. Nocardial organisms stain with difficulty in the tissues or purulent exudate and appear as delicate branching, acid-fast organisms. The purulent exudate obtained from lesions of nocardiosis contains granules that appear similar to the ray fungus of actinomycosis. Nocardiae organisms are aerobic, whereas actinomyces are anaerobic organisms, a distinction readily made by growing a culture.

Nocardial organisms disseminate and on occasions develop a

septicemic disease, which undergoes widespread dissemination. The disseminated form of Nocardosis produces a suppurative type of tissue response accompanied by widespread formation of nocardiae abscesses.

NONINFECTIVE GRANULOMAS

The noninfective granulomas comprise a heterogenous group of diseases in which the chronic granulomatous inflammatory process is apparent. These granulomas follow classical patterns, similar to those of the lesions of tuberculosis, which are produced by nonliving agents. In some instances the line between a progressive chronic granulomatous process and a neoplasia is very difficult to distinguish. Thus, for example, Hodgkin's disease is partially a chronic, granulomatous, inflammatory process, but its relationship to viral disease is not clearly understood. The following granulomas represent diseases in which infective mechanisms have not yet been demonstrated. Sarcoidosis (Boeck's sarcoid) and special foreign body granulomas.

Sarcoidosis (Boeck's sarcoid) is a chronic granulomatous inflammatory disease of obscure etiology and having highly variable but chronic clinical features. Every tissue or organ of the body may be involved; however, the most common lesions appear in the lymph nodes, skin, and larger visceral organs (lungs, liver). The eyes may be involved with iridocyclitis.

The characteristic chronic granulomatous process produces a "hard" tubercule, i.e. a granuloma composed of circular collections of epithelioid cells and multinucleated giant cells surrounding small zones of amorphous, eosinophilic material similar to fibrinoid. Caseation necrosis is absent in the tubercle of sarcoidosis. However, Schaumann bodies may be present, i.e. laminated, irregularly shaped bodies, which may be heavily calcified. A limited number of lymphocytes are present at the periphery and surround the lesion. No organism can be demonstrated in the granulomatous lesion or in adjacent tissues. The hard granuloma of sarcoidosis heals by fibrotic repair, and fibrosis results. The Kveim test is a skin test useful for the diagnosis of sarcoidosis. This skin test utilizes an antigen, i.e. sterilized material from the sarcoid lesions. It is analogous to the tuberculin reaction.

Special foreign body granulomas show resemblances to the granuloma (tubercle) of the chronic granulomatous inflammatory process. The foreign body granulomas are caused by silicon, beryllium, barium sulfate etc. The inhalation of fine particles of silica occurs frequently in miners, stone cutters, and quarry workers, and gives rise to a silicosis (a severe, fibrogenic pneumoconiosis). Silicosis produces local (focal) and diffuse necrotic lesions adjacent to the inhaled silica particles, which readily provoke a fibroblastic reaction around the silica. Extensive pulmonary fibrosis may be the final result of the fibroblastic proliferation. When silica particles become embedded into the skin in various occupations, it provokes limited necrotic foci around which epithelioid cells and giant cell multinucleated systems develop, which subsequently leads to fibrotic scarring.

Asbestosis is a foreign body granuloma similar to silicosis.

Asbestosis is caused by the inhalation of fine asbestos fibers, which stimulate a granulomatous reaction.

Beryllium produces a foreign body granuloma composed of epithelioid cells, tuberclelike lesions, and a relatively intense chronic granulomatous inflammatory response.

THERAPY FOR THE CHRONIC GRANULOMATOUS INFLAMMATIONS

Chronic granulomatous inflammations are known as very difficult diseases to treat, with an uncertain outcome in many cases. Where no specific artificial means of treatment is available to eradicate the etiologic agent, the individual is doomed to a precarious existence. The best that has been achieved in patients is a quiescence or quieting down of the symptoms of the chronic granulomatous process. The inactive lesion may become reactivated, causing further disability (leprosy) and other infective granulomatous conditions.

Advances in modern chemotherapy have produced a revolution in the management of many chronic granulomatous inflammations. The effectiveness of the chemotherapy may be altered by the following: accessibility of the organisms to the therapeutic agent, and the ease with which the therapeutic agent is able to penetrate into and destroy the organism.

In the treatment of tuberculosis, the therapeutic agent must reach the tubercle bacilli through necrotic debris and extensive caseation necrosis. It takes considerable time for a therapeutic agent to diffuse through the granulomatous mass to destroy the microorganisms. Therefore, isolated pockets of microorganisms remain viable in masses of caseous necrosis, which are not in contact with lethal concentrations of therapeutic agents (antimicrobial drugs), and thus, these areas remain as a source of future (recurrent) activity after the initial therapy has ended.

Antibiotic therapy for extensive chronic granulomatous inflammations is only of partial success. In the smaller granulomatous lesions, the antibiotics can successfully kill the microorganisms in the accessible parts of the lesion, and the macrophages absorb the inner zones and gradually eradicate the less massive granulomas. The massive type of granulomatous lesion presents a task with which it is impossible for the phagocytes to cope. Massive lesions cannot be resolved in a permanent fashion. They can be walled off by deposition of fibers around the periphery, or they may become calcified. However, there still remains the risk of viable microorganisms surviving in the depths of the granuloma. Under certain conditions, these microorganisms can be activated and cause an extension of the chronic granulomatous inflammatory process.

The three basic criteria for therapy for chronic granulomatous disease consist of the following principles:

1. A decision must be made whether antimicrobial therapy is to be utilized;

2. If chemotherapy is to be used, treatment must be rather prolonged using an adequate dosage level;

3. If a rather prolonged course of chemotherapy has not produced resolution of an area of caseation necrosis, surgical removal should be considered as the next method of achieving resolution of the necrotic lesion. A persistent or quiescent lesion composed of caseation necrosis should be removed surgically because of the probability of future recurrence of the granulomatous inflamma-

tion. Chemotherapy may be utilized to achieve a state of quiescence and can be followed by surgical removal of the persistent, cavitated, granulomatous lesions. The latter principles of therapy apply to all granulamatous inflammations, particularly to the destructive, deep mycoses.

In widely disseminated chronic granulomatous inflammations, i.e. syphilis and chronic brucellosis, surgery has no place in management of these patients. However, if effective chemotherapy is to exist, the drug must be administered in sufficient dosage, for a prolonged duration, in order to overcome the natural obstacles presented by the chronic inflammatory process.

CONCLUSION

The chronic granulomatous diseases follow a general sequence of events in the evolution of a granuloma or tubercle. The chronic granulomatous process represents a basic pattern of defensive response on the part of the body to the various noxious agents (both viable and nonviable), and the observed biologic differences between the various chronic granulomatous reactions are very superficial and minimal. The majority of findings in the granulomatous reactions described in this chapter show numerous major similarities between the various reactions, regardless of the etiologic agent. Thus, the evolution of the chronic inflammatory process subsequently creates unity out of initial diversity, and the latter is just as true for the other biological defense mechanisms in the human body.

References

Amstey, M.S. et al.: *Cancer, 32*:1321-1325, 1973.
Calmette, A., and Guerin, C.: *Ann Inst Pasteur, 38*:371, 1924.
Cohn, Z.A.: In Zeverifach, B.W., Grant, L., and McCluskey, R.T. (Eds.): New York, Acad Pr, 1965, pp. 323-353.
Denton, T.F. and DiSalvo, A.F.: *Am J Trop Med Hyg, 13*:116-122, 1964.
Fiese, M.J.: *Coccidioidomycosis,* Springfield, Thomas, 1958.
Grayston, J.T. and Furcolow, M.L.: *Am J Public Health, 43*:665-676, 1953.
Hackett, C.J.: In Brothwell D. and Sandisen, A.T. (Eds): *Diseases in Antiquity.* Springfield, Thomas, 1967, pp. 152-159.
Kean, B.H., and Childress, T.E.: *Int J Lepr, 10*:51-59, 1942.
Krogh, A.: In *Anatomy and Physiology of Capillaries,* 2nd ed. New Haven,

Yale U Pr, 1929.
Menkin, V.: In *Biochemical Mechanisms of Inflammation*, 2nd ed. Springfield, Thomas, 1965.
Miles, A.A. and Wilhelm, D.L.: *Br J Exp Pathol, 36*:71-81, 1955.
Moulder, J.W.: *CIBA lectures in Microbial Biochemistry*, 1964.
Scott, S.M., et al.: *N Engl J Med, 265*:453-457, 1961.
Sherry, S. and Coleman, R.: *Trans Assoc Am Physicians, 81*:40-48, 1968.
Straub, M. and Schway, J.: *Am J Clin Pathol, 25*:727-741, 1955.
Wilhelm, D.L.: In Zweifach, B.W., Grant, L. and McCluskey, R.T. (Eds.), *The Inflammatory Process*. New York, Acad Pr, 1965, pp. 389-425.
Wolstenholm, G.E.W. and O'Connor, M.: *Pathogenesis of Leprosy*. Boston, Little, 1963.

CHAPTER 12

VIRAL AND RICKETTSIAL DISEASES

VIRAL DISEASES

Introduction to Viral Diseases

VIRUSES ARE PARASITIC ORGANISMS that invade cells and utilize the metabolic systems of the cells to survive and reproduce. The virus may show an affinity for specific tissues. Neurotrophic viruses invade nervous tissue. Some cells are resistant to viruses and undergo proliferation while the viruses die. Other cells undergo degeneration and necrosis in the presence of viruses. Viruses multiply within cells, forming colonies in the cytoplasm or nucleus. The viral colonies appear as homogeneous granules or small bodies termed *inclusion bodies.*

Antibodies may be produced following a viremia and are responsible for immunity. However, no immunity is produced when the viral organisms remain localized on the surface of cells. The common herpetic lesion of the lips is an example of a viral disease whereby the virus is localized on the surface of cells. No viremia develops following the herpes simplex infection; therefore, no immunity is present, and the infection is recurrent as long as the virus remains in the cells. Dermatotrophic viruses, such as smallpox, affect the skin. The molluscum contagiosum dermatotrophic virus causes a proliferation of epithelial cells.

RESPIRATORY VIRUSES. Respiratory viruses affect the respiratory epithelium, producing a transient viremia and an incomplete immunity. A number of strains of viruses actually localize in the upper respiratory tract during the common cold. Immunity is nonexistent following the common cold.

Influenza viruses affect respiratory membranes, small bronchi, and the alveolar cells of the lung. Atypical interstitial pneumonia is due to a filterable respiratory virus, which is accompanied by cold agglutinins in the blood of 60 percent of individuals.

DERMATOTROPHIC VIRUSES. The dermatotrophic virus produces liquefaction necrosis and vesicle formation develops in the infected epithelium.

Smallpox virus produces areolar dermatotrophic lesions characterized by multiple macules in one generalized region. Scarring may result from the smallpox infection, producing a disfigured face.

Chickenpox is a mild dermatotrophic viral disease, producing limited skin lesions. Permanent immunity to chickenpox results after the viral infection subsides. In children, herpes zoster virus produces chickenpox, and in the adult the same virus produces herpes zoster. Infection with either chickenpox or herpes zoster virus provides immunity against the other disease.

Herpes zoster virus affects the sensory nerves and sensory ganglia of the spinal cord and the nerve trunks of the skin of the face and abdomen. The herpes zoster virus affects sensory nerves, causing a severe and disabling type of pain. Herpes zoster virus produces shingles on the skin. The lesions of herpes zoster may follow the course of the facial nerve.

Herpes simplex is a dermatotrophic viral infection producing vesicular lesions at the mucocutaneous junction of the lips and angle of the mouth. Infection does not produce an immunity to the herpes simplex virus. The virus lies dormant in the tissue; however, it may become activated.

Measles is a viral disease that produces a permanent immunity. The initial manifestations of measles appear in the oral mucosa and are termed *Koplik's spots*. Flattened lesions appear on the skin several days following the appearance of the Koplik's spots.

German measles or rubella is a mild viral disease that produces a small rash in the skin. When the viral disease occurs during pregnancy, the virus may produce fetal abnormalities. The rubella virus passes through the placenta, affecting all germ layers of the fetus.

NEUROTROPHIC VIRUSES. Neurotrophic viruses invade the cells of the brain and spinal cord and ganglia. Rabies and poliomyelitis affect the ganglion cells.

Rabies is transmitted by dogs, wolves, cats, and foxes by the inoculation of infected saliva under the skin. The relatively large rabies virus travels slowly along the route of nerves. Fortunately, the incubation period lasts from fifteen days to six months or one year. The maxillofacial region is a highly innervated anatomic region; therefore, a bite in this area is dangerous. Death will occur in ten days if the infected animal harbors the rabies virus in his brain and salivary glands. Chromatolysis of cells, destruction of cell nuclei, and negri bodies are findings in the degenerated cytoplasm of affected cells. Negri inclusion bodies are the principle basis for the histopathologic diagnosis of rabies.

In man the prodromal symptoms of rabies are excitability, muscular twitch, hydrophobia, collapse, and death. Fifteen injections of the rabies vaccine are required to produce an immunity in humans.

Poliomyelitis is due to a neurotrophic virus. Poliomyelitis virus enters the body through the nasal cavity, respiratory tract and intestinal mucosa. The virus travels along the axons of nerves and subsequently reaches the central nervous system. The virus is located in the anterior horns of the gray matter of the spinal cord, in the nuclei of the medulla oblongata, and in the motor area of the cortex. The virus stops suddenly when it passes the motor area of the cortex and enters the sensory areas of the brain.

The prodromal stage of poliomyelitis is characterized by muscular weakness and neck rigidity. When the lower neuron of the spinal cord is involved, a flaccid paralysis results. When the cord is affected above the lower neuron, spastic paralysis results.

MISCELLANEOUS VIRAL INFECTIONS. Mumps differs from the latter viral diseases because of the acute suppurative character of the exudate. Infectious mononucleosis is an acute infectious disease of unknown origin, producing enlarged cervical lymph nodes. The disease produces atypical lymphocytes. The disease is characterized by oral and pharyngeal lesions. Laboratory find-

Viral and Rickettsial Diseases

ings include the following: leukocytosis (10,000 to 25,000), lymphocytosis (50 to 90%), and atypical lymphocytes. Heterophil antibodies are present in the circulating blood. Yellow fever is a viral disease transmitted by the mosquito. The disease produces necrosis of hepatic cells and periportal inflammation.

RICKETTSIAL DISEASES

Rickettsial organisms produce toxins and a proliferation of cells at the site of inoculation. A good immunity results following infection because of the presence of a rickettsemia and the production of antibodies.

TYPHUS GROUP. Epidemic typhus is due to *Rickettsia prowazekii*. The lumen of infected vessels may be blocked by *Rickettsia prowazekii* organisms. A cutaneous rash develops, characterized by a poorly defined erythema of the skin. Hemorrhages occur in the skin. Endemic typhus is due to infection by *Rickettsia typhi*. This disease has a milder course than epidemic typhus.

Brill's disease is a mild form of epidemic typhus. A partial immunity follows the initial infection. Epidemic hemorrhagic fever follows a rapid clinical course with high fever, toxic and extensive hemorrhagic manifestations. Mucosal, skin, esophageal, and gastric mucosal hemorrhages are present.

SPOTTED FEVER GROUP (TICKS). Rocky Mountain spotted fever is due to infection by *Rickettsia rickettsii*. Hemorrhage is characteristic of Rocky Mountain spotted fever. Petechiae and ecchymosis are numerous on the skin and capsular surface of the kidney. Boutonneuse fever is a variety of spotted fever that occurs in the Mediterranean region.

Tsutsugamushi fever or scrub typhus is due to *Rickettsia tsutsugamushi*. The eschar lesion at the portal of entry is a crusted lesion. A small ulceration develops at the site of inoculation. Perivasculitis is present and a rash develops on the skin surface. Q fever is produced by *Rickettsia burneti* and is transmitted by ticks or by direct contact resulting in an interstitial pneumonitis and cyanosis.

Rickettsial pox is a self-limiting, acute febrile disease caused by *Rickettsia akari*. Rickettsial pox is characterized by an initial lesion at the site of infection, fever persisting for approximately one week, and a papulovesicular rash. The lesions of rickettsial pox are discrete, abundant, or scanty in distribution. Papules and vesicles are observed on the skin and tongue.

PROTOZOAL INFECTIONS

LEISHMANIASIS. Leishmaniasis is caused by *Leishmania donovani*, which produces a recurrent fever, anemia, and leukocytopenia. The clinical manifestations of leishmaniasis are chronic ulcers with sharply demarcated borders. Secondary infection is common.

References

Andrews, C.H.: *Med Clin North Am, 51*:765, 1967.
Arean, V.M.: In Summers, S.C. (Ed.): *Pathology Annual*, New York, Appleton-Century-Crofts, 1966, vol.I.
Armstrong, R.W., et al.: *N Engl Med, 283*:1182, 1970.
Baker, R.D. (Ed.): *Human Infection with Fungi, Actinomycetes, and Algae*, New York, Springer-Verlag, 1971.
Baum, G.L. and Schwartz, J.: *Am J Med Sci, 238*:660, 1959.
Beck, J.W. and Barrett-Conner, E.: *Medical Parasitology*, St. Louis, Mosby, 1971.
Blumberg, B.S. and Melartin, L.: *Arch Intern Med, 125*:287, 1970.
Del Prete, S., et al.: *Lancet, 2*:579, 190.
Dudgeon, J.A., et al.: *Br Med J, 2*:155, 1964.
Emmons, C.W., Binford, C.H. and Utz, J.P.: *Medical Mycology*, 2nd ed. Philadelphia, Lea and Febiger, 1970.
Enders, J.F., et al.: *N Engl J Med, 261*:875, 1959.
Henle, G. and Henle, W.: *Hosp Pract, 5*:33, 1970.
Hersh, T., et al.: *N Engl J Med, 285*:1363, 1971.
Hirshaut, Y., et al.: *N Engl J Med, 283*:502, 1970.
Ho, M.: *N Engl J Med, 283*:1222, 1970.
Hutter, R.V.P.: *Cancer, 12*:330, 1959.
Krugman, S. and Giles, J.P.: *JAMA, 212*:1019, 1970.
Krugman, S., et al.: *JAMA, 217*:41, 1971.
Landers, J.J., et al.: *N Engl J Med, 285*:303, 1971.
London, W.T., et al.: *N Engl J Med, 281*:571, 1969.
Melnick, J.L. and Rawls, W.E.: *Hosp Pract, 4*:37, 1969.
Naji, A.F.: *Arch Pathol, 68*:282, 1959.
Neva, F.A.: *N Engl J Med, 277*:1241, 1967.

Rhodes, A.J. and van Roogen, C.E.: *Textbook of Virology,* 5th ed. Baltimore, Williams and Wilkins, 1968.
Sanger, P.W., et al.: *JAMA, 181:*88, 1962.
Suringa, D.W.R., et al.: *N Engl Med, 283:*1139, 1970.
Tamm, I.: *Am J Med, 38:*649, 1965.

CHAPTER 13

DISEASES DUE TO PHYSICAL INJURIES, CHEMICAL POISONS, AND THERMAL AND IRRADIATION INJURIES

DISEASES DUE TO PHYSICAL INJURIES (TRAUMA)

TRAUMA IS THE RESULT of mechanical forces, and the lesions produced are wounds. Physical injuries (traumas) include the following: contusion, abrasion, laceration, fracture, sprain, and concussion. A contusion is defined as a wound in which the skin surface is intact but the underlying blood vessels are torn. An abrasion is defined as a wound in which the surface epithelium is lost due to trauma. A laceration (cut) is a wound whereby the soft tissues are severed or cut. A fracture is a break in the continuity of a bone. A sprain is the tearing of a ligament, tendon, or muscle. Concussion is marked jolting of the brain within the skull and is defined as momentary loss of consciousness resulting from the rocking movement of the brain within the cranium. Concussion is associated with a transient amnesia present at the time of the trauma.

The greater the physical force applied to the body and the smaller the area, the deeper will be the penetration of the force and the greater will be the tendency for rupture or tearing of tissues. When physical forces are exerted in resilient tissues, the elasticity of the specific tissue may be an important factor in preventing its rupture. The same force applied to a bone (having rigidity) will produce a fracture, whereas the elastic tissue is unharmed. Trauma to the abdomen or chest may rupture the intestines, liver, and lungs in the absence of any surface pathology or involvement of superficial tissues.

The area of damage resulting from a physical injury or trauma is related to the site of impact. Physical injuries may be localized to the site of impact or they may be transmitted through the body due to fluid waves, bony leverage, and muscle pull to a site distant from the impact.

Physical injuries or traumas generally cause secondary alterations within the body. Hemorrhage is a common complication of physical injuries. Hemorrhage readily follows damage to blood vessels. A severe hemorrhage resulting from a massive trauma may prove to be fatal as follows:

1. By loss of one-third of the volume of blood within several hours, leading to fatality;

2. By slow progressive reduction in blood volume, leading to irreversible shock; and

3. By the rapid accumulation of blood in the pericardium, causing tamponade, in the cranial cavity, causing increased intracranial pressure, or in the renal pelves, causing blockage of urinary excretion and uremia.

The injury caused by trauma is generally nonselective in nature. The injured organ is generally the organ that receives the mechanical force or trauma. However, exception occurs since, in the case of trauma to the abdominal wall (resilient tissues), the bowel may rupture by bursting, but no signs are present of the direct force to the abdominal wall. Trauma to a hollow, viscus organ causes an increased hydrostatic pressure in the organ, which is the cause of its rupture. Severe forces to a rigid bone cause fractures by the direct trauma. It is also possible for a fracture of the bone to develop at some distant site from the initial point of contact due to the leverage exerted by bone tissue. Veins and arteries may rupture some great distance from the initial site of injury because of transmission of hydrostatic pressure.

Physical injuries may predispose normal tissues and organs to infection. Post-traumatic infections are based upon the following predisposing factors:

1. Degenerated tissues or coagulated blood, which produces a culture medium for microorganisms;

2. Introduction of a foreign body (exogenous nature) or an endogenous foreign body (bone fragment);

3. Rupture of the normal lines of tissue resistance and barriers to spread of microorganisms;

4. Certain types of physical injuries (human bites, rabid dog bite) predispose to infection; and

5. Criminal abortion accompanied by streptococcal or staphylococcal infection of genital tract.

Traumatic injuries may, therefore, be complicated by hemorrhage, shock, infection, fracture, nerve injury, and rupture of viscus organ. Infections following traumatic injuries are very dangerous in the patient with diabetes mellitus, since they may pass into diabetic coma following an abscess superimposed on wounds. The bites of cats and rats may cause cat scratch fever and rat bite fever respectively, and secondary infection may develop in these wounds.

Selye (1950) described the general adaptation syndrome. This syndrome is a secondary defensive mechanisms of the body, which comes into play during severe physical injuries or trauma, infections, and following extended exposure to cold, strenuous exercises, pregnancy, and major surgery. The general adaptation syndrome consists principally of a hyperfunctioning of the adrenal-pituitary axis. There is an increase in the secretion of adrenalin, constriction of peripheral blood vessels, and mobilization of glucose from the liver and leukocytes from the spleen.

The principal alterations in the body during the general adaptation syndrome include the following: (1) an initial mobilization of glucose and leukocytes by the adrenalin; (2) a shift in the fluid and electrolyte balances; (3) a shift in protein and carbohydrate metabolism; (4) alterations in the blood cell count and serum proteins; and (5) reinforcement of the endothelium of capillaries and of the matrix of connective tissue (anti-inflammatory effect).

The general adaptation syndrome consists of an immediate and a delayed response. The immediate response occurs within minutes and produces both local and systemic effects. The local effects include the following: damage or death of tissue with release of painful stimuli and alarming substances (histamine, choline); and action directly on the adrenal medulla to release epinephrine. The systemic effects include the following: peripheral vasoconstriction; tachycardia; leukocytosis; and hyperglycemia through glycogenolysis in the liver.

The delayed response of the general adaptation syndrome occurs from several hours through a period of several days. The local effects of the delayed response are prolongation of painful stimuli and the continued release of alarming substances, and action through the hypothalamus to release ACTH from the adenohypophysis, which in turn releases adrenal cortical hormones. The systemic effects of the delayed response include the following:

1. Retention of sodium chloride and water, and increased excretion of potassium, uric acid, histamine, and nitrogenous wastes;

2. Increased glyconeogenesis from protein plus increased hepatic storage of glycogen;

3. Increased destruction of lymphocytes and eosinophiles, increased fibrinogen and immune globulins from the liver and reticuloendothelial system, and increased numbers and stickiness of the platelets; and

4. Increased capillary resistance to rupture and histamine, and inhibition of fibroblastic proliferation.

Hemorrhage is a form of secondary alteration associated with physical injuries or trauma to blood vessels. Hemorrhage is a very common complication of wounds due to trauma. The physical injury and mechanical forces readily severe blood vessels. Internal as well as external hemorrhage is the result of mechanical forces or trauma. Internal hemorrhages are hemorrhages that are localized and surrounded by a capsule within the tissue. External hemorrhages are hemorrhages whereby blood escapes from the surface of the body.

Rapid loss of one-third of the blood volume from the human body following a physical injury to a major blood vessel is fatal. Loss of one-half of the blood volume over a prolonged period of time will also prove to be fatal. Hemorrhage into a closed body cavity may possibly cause death due to compression of vital organs and structures. Blood may accumulate in the pericardium, as a hemopericardium, and cause compression of the heart with fatal ventricular arrest, i.e. cardiac tamponade. Bilateral hemorrhage into the renal pelves occur during leukemia and blood dyscrasias due to an interference with blood clotting. Uremia develops when the urinary outflow is blocked.

When hemorrhage is severe in nature, the pressure in the right auricle begins to fall, which is directly proportional to the volume of the hemorrhage. Venous return to the heart becomes decreased, and there is a fall in the output of the heart and a decrease in the peripheral arterial blood pressure. Delayed shock (hypovolemic shock) is accompanied by the mechanism termed *hemodilution*. Delayed shock caused by hemorrhage is accompanied by loss of circulating blood volume through blood loss or passage of fluid and plasma into the traumatized tissue. Delayed shock produces a diminished venous return of blood to the right heart, decreased output from the heart, and a decrease in arterial blood pressure with anoxia of the capillary bed.

Neurogenic (primary) shock is not due to hemorrhage but may follow a severe physical injury because of the presence of painful stimuli. In primary shock a reflex vasodilatation develops rapidly, within seconds, following a physical injury and is accompanied by a drop in blood pressure, resulting in loss of consciousness. Primary or neurogenic shock following trauma is generally transient in nature; however, it is possible for severe physical injuries with severe hemorrhage to produce a state of delayed shock.

Traumatic or physical injuries to the brain and spinal cord are capable of producing (most severe to less severe) the following: concussions, contusions, lacerations and penetrating injuries, and crushing. The most severe injury is the concussion and the least severe injury is crushing. Concussion is defined as the interruption of the physiology of the brain in the absence of any structural alterations. Concussion is not commonly found in athletes and those engaging in physical tasks. It is common in sedentary individuals. The patient with concussion may have varying degrees of consciousness, from no memory of injury to coma. The concussion may cause unconsciousness at injury with a return to complete consciousness for several days followed by a return to unconsciousness. Concussion primarily causes unconsciousness, shock, and return to consciousness in fifteen to twenty minutes. Concussion produces changes in the large neurons of the brain stem, followed by a disappearance of these cells. Some edema is also present in the brain during concussion.

Contusion of the brain follows physical injuries and may be accompanied by coma and symptoms of edema of the brain. Petechial hemorrhage may be scattered diffusely in areas of the brain distant from the site of physical injury. The petechial hemorrhages are termed traumatic cerebral purpura.

Laceration and crushing of the brain and spinal cord may follow physical injuries due generally to penetrating injuries or where a fractured skull or spinal cord pushes the bone into the neural tissues. Little or no hemorrhage occurs in the penetrating injury since spasms of the severed arteries seal them to the flow of blood. Softening of brain tissues occurs distal to the penetrating wound due to ischemia and the arterial spasm. When the spinal cord is severely injured, the immediate area of injury becomes edematous, hemorrhage is present, and the brain has a semifluid appearance.

Fracture is defined as a break in a bone or surface of a joint. Dislocation is a displacement of a bone from its articulating counterpart. A sprain is defined as tearing of a ligament, tendon, fascia, or muscle surrounding a joint. Subluxation is defined as an incomplete displacement of a bone from its articulating counterpart. Simple fractures occur when the break in a bone is the result of a physical injury. When the break in a bone is preceded by a pathologic process in the bone tissue, which is responsible for weakening the bone, the fracture that results is designated a pathologic fracture. If the physical injury breaks the bone but also lacerates the tissue, causing bony fragments to become exposed, the fracture is called a compound fracture. If the broken bone is divided into two or more portions, the fracture is called a comminuted fracture. When the fracture extends only partially through the bone, the fracture is called a greenstick (incomplete) fracture.

Fracture of a bone produces bone spicules and hemorrhage,

tearing of the muscle and adjacent soft tissues, and damage to the bone marrow present in the cancellous spaces of the bone. Necrosis of muscle, degeneration of fatty bone marrow, and destruction of small fragments of bone occur in one to several weeks after the fracture occurs.

Healing of fracture of a bone goes through the following steps: coagulation of the hematoma present at the site of fracture; organizaton of the thrombus during the first week after fracture; formation of a fibrous callus; fibrous callus is replaced subsequently by a periosteal callus within two weeks; ossification of the periosteal callus develops in three to four weeks. The periosteal (anchoring) callus remains for one month or more and is replaced by new bone. The new bone formation is remodeled within six to twelve months.

Malunion of a fracture indicates that the fragments of bone have healed in an abnormal (poor) position. Fibrous union means that the fractured bone has been united only with fibrous tissue. If the fractured ends of a bone fail to unite, generally due to poor blood supply and nutrition, it is called a nonunion. When nonunion occurs, the fragment of the fractured bone may undergo resorption.

Nerve injuries may result from physical forces. Physical injuries to the extremities may cause cuts, tears, or contusions to peripheral nerves. Such injury may occur directly from the physical force or secondarily because of pressure exerted from scar tissue or a hematoma. Physical injury to a peripheral nerve may cause the nerve to be severed. The distal end of the severed nerve undergoes degeneration, i.e. the myelin and axis cylinders are destroyed; however, the sheath of Schwann remains intact. The degeneration of peripheral nerves is called Wallerian degeneration. Physical forces may produce complete interruption of peripheral nerves accompanied by paralysis of the muscles, and regional anesthesia occurs in the area supplied by the sensory fibers. The affected muscle soon appears flaccid, and atrophy is prominent. If severe compression occurs in a peripheral nerve, the symptoms are identical to those of complete severance. Mild compression of a peripheral nerve resulting from a contracting scar located around the nerve produces symptoms of irritation, partial paralysis, and sensory disturbances.

Rupture of the internal visceral organs may be due to physical injuries (automobile accidents). For instance, rupture of the liver may follow physical injuries, producing tears of the liver, subdiaphragmatic hematoma, or intraperitoneal hemorrhage. The lacerated liver heals with scar formation. The kidney may be rarely ruptured by physical forces with extravasation of urine into the retroperitoneal spaces after laceration of the pelvis. Rupture of the spleen may occur following splenomegaly. Enlargement of the spleen predisposes it to rupture. Fracture of a lower left rib is a predisposing factor to rupture of the spleen. When the spleen is ruptured, acute abdominal pain develops, radiating to the back. The fragments of splenic tissue separated by the physical injury may grow as autotransplants, which mature and develop into accessory spleens. The pancreas may be lacerated by blunt injuries to the abdomen associated with intersititial hemorrhage, hematoma, and cystic structures following resorption of the hemorrhage.

Rupture of an internal viscus containing air may occur during underwater blasts. The gas is compressed in the viscus, then expands and causes a rupture of the lungs, stomach, or colon. The ruptured viscera are associated with shock of a severe character, with a high mortality. Frequently, rupture of internal viscera is multiple following a severe traumatic accident.

Altitude sickness or injury occurs in pilots and mountain climbers because the individual has been subjected to increased atmospheric pressure or is suddenly released from normal atmospheric pressure. Caisson disease occurs in deep sea divers who are suddenly released from deep water with the formation of air emboli.

CHEMICAL POISONS

Poisons are defined as chemical substances capable of blocking physiologic cell functions plus producing devitalization of living tissues by reacting with protoplasm. Some types of poisons are generally harmful to all tissues in the human body. However, other poisons demonstrate high selectivity and thus alter only certain organs. Universal poisons that injure all tissues are called protoplasmic poisons. Some examples of universal poisons are corrosives, i.e. sulfuric acid, caustic potash, phenol, and formaldehyde. The heavy metals also affect a very wide range of different tissues and organs. The heavy metals include arsenic, phosphorus, zinc, antimony, nickel, silver, gold, lead, and radioactive metals (uranium, thorium and radium).

Protoplasmic Poisons

The protoplasmic poisons, i.e. the corrosives and heavy metals, are generally inorganic chemical compounds. Another group of protoplasmic poisons is the poisonous or irritant gases, which encompasses the halogens, hydrogen sulfide, nitric oxide plus the war gases (mustard gas, phosgene, lewisite, and hydrocyanic acid).

All protoplasmic poisons (corrosives, heavy metals, and irritant gases) have the following characteristics:

1. They destroy tissues or organs upon contact;

2. The primary damage produced is parenchymatous necrosis;

3. They are nonselective, thus producing death of tissues at the portal of entry (ingested or inhaled) and also in the organs of excretion (bowel, kidney, and bladder);

4. They produce painful irritations of the tissue and are not ingested for therapeutic results but are ingested in large doses by accident or for suicidal or homicidal reasons (acute poisoning); and

5. The chemical must be artificially manufactured and is not present in nature.

Protoplasmic chemical poisons produce coagulation necrosis of the epithelium of the mucous membranes and skin. Within twenty-four hours an inflammatory defensive reaction occurs to the destroyed epithelium. The disintegrated epithelium is sloughed off and ulceration results, accompanied by secondary infection. If the individual recovers, scarring occurs in direct proportion to the quantity of tissue injured by the poison. In the visceral organs, i.e. liver, brain, and kidneys, the degenerated and necrotic cells are dissolved and hemorrhage occurs, followed by postnecrotic scarring in the liver. Atypical bile ducts and lobular regeneration also occur in the postnecrotic liver. Gliosis takes place in the brain, and tubular cells regenerate in the kidney of the living patient.

Naturally occurring poisons are derived from animals and vegetables and include the following: bacterial and zootic toxins (tetanus, diptheria, botulinus toxin, snake and spider venoms); and poisonous mushrooms and alkaloids (drug substances obtained from vegetables). Examples of alkaloids are morphine, quinine, physostigmine, pilocarpine, cocaine, digitalis, strychnine, ipecac, and atropine. The alkaloids primarily affect the nervous and circulatory systems.

Organic solvents represent another major class of poisons. Examples of this group include the following: carbon tetrachloride, methyl alcohol, chloroform, acetone, phenol derivatives (toluene and benzol). The latter solvents are either prepared synthetically or are made by distillation from either wood or coal. Organic solvents primarily cause poisoning of the kidney, liver, bone marrow, and central nervous system.

Corrosive Poisons

Corrosive acid and alkali may produce damage to the mucous membranes of the eye, oral cavity, throat, gastrointestinal tract, and skin. Excretion of corrosives produces damage to the kidneys. Corrosives produce anemia in the living patient. Corrosive acids or alkalis may be inhaled (fumes from nitric acid or ammonia) and cause damage to the pulmonary alveoli, including injury to the capillary bed. Acute pulmonary edema and severe pulmonary congestion or pneumonia may develop, leading to death. When an acute massive quantity of a corrosive is ingested, it acts upon the tissues similarly to a very severe burn, and death may ensue following shock.

Ingestion of sulfuric, nitric, and hydrochloric acids causes rapid necrosis of the mucous membranes of the body. Sulfuric acid ingestion produces red brown to black lesions on the mucous membranes of the lip, oral cavity, pharynx, esophagus, and stomach. Nitric acid ingestion produces yellow brown lesions of the mucous membranes. Hydrochloric acid ingestion causes gray white lesions of the mucous membranes. Corrosives produce extensive damage to the stomach and intestines. Sulfuric acid ingestion causes a hard, rough, or dry gastric mucosa. Nitric acid ingestion produces severe ulcerations and sloughing of gastric mucosa. Hydrochloric acid causes a shrivelled gastric mucosa. The corrosives cause the blood to produce hematin, which in turn is responsible for a brown black pigmentation of the visceral organs. Ingested alkali, e.g. lye, causes a soapy gastric mucosa accompanied by softening and necrosis with ulceration. Healing results in severe fibrosis with strictures of the upper one-third of the esophagus in the living patient. Solutions of lye that are splashed into the eye produce a severe conjunctivitis, ulceration, and necrosis of the conjunctiva and cornea. Corrosive alkali (lye) produce lesions in the eye much more severe than the lesions produced by corrosive acids.

Ingested phenol (carbolic acid) causes fixation with partial detachment of the mucous membranes. Phenol causes a brown, parched mucosa. Systemic absorption of phenol produces cerebral edema, cardiac dilatation, glomerular and tubular degeneration of the kdineys, and central necrosis of the liver. Secondary infection is common.

Heavy Metal Poisons

Heavy metals are capable of producing systemic effects following ingestion and poisoning. Heavy metals produce damage to the gastrointestinal tract at their site of entry and at their site of excretion (kidneys).

If arsenic is placed upon the skin in a high concentration, ulceration develops locally, and systemic effects result from absorption. Arsenic produces conjunctivitis, palpebral edema, keratitis, and ulceration of the cornea. Ingestion of arsenic produces acute arsenical poisoning. Inhalation of arsenic dust or fumes in industry causes an acute pharyngitis, pulmonary hemorrhages, and pulmonary gangrene. Arsenic poisoning may involve the central nervous system with paralysis of the peripheral motor nerves, muscular atrophy, muscular contractions, and an abnormal position of the limbs.

The effects of ingested bichloride of mercury are directly proportional to the dosage and length of survival time. Acute mercury poisoning corrodes the mucosa of the stomach and duodenum. The mucosa turns white and opaque. Mercury in a metallic form (broken thermometer) may be absorbed through the lungs, skin, and gastrointestinal tract. Metallic mercury toxicity is caused from chronic industrial exposure. Granulomas form and are composed of a mobilization of macrophages around small globules of mercury present in the tissues. Teeth become black, fragile, and loose in their alveolar sockets. Metallic mercury is highly volatile and readily absorbed in the form of fumes. Endarteritis of small blood vessels, nephritis, and death may be observed. Mercuric chloride, i.e. calomel, may cause dermatitis if repeated topically very often. Systemic poisoning with mercuric chloride causes purpura and petechial hemorrhage and discoloration of fingernails.

Lead salts cause poisoning when ingested or inhaled (dust or fumes) or absorbed through the skin. Chronic lead poisoning is characterized by the following: intestinal colic; impaired renal and hepatic function; weakness of extensor musculature; blue line in the gingiva; and anemia with stippling of the red blood cells. Chronic lead poisoning (plumbism) is common as an industrial disease. Acute lead poisoning develops in children who chew lead paint.

Antimony poisoning produces skin eruptions, which initially appear as small vesicles but later form pustules. Acute poisoning produces pustular stomatitis, severe gastric lesions, and toxic hepatitis. Death may result from respiratory and circulatory failure.

Nickel salts produce skin irritations with dermatitis or necrosis. Permanent kidney damage results from nickel poisoning.

Gold salts are used as therapeutic agents in the treatment of arthritis and lupus erythematosus. Large doses of gold salts cause toxic reactions as follows: urticaria, stomatitis, purpura, maculopapular rashes and pruritis, lymphadenopathy, gastrointestinal disturbances (ulcerative enteritis and diarrhea), renal injury, and massive toxic necrosis of the liver.

Thalium poisonings are rare industrial poisonings. Acute

thalium poisoning causes severe gastroenteritis, tachycardia, increased blood pressure, and myocardial damage. Chronic rare poisoning with thalium or suicidal ingestions causes impaired endocrine glands.

Zinc toxicity causes skin eruptions and inflammation of hair follicles due to repeated topical applications to the skin. Inhalation of zinc chloride fumes causes a severe respiratory tract irritation and inflammation. Acute zinc poisoning produces tracheitis, bronchitis, and rarely, penumonia. Suicidal zinc chloride ingestion is fatal in 50 percent of instances. It is accompanied by severe gastritis, nephritis and albuminuria, hemoglobinuria, and casts. Death follows shock or a perforated gastrointestinal tract ulcer with peritonitis.

Phosphorus (yellow) is a protoplasmic poison, which burns the skin upon contact. Acute phosphorus poisoning damages the myocardium, liver, and kidneys with shock and death. If the patient survives, juandice is present due to the presence of hepatic necrosis. Chronic phosphorus poisoning produces ulcerative stomatitis, severe osteitis, leukopenia, and anemia. If the patient survives the chronic poisoning hepatic cirrhosis develops.

Halogens and Gaseous Poisons

Halogens, i.e. chlorine, bromine, fluorine, and iodine, are poisons that cause an irritation and inflammation in the gastrointestinal tract, skin, and lungs. High dosages or prolonged ingestion or inhalation of the halogens affect the bone marrow and central nervous system. Fluorine is a highly irritating element, which causes damage to all vital organs when present in high concentrations. Fluorine is stored in the bones and teeth. Large dosages of fluoride are capable of producing osteosclerosis of the skeleton. Fluoride ingestion may produce nephritis and hepatic injuries. Ingestion of iodine is accompanied by severe abdominal pain, diarrhea, collapse, and hemorrhagic nephritis if it is a severe poisoning. Chronic iodine overdosage causes irritation to the ocular, nasal, and oral mucous membranes plus anemia. Chlorine in contact with the eyes cause irritation and inflammation of the ocular mucous membrane of the eye, with ulceration of the eyelids and the cornea. Inhalation of chlorine results in a spasmodic cough, and it may be accompanied by blood in the sputum.

Gaseous poisons are synthetic gases used in industry. They are all volatile and irritating substances primarily to the lungs and central nervous system. Carbon monoxide is a respiratory gaseous poison, which produces asphyxia because of its strong affinity for hemoglobin. Carbon monoxide also causes areas of softening or hemorrhages in the brain in those cases that become fatal. Other volatile gaseous poisons are phosgene, mustard, lewisite, and hydrocyanic acid gases, again producing their irritant effects to the lungs and central nervous system.

All protoplasmic poisons (corrosives, heavy metals, halogen gases) produce tissue necrosis and local tissue destruction within thirty minutes to several hours following exposure. An inflammatory defensive reaction occurs in twelve to twenty-four hours. Resolution takes place in three to four days, followed by regeneration and repair by fibrosis.

Alkaloids and Poisonous Mushrooms

Alkaloids are useful in medical therapeutics. All of the latter are central nervous system poisons in high dosages, which produce coma, convulsions, and death. Alkaloids, as poisons, have a tendency to cause paralysis of the cardiac and respiratory medullary centers. Death results from terminal pneumonia when respiratory depression is severe. Aconite, strychnine, ergot, and quinine in high dosages have an effect upon the heart, kidneys, and gastrointestinal tract. Atropine poisoning may injure the fetus in the pregnant female. Atropine produces a rapid pulse and respirations followed by coma and death.

Mushroom poisoning *(Amanita phalloides)* causes acute symptoms of gastrointestinal disorders. Fatty degeneration occurs in the liver, which is followed in time by massive hepatic necrosis. Fatty degeneration also occurs in the heart, kidneys, and voluntary muscles, with necrosis of ganglion cells in the brain.

Bacterial and Zootic Toxins

Bacterial and zootic toxins include the following: tetanus, diphtheria, botulinus toxins, and venoms. Botulinism is caused by the ingestion of foods contaminated by *Clostridium botulinus*, which produce a poisonous exotoxin. The principal effect of the exotoxin is on the central nervous system. Cranial nerve palsies and death are due to asphyxia. Scattered hemorrhages are present in the brain and spinal cord along with general vasodilatation of blood vessels.

Animal venoms are poisons produced by snakes, jellyfish, scorpions, spiders, and lizards. The common poisonous snakes are the coral, cobra, copperhead, water moccasin, and rattlesnake. The poisonous snakes produce neurotoxins. Following a bite, the toxin paralyzes the medullary motor centers and act as poisons to the vascular system, causing death of endothelial cells and hemolysis of red blood cells. Rattlesnakes, copperheads, and water moccasins secrete a hemolytic venom by biting an individual. The endothelial cells are damaged or destroyed, and the red blood cells are lyzed. Swelling follows as blood flows into the tissues. Blood passes from the oral cavity, conjunctiva, and stomach, and blood is excreted in the urine. Coma and death may result from the most powerful neurotoxins in animal venoms.

Spiders may also secrete poisons following a bite. The poisonous material causes local edema, hemorrhage in the tissue, and inflammation. If the area of the bite and local adjacent tissue become secondarily infected, death may result. The black widow spider is the most poisonous United States spider. A bite by a black widow spider causes severe and dangerous signs and symptoms, i.e. dilated pupils, depression of respiration, cyanosis, skin eruption, edema of the face and extremities, lymphangitis and lymphadenitis, and vascular lesions of the visceral organs.

Insects, i.e. wasps, bees, hornets, ants and bedbugs, secrete poisonous substances as they bite or sting an individual. The sting of a bee, wasp, or hornet may be highly dangerous in hypersensitive individuals. Laryngeal edema and death have been reported in allergic subjects.

Alcohols and Barbiturates

Alcohol is a variety of poisoning in modern civilized man. Alcohol intoxication is defined as affecting temporarily the individual's ability to control his or her physical and mental powers. Alcohol is a habit-forming poison, which may lead to addiction. Alcohol acts by depressing the central nervous system.

Acute alcohol poisoning due to an overdose results in respiratory failure and death. A blood level of alcohol greater than 0.5 percent generally causes death. The brain becomes congested, the medullary centers are suppressed, and ganglion cells are destroyed by macrophages. Chronic alcohol intoxication produces atrophic gastritis, fatty liver, and hepatic cirrhosis. The liver is enlarged with varying degrees of fibrosis. The brain is decreased in size, ventricles dilated, edema is present in the pia mater, and there is thickening of the meninges.

Chronic barbiturate poisoning causes degeneration of thousands of neurons in the forebrain and perivascular edema of the central nervous system. No liver damage is present. Skin eruptions with urticarial or maculopapular lesions develop on a hypersensitivity basis.

Solvents As Poisons

The most important solvents that act as poisons are carbon tetrachloride, benzol, methyl alcohol, methyl chloride and carbon disulfide. The latter solvents are irritating substances to the lungs, but poisonous chemicals to the central nervous system. They are also poisonous to the liver, kidneys, and bone marrow.

Carbon tetrachloride produces hemorrhagic centrilobular necrosis of the liver plus severe tubular necrosis of the kidneys, causing death from hepatic or renal failure. Kerosene, gasoline, and petroleum products injure the central nervous system and cause bronchopneumonia with a hyaline membrane in the lungs. Chronic benzene poisoning by ingestion produces hemorrhages in the skin and mucous membrane of nose, gingiva, and gastrointestinal tract, and irregular menstruation.

THERMAL AND IRRADIATION INJURIES
Thermal Injuries

Damage occurs to the human body from the following: electric currents of high voltage, temperature extremes or intense forms of radiant energy. The primary lesion is a burn on the exposed surface of the body.

A burn results if intense heat (dry heat, hot water, fire, steam) is applied to the body. A first degree burn is referred to as hyperemia. A second degree burn produces vesication. A third degree burn causes deep dermal necrosis with eschar formation. A fourth degree burn means that the tissue is charred for a considerable depth.

The systemic effects of severe burns include the following:

1. Loss of fluid, hemoconcentration, shock, and renal ischemia;

2. Renal damage produced by ischemia and excretion of the decomposition products of hemoglobin and myoglobin that forms within the renal tubules;

3. Necrosis of germinal centers of lymph nodes and spleen;

4. Elevation of the blood sugar due to release of adrenalin and increase of serum potassium; and

5. Ulcerations of the duodenum caused by histamine release, which in turn stimulates increased secretion of gastric hydrochloric acid.

Frostbite represents a form of necrosis of tissue in peripheral organs (fingers, toes, ears, tip of nose) following exposure to cold. The latter sites become anoxic due to spasm of arterioles that result in dilatation of capillaries and slowing of the blood flow. If exposure to extreme cold is prolonged, toxic products develop, and the absence of oxygen leads to cell death. Freezing of tissue causes death when the body temperature is below 20°C. The blood vessels show stasis, damage endothelium, and thrombosis. High temperatures kill tissues when the body temperature is above 50°C (112°F). The tissues show liquefaction and coagulation necrosis. Inflammatory response occurs to the damaged tissue and secondary infection is common. Hemoconcentration, shock, renal ischemia, duodenal ulcers, coma, and death are the sequence of events in high temperature burns.

Radiation Injuries

The forms of radiation injury may be classified in the following ways: heat waves (infrared rays), electrical waves, radio waves, ultraviolet radiation, and ionizing radiations of very short wave lengths (roentgen rays, gamma rays, and cosmic rays). Radioactive particles may be classified as electrons, alpha particles (the helium nuclei), protons, and neutrons.

Serious injuries to the body may result from electric currents. Electrical shock produces serious injuries if the body is grounded for the transmission of the electric current. Wet skin aids in the passage of an electric current through the body. The injuries produced by the electric shock are determined by the path that the current takes once it enters the body, by the duration of time that the current passes through the body, and by the kind and intensity of the current. For instance, brief electrical shocks are withstood, whereas longer duration shocks are not. If the electric current should penetrate the heart or brain or vital organs, death is more likely to occur due to fibrillation or myocardial arrest or by damage to the nerve cells of the medulla. Fifty volts of electricity could prove fatal if it passed through the heart or brain. Also, passage of alternating current rather than direct current is more dangerous, and high frequency currents have a high capacity for causing tissue destruction. Alternating currents generate heat, and it is the heat that produces the injury to tissue. Direct current also produces heat; however, they produce destructive electrolytic pathologic process with gases within the tissues.

Electric currents may burn the skin at the sites of entry and exit. The dermal structures are coagulated by heat. After the tissue is injured, it dies and undergoes autolysis followed by sloughing of the necrotic tissue. Deep necrotic lesions may develop in the skin and subcutaneous tissues if the electrical contact has been with a large body surface. Electrical injury and necrosis may result without the production of inflammation since the blood vessels are thrombosed and damaged.

Ultraviolet Irradiation

Exposure of the body to ultraviolet light from the sun or ultraviolet light lamps may produce injurious effects to the skin and conjunctiva and also may cause sunstroke. Ultraviolet light rays do not penerate the skin or conjunctiva to any depth; therefore, they produce injury to the more superficial tissues. Sunburn is due to exposure to ultraviolet light rays and heat from infrared rays. The ultraviolet light has a latent period of two to twelve hours prior to producing adverse effects so that clinical symptoms occur sometimes after sunset has taken place. Infrared rays cause redness of the skin that is of a transient nature. Sunburn is associated with erythemia of the skin, blisters that remain for a few days, and finally, the presence of melanin in the epidermis and clinical suntan. The most superficial layer of the epidermis is destroyed and is desquamated. Systemic effects accompany the sunburn and include the following: headache, fever, nausea, prostration. Excessive exposure of the eyes to ultraviolet light rays may result in cataracts and ulcers of the cornea. In normal individuals (farmers, sailors, fishermen), prolonged exposure to ultraviolet light rays for years will result in hyperpigmentation, keratoses or benign and malignant tumors of the epidermis of the skin.

Ionizing Radiation

Ionizing radiations effect human tissues by producing ionization in the tissues. Ionizing radiations include beta, gamma, and roentgen radiations, alpha particles, neutrons, deutrons, and protons. The unit of measurement for the ionizing radiations is the roentgen. The roentgen is defined as the amount of radiation that is capable of ionizing a cubic centimeter of air. The roentgen carries one electrostatic unit of charge. Ionizing radiation is customarily measured in roentgens per minute.

The effects of ionizing radiation are the same for all forms described above and are directly proportional to the quantity of radiation absorbed by the specific living tissues. Ionizing radiation produces penetrating rays, which strike molecules of individual cells and molecules of extracellular fluid. Some ionizing radiations may pass through tissues without any absorption. Absorbed ionizing radiations either jolt electrons from their orbits or collide with some electrons and drive the electrons out of their orbit. One roentgen of radiation is sufficient to denature protein molecules, form peroxides in the tissue fluid, and inactivate enzymes. Mitosis (cell division) is blocked in cells, and numerous disturbances are manifested in affected cells. The result is premature death of cells, a decrease in the blood count, increased permeability of the tissue membranes, and systemic effects (radiation sickness). Radiation sickness includes gastrointestinal disturbances. Eight hundred roentgens administered as a single exposure of ionizing radiation in less than one day will prove to be fatal.

The effect of the ionizing radiation is directly proportional to the quantity of roentgens divided by the time of absorption by the tissues. The safe allowable dosage for radiation technologists and x-ray workers is 0.1 roentgen per day. Therapeutic ionizing radiation for cancer is generally 250 roentgen daily, through alternate areas of the skin, for up to a total of 5,000 to 10,000 roentgen. The greater the field exposed to ionizing radiation, the greater will be the effect. An increase in the mass of the tissue irradiated increases the backscatter or effects from secondary irradiation. The shorter the wave length of the ionizing radiation, the greater the tissue penetration, and in turn the less damage to the skin. X-rays and gamma rays have short wave lengths and, therefore, high penetrating ability. Alpha particles, i.e. helium nuclei, are approximately 100 times more damaging than beta rays, i.e. electrons. Alpha particles and beta rays are both screened out by means of filters. Protons, i.e. hydrogen nuclei, are similar irradiations to alpha particles.

Ionizing radiations produce biologic effects in the human body. They cause denaturing of proteins, formation of peroxides, and blocking of enzymes systems in body fluids. They cause arrest of mitosis, delayed mutations, and pyknosis or karyorrhexis of nuclei of cells. They cause inhibition of phagocytosis, increased membrane permeability, vacuolization of cytoplasm, and inhibition of secretion on the cytoplasm of cells.

Tissue reaction to ionizing radiation is related to the modification of cell function and structure. For instance, reproduction (mitosis) of cells may be stopped. Motility of normal leukocytes and sperm cells is suppressed, and growth of immature cells is restricted. The nucleus is destroyed, and the permeability of cell membranes is increased. Glandular secretion may be suppressed. Toxic products are liberated in the tissues due to cellular decomposition. Recovery of irradiated tissues is partially the result of tissue regeneration replacing the destroyed cells.

Radiosensitivity of Cells

Immature cells are more radiosensitive than mature (adult) cells. Tissues have been classified (Warren) into three major groups based on relative radiosensitivity. Group I consists of radiosensitive tissue; 2,500 roentgens or less will kill or injure the following cells: lymphocytes and lymphoblasts; myeloblastic and erythroblastic cells of the bone marrow; epithelium of the stomach and intestines; and germ cells of the ovary and testes.

Group II consists of radioresponsive tissues; from 2,500 roentgens but less than 5,000 roentgens will kill or injure the following cells: epithelium of the skin plus skin appendages; endothelium of the blood vessels and cells of the lung, salivary glands; cells of growing bone and cartilage; cells of the conjunctiva, cornea, and lens of the eye; and collagen and elastic tissue (fibroblasts are highly resistant).

Group III consists of radioresistant tissues; over 5,000 roentgens will kill or injure the following cells: cells of the kidney; cells of the liver; cells of the thyroid, pancreas, pituitary, adrenal, and parathyroid glands; mature cells of cartilage and bone tissue; cells of all types of muscles; and brain cells and cells of other nervous tissue.

References

Adelman, L.S. and Aronson, S.M.: *Bull NY Acad Med, 45*:225, 1969.
Anderson, R.E.: *Hum Pathol, 2*:515, 1971.
Baden, M.M.: In Wecht, C.H. (Ed.): *Legal Medicine Annual.* New York, Appleton-Century-Crofts, 1971.
Bainborough, A.R. and Jericho, K.W.F.: *Can Med Assoc J, 103*:1297, 1970.
Citron, B.P., et al.: *N Engl J Med, 283*:1003, 1970.

Dublin, W.B.: *Fundamentals of Neuropathology.* Springfield, Thomas, 1954, p. 331.
Edholm, O.H.: The effects of hemorrhage on the cardiovascular system in man. In *Lectures on the Scientific Basis of Medicine.* London, The Athlone Press, 1953, vol. I, 1951-52.
Edland, J.F.: *Hum Pathol, 2*:75, 1972.
Epstein, S.S.: *Am J Pathol, 66*:352, 1972.
Fairhall, L.T.: *Industrial Toxicology.* Baltimore, Williams and Wilkins, 1949.
Froede, R.: *Hum Pathol, 3*:23, 1972.
Gill, W.G. and Hay, C.P.: *Br J Surg, 31*:67, 1943.
Gleason, M.N., et al.: *Clinical Toxicology of Commercial Products, Acute Poisoning (Home and Farm).* Baltimore, Williams and Wilkins, 1957, p. 152.
Gonzales, T.A., et al.: *Legal Medicine—Pathology and Toxicology,* 2nd ed. New York, Appleton-Century-Crofts, 1954, p. 785.
Goyer, R.A.: *Am J Pathol, 64*:167, 1971.
Grace, W.H., et al.: *Lancet, 2*:102, 1940.
Helpern, M.: *N Engl J Med, 284*:113, 1971.
Hicks, S. and Warren, S.: *Introduction to Neuropathology.* New York, McGraw, 1950, p. 240.
Kark, R.A.P., et al.: *N Engl J Med, 285*:10, 1971.
Key, C.R.: *Hum Pathol, 2*:475, 1971.
Kotin, P.: *Am J Pathol, 64*:165, 1971.
Moritz, A.R.: *The Pathology of Trauma,* 2nd ed. Philadelphia, Lea & Febiger, 1954.
Murphy, R.L.H., et al.: *N Engl J Med, 285*:1271, 1971.
Murray, R.M., et al.: *Br Med J, 2*:479, 1971.
Naffziger, H.C. and McCorkle, H.J.: *Ann Surg, 118*:594, 1943.
Nielsen, J.M.: *A Textbook of Clinical Neurology,* New York, Hoeber, 1943.
Sargent, J.C.: *J Urol, 53*:381, 1945.
Schaller, W.F.: *Arch Neurol, 37*:1048, 1937.
Selye, H.: *Stress,* 1st ed. Monteral, Acta, 1950, p. 773.
Siegal, H.: *Hum Pathol, 2*:55, 1972.
Solitare, G.B.: *Hum Pathol, 2*:85, 1972.
Steenrod, E.J.: *Am J Surg, 49*:129, 1940.
Thienes, C.H. and Haley, T.J.: *Clinical Toxocology,* 3rd ed. Philadelphia, Lea & Febiger, 1955, p. 170.
Von Oettingen, W.F.: *Poisoning.* New York, Hoeber, 1952.
Wallace, J. and Sharpey-Schafer, P.: *Lancet, 2*:393, 1941.
Weinmann, J.P. and Sicher, H.: *Bone and Bones.* St. Louis, Mosby, 1947, p. 290.
Windle, W.F., et al.: *J Neurosurg, 3*:175, 1946.

Wright, L.T., et al.:   *Arch Surg, 54*:613, 1947.
Wunternitz, M.C.:   *Pathology of War Gas Poisoning.*   New Haven, Yale U Pr, 1920.
Wyatt, J.P.:   *Am J Pathol, 64*:197, 1971.
Young, F.G.:   Adrenal hormones and ACTH.   In *Lectures on the Scientific Basis of Medicine.*   London, The Athlone Press, 1953, vol.I, 1951-52.

CHAPTER 14

NUTRITIONAL DEFICIENCY

INTRODUCTION

NUTRITIONAL DEFICIENCIES REPRESENT negative agents of injury compared to the positive agents of injury described under poisons or microorganisms, which persist in the tissues and are identified as the cause of a disease. Seventeen or eighteen out of ninety-odd elements, fifteen vitamins, ten out of twenty-odd amino acids, and three unsaturated fatty acids are essentials to normal growth (Follis, 1948). The absence of one or more of these latter substances is capable of producing disease as a negative agent of injury.

Essential nutrients may be classified as mineral and organic substances. The minerals of the body essential for normal growth and well being are calcium, magnesium, iron, iodine, and the trace elements (copper, cobalt, zinc, and manganese. The essential organic substances are vitamins, several amino acids, and fatty acids.

When an essential organic or mineral substance is absent (negative agent of injury), it produces a selective alteration or impairment in tissues that must utilize the essential metabolic substance. Functional alteration of the tissue may occur as a relatively late finding; an example is hyperirritability of the musculature in deficiency of calcium or paralysis of nerves caused by deficiency of vitamin B_1. Morphologic impairment, however, may be present early and stimulate a compensatory proliferation of new cells. For example, in calcium deficiency, demineralization of bone takes place with a compensatory proliferation of osteoblasts. In iron deficiency, the number of red blood cells are diminished; however, there is a compensatory hyperplasia of bone marrow. In iodine deficiency there is a compensatory hyperplasia of the thyroid gland.

Nutritional deficiencies may occur by deprivation (inadequate intake in the diet; defective absorption or metabolism), and increased loss or use (loss through hemorrhage, vomiting, or excessive excretion; increased utilization during growth and pregnancy).

MINERAL DEFICIENCIES

Iron is present in the blood in between 45 and 50 mg percent; 98 percent is present in the hemoglobin, which has 75 percent of the iron in the body. If the storage of iron in the body is low, it is rapidly absorbed from ingested foods. The acidity of the gastric juices aids the absorption of iron; however, if achlorhydria exists, hypochromic anemia may develop because iron is only poorly absorbed from alkaline gastric juices. Iron is not excreted or is excreted in very minimal amounts. Iron is, therefore, a one-way mineral.

Ferric iron is converted to ferrous iron by reducing substances present in the diet. The ferrous iron is absorbed through the mucosal cells of the duodenum and jejunum. Apoferritin (protein compound) is located in the mucosa of the intestines and unites with ferrous iron, forming ferritin. Ferritin releases iron to the plasma, reverting to apoferritin in the process so that apoferritin can be reutilized in the body to combine with more ferrous iron. Iron is transported in the blood and stored in the liver as ferritin only in physiologic quantities. Excess amounts of ferritin are phagocytized as hemosiderin.

Iron is present in hemoglobin, and when the red blood cell disintegrates, the iron is reabsorbed from the bile in the alimentary tract. Very insignificant quantities of iron may be lost in the urine, bile, and from the intestinal tract. Iron deficiency produces a microcytic, hypochromic anemia. The red blood cells are small and reduced in number, containing decreased quantities of hemoglobin. Iron deficiency is caused by chronic hemorrhage or the defective absorption of iron due to low gastric acidity. There are greater demands for iron during pregnancy and adolescence,

Nutritional Deficiency

thus deficiencies may occur. Patients with iron deficiency have a sore tongue, dysphagia, sore mouth, and predisposition to carcinoma of the esophagus in females and the Plummer-Vinson syndrome. Iron deficiency produces spoon nails, i.e. ridges and flattened finger nails, anemia, and hyperplasia of the bone marrow. Iron therapy reverses the alterations and restores a normal red blood cell count.

Hemochromatosis is an inherent defect in iron metabolism, whereby the total body iron is greater than 50 gm compared to 4.5 gm for the normal total body iron. The iron may occur as hemosiderin and is phagocytized by macrophages. This disease produces degeneration of hepatic and pancreatic tissues, resulting in cirrhosis of the liver and diabetes mellitus. Excessive iron may be stored in the skin and endocrine glands.

Hemosiderosis is an exogenous defect in iron metabolism or exogenous hemochromatosis. It is caused by administration of large quantities of iron either orally or by transfusions, resulting in excess deposition of iron as hemosiderin.

Calcium (98%) is present in the skeletal system where it represents a reserve from which to supply the serum calcium, necessary for the blood clotting mechanism. Calcium is present in the muscles and is necessary for contraction and control of membrane permeability. The calcium present in the body is maintained at a physiologic level by intake of food and drink and by the presence of optimal vitamin D in the diet. Vitamin D aids in the absorption of calcium in addition to the effect of digestive juices and of the parathyroid glands.

Calcium is absorbed through the intestinal tract in the presence of vitamin D and passes into the circulation. Calcium (85%) is transported to the tissues in one hour; 75 percent is transported to the matrix of bones in two hours. Calcium (20%) is lost by excretion by the urinary tract and bowel in twenty-four hours. The quantity of calcium retained by the bones of the body is directly related to the amount of protein matrix. The protein matrix is increased by administering steroid sex hormones (estrogen, testosterone) and decreased by administering cortisone, since it converts the protein matrix into sugar.

When there is an increase in the amount of parathyroid hormone in the serum, the urinary excretion of phosphate is increased and calcium ions are removed from the bones. Hyperfunction or hyperplasia of the parathyroid glands is a mechanism to maintain serum calcium in the face of decreased absorption due to pancreatic steatorrhea or biliary disease. The parathyroid glands undergo secondary hyperplasia during renal disease, whereby the kidney cannot excrete phosphate. The phosphate passes through the bowel with the calcium.

Bones may lose calcium but retain their normal matrix of protein. The latter disorder is termed *rickets* or *malacia*. When the bones lose their calcium due to a prior loss of protein matrix, the condition is described as bone atrophy.

Abnormal calcium metabolism is the result of deficient absorption of calcium. Improper calcium absorption is due to the following: (1) deficient dietary calcium; (2) absence of vitamin D; and (3) trapping calcium in the bowel by undigested fat. Calcium is lost excessively in the following situations. (1) in renal diseases whereby phosphate is excreted by the bowel rather than by kidneys; and (2) in primary and secondary hyperparathyroidism where there is increased urinary excretion of calcium and phosphorus. Calcium is lost from the bones in both primary and secondary hyperparathyroidism, with loss of the protein matrix of bones, with senility, and with immobilization of the extremities due to the presence of a cast. Degeneration of the protein matrix of bone occurs in hyperthyroidism, in females at the menopause, and in severe skeletal diseases (multiple myeloma, metastatic carcinoma to bone).

When the serum calcium is reduced from 10 mg percent to 5 mg percent, the muscles are affected by tetany. Tetany is the presence of cramps and spasms in the muscle. During very low serum calcium, the heart will pass into systolic arrest. Increased serum calcium initially stimulates but later depresses the heart.

Magnesium is present in the tissues and in very minimal amounts in the plasma. Magnesium has the function of regulating nerve impulses. Excessive concentratons of magnesum result in tissue necrosis, and deficient magnesium results in hyperirritability. Magnesium deficiency in man leads to muscle tremors and tetany.

Iodine deficiency is associated with the production of goiters. Goiters develop in land-locked regions where iodine is absent in the diet. Iodine deficiency causes hyperplasia of the thyroid gland and involution with increased storage of colloid. If iodine becomes available after the latter changes have taken place, a colloid goiter develops.

Proteins are essential to every tissue of the human body and function as an aid in the body's growth, maintenance, and repair. The proteins ingested in the diet break down into amino acids, which are absorbed through the intestinal wall. If not used by the tissues, proteins are broken up into urea, fatty acids, or converted to glucose. When fats and carbohydrates are deficient in the diet, proteins are used as energy supplies. Two kilograms of protein are stored in protein storage deposits of the body to be used during starvation.

Deficiency of dietary protein is due to starvation or gastrointestinal tract diseases with or without diarrhea. Protein deficiency is characterized by edema, delayed wound healing, anemia, loss of weight and strength, and cirrhosis of liver (severe protein deficiency). Patients who are bedridden lose stored protein; hyperthyroidism also causes a loss of body protein. Low protein leads to vitamin B complex deficiency states (tryptophane deficiency). Severe liver damage results in lower plasma proteins. Protein deficiency lowers the individual's resistance to infection and his immunity.

Fats occur in the human body in the following forms: glycerol esters of fatty acids (neutral fats); steroids or waxes (cholesterol); and phospholipids (lecithins and cephalins). Fat has a high caloric value and is used for energy by the body. Fat is absorbed by the small intestines in the presence of bile acids (emulsification) and lipase (hydrolysis) from the pancreatic juice. Fat droplets are present in the mucosal cells of the intestines and are then transported to the lymphatics.

Absorption of fat (fatty acids and glycerols) may be altered by the following: (1) pancreatic disease; (2) liver and biliary tract diseases; and (3) anomalies of the lymphatics. Disturbances of lipids reduce the absorption of the fat-soluble vitamins, i.e. vitamins A, K, and D, and the absorption of calcium.

The rate of absorption of fats by the mucosal cells of the small intestines depends upon age, i.e. young children and the aged have a lower rate of absorption than adults. The essential unsaturated fatty acids should represent one percent of an individual's daily calories, and the total fat consumed should be 20 percent for adults and 30 percent for growing children.

The essential fatty acids include linoleic acid, linolenic acids, and arachidonic acid. Linoleic acid and linolenic acids are present in vegetable oil. Arachidonic acid is present in animal fat. There is evidence that fatty acids are essential in the diet of adults.

During pancreatic and biliary diseases, fat is lost in the stool in addition to calcium and fat-soluble vitamins A, K, and D. Obstruction of the common bile duct results in a 25 to 75 percent loss of ingested fat. Endocrine disorders (diabetes mellitus and hyperthyroidism) are accompanied by excessive quantities of fat in the blood stream (hypercholesterolemia). Blood cholesterol is increased in von Gierke's disease (glycogen storage disease), where the stored glycogen cannot be transformed into sugar.

The xanthomatoses are a group of disorders caused by disturbances in the metabolism of complex lipids. Niemann-Pick's disease and Gaucher's disease, forms of xanthomatoses, are inherited anomalies of metabolism. Christian's disease, another form of xanthomatoses, is not a metabolic disorder in the metabolism of lipids but a variety of granuloma. In the xanthomatoses, storage of lipid substances occurs in the macrophages present in the bones, liver, and spleen. Thus, bony defects and hepatosplenomegaly are evident.

Carbohydrate is the major fuel for the human body. Carbohydrate is stored in the body as glycogen, but only in small amounts. Therefore, it must be constantly ingested in the diet or it will be converted from the stores of fat and protein into carbohydrate. Carbohydrates are digested along the entire alimentary tract. The majority of carbohydrates are, however, digested in the small intestines and require pancreatic amylase plus intestinal enzyme capable of converting carbohydrate to simple monosaccharides. The sugar is stored in the liver and in muscles in the form of glycogen. When it is required, glycogen is converted to glucose and transported to the tissues from the storage depots of glycogen.

Carbohydrates metabolism is under the control of the following: islet cells of the pancreas; pituitary growth hormone and by both adrenal and thyroid hormones. In von Gierke's disease, glycogen is easily stored but cannot be converted to glucose and utilized by the tissues. Therefore, we find excessive accumulations of glycogen in the liver cells, cardiac cells, kidney cells, voluntary muscle cells, and also in smaller quantities in the spleen and adrenal glands. These individuals have a low blood sugar, which refuses to rise in the presence of epinephrine.

Glycogen and glucose are the primary forms of carbohydrate in the body; however, minor quantities of galactose and pentoses are present.

FAT-SOLUBLE VITAMINS

Vitamin A is a fat-soluble vitamin that occurs in plants (particularly in carrots as carotene) and in the livers of both fish and animals. Provitamin A (carotene) is transformed into vitamin A in the liver. Vitamin A is absorbed in the small intestines when fat and pancreatic juices are present, and it is stored in the liver. Vitamin A is necessary for normal growth in young children and for maintaining the corneal epithelium. Absence of the vitamin causes xerophthalmia. Night blindness may occur in individuals with cirrhosis of the liver, due to inadequate vitamin A.

Vitamin E (tocopherol) shows a relationship with and is similar to vitamin A. Vitamin E functions by protecting and stabilizing vitamin A. Vitamin E occurs in soy beans, wheat germ, cottonseed and corn oil. It is stored in the fatty deposits of the body. No human deficiency states have been observed in man.

Vitamin K is present in leafy vegetables and alfalfa. It is synthesized by the microorganisms in the normal human intestines. Vitamin K is essential for the liver, which synthesizes prothrombin. Deficiency of vitamin K produces a decrease in the normal plasma prothrombin and impairment of blood clotting. A physiologic supply of bile salts is required for the absorption of vitamin K through the small intestines. Vitamin K is apt to be deficient in subjects with biliary diseases. Extended and prolonged antibiotic therapy reduces the number of vitamin K producing microorganisms, producing vitamin K deficiency.

Vitamin D is a fat-soluble vitamin related to cholesterol. Vitamin D is necessary for normal calcium metabolism and adequate mineralization of bones. Vitamin D is present in cod liver oil, egg yolk, butter, and fish oils. Vitamin D deficiency in man is caused by an inadequate intake or lack of sunshine. The calcium and phosphorus levels are under 40 mg percent in rickets compared with 60 mg percent in normal subjects. Rickets develop primarily in infants from four months to two years of age. The failure of deposition of calcium salts in bone tissue results in the following disturbances and deformities: (1) enlarged epiphyseal junctions of ribs (beaded ribs); (2) softening of bones (bending); (3) stunted growth of the skeleton; (4) formation of osteoid, not bone tissue, in the bony metaphysis of long bones; (5) new bone formation is subperiosteal osteoid tissue; (6) delayed ossification of the cranial bones; (1) wide and saucer-shaped epiphyseal lines in long bones; (8) generalized weakness and irritability; and (9) hypotonia of muscles and excessive perspiration.

Physiologic ossification consists of resorption of old bone and apposition of new bone side by side. During rickets there is resorption of old bone, but in place of new bone there is deposition of osteoid tissue, which is uncalcified.

Hypervitaminosis D may occur if large quantities of vitamin D plus alkaline salts are ingested. Renal calcification (metastatic) is related to ingestion of excessive vitamin D.

VITAMIN B DEFICIENCIES

Vitamin B complex includes the following water-soluble vitamins essential to normal health: B_1 (thiamine); B_2 (riboflavin); B_6 (pyridoxine); B_{12} (antianemic factor); folic acid; niacin; and pantothenic acid. Vitamin B complex is present in the liver, brewer's yeast, whole grains, and dairy products. Deficiencies of the major components of the vitamin B complex produce the following nutritional diseases: polyneuritis or beriberi due to thiamine deficiency; pellagra due to niacin deficiency; and pernicious anemia due to vitamin B_{12} deficiency.

Beriberi (thiamine deficiency) is accompanied by the following symptoms: polyneuritis, muscle weakness, dyspnea, edema, anorexia, tachycardia, insomnia, and constipation. Beriberi develops in malnourished patients, alcoholics, and persons with diabetes mellitus. Cardiac muscle is flabby, fibers are shrunken, and edema fluid is present in the interstitial spaces. Peripheral nerves undergo myelin degeneration, and fatty droplets appear. Axons become fragmented. There is degeneration of ganglion cells and swelling of the brain.

Thiamine (vitamin B_1) is important in the oxidation of glucose to carbon dioxide and water since it acts as cocarboxylase. The latter oxidation is important to the metabolism of the peripheral nerves and brain tissue. Individuals with viatmin B_1 deficiency have a blood sugar level similar to that of diabetics. Pellagra, beriberi, and alcoholism are all accompanied by polyneuritis and an inadequate intake of vitamin B_1. Patients with sprue and pernicious anemia have poor absorption of vitamin B_1 accompanied by paresthesia. In patients with hyperthyroidism, pregnancy, and fever there may be a deficiency of vitamin B_1 caused by the enhanced metabolism of carbohydrates.

Niacin deficiency or nicotinic acid deficiency is responsible for production of pellagra in the poor and in alcoholic patients. The neurological symptoms (early) of this syndome are lethargy, insomnia, vertigo, and apprehension. The gastrointestinal early symptoms of this syndrome are anorexia, diarrhea and flatulence. Later symptoms of the pellagra syndrome include the following: dermatitis of hands and feet; glossitis, gastritis, proctitis, diarrhea, and mental symptoms such as mania and hallucinations.

Pathological alterations develop in the skin and gastrointestinal tract during the pellagra syndrome. The epidermis of the skin becomes hyperkeratotic, the dermis becomes edematous, the tongue is red, bald, and ulcerated in its lateral margins, there is atrophic esophagitis and gastritis; and there is degeneration and loss of ganglion cells and edema of the brain.

The pellagra syndrome is due to multiple deficiencies rather than to simply a deficiency of vitamin B_1, which is responsible for neuritis. Vitamin B_6 (pyridoxine) is also deficient during pellagra and is responsible for irritability and pain on walking. Pellagra subjects excrete no nicotinic acid, whereas normal subjects excrete up to 50 mg of nicotinic acid daily.

Folic acid is present in the diet—leafy vegetables, cereals, cauliflower, liver, kidney, and muscle (meat)—as a water-soluble chemical compound. Folic acid is absorbed through the upper and lower portion of the gastrointestinal tract, and may be synthesized by intestinal microorganisms.

Deficiency of folic acid produces impairment in development of the erythrocytic and granulocytic tissues of the bone marrow. Folic acid is necessary for normal metabolism of vitamin B_{12}, ascorbic acid, and some amino acids.

Pernicious anemia is characterized by achlorhydria, atrophic gastritis, and failure to absorb vitamin B_{12}, resulting in macrocytic anemia with pallor, weakness, dyspnea, a sore tongue, and lemon-colored tongue. Gastric secretion is described as the intrinsic factor, and an absorbed dietary factor (extrinsic factor) is vitamin B_{12}. The extrinsic factor (B_{12}) is necessary for the maturation of red blood cells. Pernicious anemia is a hereditary disease common in Scandinavia and Germany. The red blood cells in pernicious anemia are irregular in shape, of extra large size, contain normal or increased hemoglobin, and a leukopenia develops. There is hyperplasia of the bone marrow. Administration of vitamin B_{12} causes a reversal of pernicious anemia with red blood cell regeneration. Patients with pernicious anemia show spinal cord changes, ataxia, hyper-reflexia, and psychoses. Recovery is rapid when the neurological symptoms are treated early in the disease with vitamin B_{12}.

Riboflavin deficiency is termed *ariboflavinosis,* which is accompanied by the following: purple sore tongue and glossitis; conjunctivitis with photophobia; lacrimation and blurred vision; cheilosis with fissures at the corner of the mouth and cracked lips; and scaly dermatitis of skin surfaces, which are normally moist. Riboflavin is present in meat, dairy foods, and yeast.

Pyridoxine deficiency (vitamin B_6 deficiency) alters the metabolism of unsaturated fatty acids. Vitamin B_6 aids in the metabolism of some amino acids and is responsible for macrocytic, hypochromic anemia. Vitamin B_6 relieves abdominal pain, irritability, and weakness when walking in individuals with the pellagra syndrome. Pyridoxine is present in green vegetables, soy beans, and wheat germ.

Choline and methionine prevent the formation of fatty livers and are described as lipotropic substances preventing cirrhosis of the liver. However, in patients with fatty and cirrhotic liver, bed rest and a high protein diet cause recovery similar to the administration of choline and methionine. Large quantities of choline are present in eggs, meat, fish, and cereal. Methionine reverses a choline-deficient diet since it aids the body in synthesizing choline.

Biotin has growth-stimulating properties. It occurs in the soil, microorganisms, and foods. Biotin reverses the injury to the body caused by a diet of egg whites or raw eggs. Symptoms of biotin deficiency are dermatitis, pain in the musculature, anorexia, nausea, and anemia. No therapeutic application has been found for biotin in man.

VITAMIN C

Vitamin C is present in citrus fruits, tomatoes, berries, and green vegetables (peppers, cabbage). Deficiency of vitamin C causes scurvy. The recommended daily requirement for vitamin C from foods is 75 to 100 mg (Food and Nutrition Board, National Research Council). Vitamin C daily requirements should be increased during pregnancy and lactation.

Vitamin C is necessary for normal development and maintenance of the matrix of connective tissue, bone, cartilage, and endothelium of capillaries. Vitamin C is present in a high concentration in the adrenal cortex. Vitamin C, present in the adrenal cortex, falls during stress with a high level of cortical secretion. ACTH, which stimulates secretion of the adrenal cortical hormone, decreases with vitamin C. Vitamin C is essential for repair of wounds.

Vitamin C deficiency of severe degree leads to scurvy, which is associated with anemia, edema, pain in the bones, hemorrhage and swelling of the gingiva, and subcutaneous hemorrhages. During scurvy there is an inability of the mesenchymal tissues of the body for production of the intracellular substance of connective tissue, cartilage, bone, and capillaries. This results in defective capillaries, with capillary fragility and hemorrhages. The formation of collagen and hyalin matrix for fibrous tissue, cartilage and bone is defective and disrupted. There is delayed wound healing and fragmentation of muscle fibers during scurvy.

Vitamin C deficiency (scurvy) is caused by an inadequate intake or increased requirements for vitamin C during pregnancy, lactation, in infectious diseases, in rheumatic fever and rheumatoid arthritis, in patients with peptic ulcers, and in fast-growing children.

Pathologic findings of scurvy are readily found in the growing bones of the body. Cartilage and osteoid tissue fail to produce adequate intracellular substances. Bony trabeculae are small and narrow and are arrested in normal growth. The cortical plate of bone is very thin. Failure of formation of collagen fibrils causes cellular connective tissue (not collagen) to develop about the epiphyseal line of long bones. Bones may be separated at the epiphysis due to absence of tensile strength present in normal collagen fibrils. During scurvy there are atrophic changes of the adrenal cortex and lymphoid tissue. Ascorbic acid administration reverses the pathologic finding in growing bones and in the capillaries.

References

Alfin-Slater, R.B., et al.: *Arch Biochem Biophys, 52*:180, 1954.
Arbeter, A., et al.: *Fed Proc, 30*:1421, 1971.
Balsley, M. and Speckmann, E.W.: *J Okla State Med Assoc, 64*:482, 1971.
Barlow, T.: *Med Chir Trans, 66*:159, 1833.
Baylis, E.M., et al.: *Lancet, 2*:62, 1971.
Beaton, G.H. and Whalen, S.: *Can Med Assoc J, 105*:355, 1971.
Bernstein, L.H., et al.: *Am J Med, 48*:570, 1970.

Berry, L.J., et al.: *J Lab Clin Med, 30*:684, 1945.
Bethell, F.H.: Petroyglutamic acid in man. In Sebrell, W.H. and Harris, Robert S. (Eds.): *The Vitamins.* New York, Acad Pr, 1954, vol.III, pp. 215-216.
Brickman, A.S., et al.: *N Engl J Med, 287*:891, 1972.
Brown, W.R., et al.: *J Nutr, 16*:511, 1938.
Burnell, J.M. and Scribner, B.H.: *JAMA, 164*:959, 1957.
Connor, C.L.: *JAMA, 112*:387, 1939.
Dameshek, W.: *Blood, 4*:168, 1949.
DeLuca, H.F.: *Nutr Rev, 29*:179, 1971.
Deuel, H.J.: In Wohl, Michael G. and Goodhard, Robert S. (Eds.): *Modern Nutrition in Health and Disease.* Philadelphia, Lea & Febiger, 1955, p. 200.
Deuel, H.J.: The lipids. *Biochemistry, Digestion, Absorption, Transport and Storage,* New York, Interscience, 1955, vol.II.
du Vigneaud, V.: *Harvy Lectures 38, 39,* 1942 and 1943.
Enklewitz, M. and Laster, M.: *J Biol Chem, 110*:443, 1935.
Farber, S.: *Blood, 4*:160, 1949.
Follis, R.H.: *The Pathology of Nutritional Disease.* Springfield, Thomas, 1948.
Galante, L., et al.: *Lancet, 2*:985, 1972.
Geschickter, C.F. and Copeland, M.M.: Radiophosphorus and radio-iodine. In Behrens, Charles F. (Ed.): *Atomic Medicine.* Baltimore, Williams and Wilkins, 1953, p. 433.
Ginter, E.: *Lancet, 2*:1198, 1971.
Gitlin, D.: *Bull NY Acad Med, 31*:359, 1955.
Goldsmith, G.A.: *JAMA, 216*:337, 1971.
Granick, S.: *Blood, 4*:401, 1951.
Granick, S.: *Bull NY Acad Med, 30*:81, 1954.
Hahn, T.J., et al.: *N Engl J Med, 287*:900, 1972.
Hallbook, T. and Lanner, E.: *Lancet, 1*:780, 1972.
Hartroft, W.S.: Experimental hepatic injury. In Schiff, Leon (Ed.): *Diseases of the Liver.* Philadelphia, Lippincott, 1956, pp. 92-124.
Heath, C.W.: *JAMA, 120*:366, 1942.
Hellstrom, L.: *Lancet, 1*:59, 1971.
Himsworth, H.P.: *The Liver and Its Diseases,* 2nd ed. Cambridge, Harvard U Pr, 1950.
Hodges, R.E., et al.: *Am J Clin Nutr, 24*:432, 191.
Iseri, O.A., et al.: *Lab Invest, 27*:226, 1972.
Kagan, B.M. and Waller, L.: Vitamin K. In Wohl, Michael G. and Goodhard, Robert S. (Eds.): *Modern Nutrition in Health and Disease.* Philadelphia, Lea & Febiger, 1955, p. 290.
Keenen, W.J., et al.: *Am J Dis Child, 121*:271, 1971.

Klatskin, G.: *Ann NY Acad Sci, 57*:909, 1954.
Landsteiner, K.: *The Specificity of Serological Reactions,* 2nd ed. Cambridge, Harvard U Pr, 1945.
Leonard, P.J. and Losowsky, M.S.: *Am J Clin Nutr, 24*:388, 1971.
Lipschitz, D.A., et al.: *Br J Haematol, 20*:155, 1971.
Machado, E.A., et al.: *Lab Invest, 24*:13, 1971.
Mayer, R.L.: *J Allergy Clin Immunol, 28*:191, 1957.
McCombs, H.L. and Gershoff, S.N.: *Lab Invest, 26*:515, 1972.
Moir, A.T.B., et al.: *Lancet, 2*:798, 1971.
Page, I.H.: *JAMA,* p. 454, Feb. 9, 1957.
Quaife, M.L. and Dju, M.Y.: *J Biol Chem, 180*:263, 1949.
Raisz, L.G.: *N Engl J Med, 287*:926, 1972.
Recommended Dietary Allowances, Food and Nutrition Board, National Research Council Circ. No. 129, 1948, p. 17.
Rhead, W.J. and Schrauzer, G.N.: *Nutr Rev, 29*:262, 1971.
Roe, D.A.: *NY J Med, 1*:270, 1971.
Rotruck, J.T., et al.: *J Nutr, 102*:689, 1972.
Sahud, M.A. and Cohen, R.J.: *Lancet, 2*:937, 1971.
Sealock, R.R., et al.: *J Biol Chem, 196*:761, 1952.
Smith, C.A.: *The Physiology of the Newborn Infant,* 2nd ed. Springfield, Thomas, 1951.
Statland, H.: *Fluid and Electrolytes in Practice,* 2nd ed. Philadelphia, Lippincott, 1957.
Stern, J.J.: In Wohl, Michael G. and Goodhard, Robert S. (Eds.): *Modern Nutrition in Health and Disease.* Philadelphia, Lea & Febiger, 1955, p. 872.
Sullivan, M. and Evans, V.J.: *Arch Dermatol, 49*:33, 1944.
Thomas, R.O., et al.: *Am J Physiol, 169*:568, 1952.
Thomas, R.O., et al.: *Am J Physiol, 176*:381, 1954.
Vilter, R.W.: Symposia on Nutrition, vol.I., *Nutritional Anemia,* published by Robert Gould Research Foundation, 1957.
Vilter, R.W.: Vitamin C. In Wohl, Michael G. and Goodhard, Robert S. (Eds.): *Modern Nutrition in Health and Disease.* Philadelphia, Lea & Febiger, 1955, p. 351.
Wasserman, R.H. and Taylor, A.N.: *Ann Rev Biochem, 41*:179, 1972.
Wohl, M.G., et al.: *Arch Intern Med, 83*:402-415, 1949.
Wolbach, S.B. and Bessey, O.A.: *Physiol Rev, 22*:233, 1942.
Woodhouse, N.J.Y., et al.: *Lancet, 2*:283, 1971.

CHAPTER 15

DISTURBANCES IN GROWTH AND NEOPLASIA

DISTURBANCES IN THE GROWTH OF CELLS

Cell Metamorphosis

ATROPHY IS AN ACQUIRED REDUCTION in the size of the units of a tissue that has attained the adult functioning size. Atrophy of the intercellular tissue indicates that a reduction is present in the amount of tissue forming cartilage, bone, and ligaments. Atrophy results following infection with the poliomyelitis virus. Atrophy of muscles occurs in rheumatoid arthritis. In atrophic parotid glands, fatty ingrowth may produce a normal clinical picture.

In cellular atrophy the reduction occurs at the expense of the cytoplasm of cells. Malnutrition, inanition, abnormal pressure, and irradiation are some of the factors responsible for initiating atrophy of cells. During starvation, an extreme degree of generalized atrophy takes place. Local atrophy of tissues is due to impairment of vessel walls. Atrophy of tissues may be induced by excessive pressure. When excessive pressure is present, the blood supply to the tissue is reduced, resulting in atrophy and the production of an ulcer. In organs with ductal excretory systems, an obstruction of the ductal system causes an increase in pressure, resulting in atrophy. In salivary glands, an obstruction causes dilatation of the major excretory ducts, resulting in atrophy.

The atrophy that accompanies aging of tissues is due to a reduction in the caliber of arteries. Atrophy is a reversible change in cells. However, atrophy may remain as a permanent state or lead to the death of cells.

Hypertrophy is an acquired increase in the size of tissues due to an increase in the size of individual cells comprising the tissue. Compensatory hypertrophy is an acquired increase in the size of an organ due to the loss of one member of a paired organ system. The individual cells in the remaining organ undergo an increase in size. Hypertrophy of the skin and mucous membranes is an increase in the size of cells associated with increased function or frictional forces. Hyperplasia is more common than hypertrophy in the mucous membranes. Muscular hypertrophy is an increase in the size of muscle cells due to increased functional demands. Dystrophy refers to alterations due to a lack of nutrition and is associated with additional factors. During dystrophy of muscles there is a decrease in the size of muscle cells in addition to necrosis of cells.

Agenesis, Plasia, Aplasia, Hypoplasia, Hyperplasia and Metaplasia of Cells

Agenesis indicates that a tissue was never formed. Plasia is multiplication of individual units. Aplasia is the minimal development of a tissue lacking complete maturation and development to an adult functioning unit. Hypoplasia is present where there has been inadequate proliferation of cells, but greater proliferation than minimal development of the tissue. The tissue is reduced in size during hypoplasia. Hyperplasia is an excessive multiplication of component cells. Reactive hyperplasia occurs in callus formation during the healing of a fracture. Hyperplasia occurs in the skin and mucous membranes. Hyperplasia may occur in the keratinized layer of the skin. The latter represents physiologic hyperplasia. Hyperplasia may take place in the basal cell layer of the epithelium of the skin and mucous membrane and represents pathologic hyperplasia.

The keloid is hyperplasia of the connective tissue of the corium of the skin. The keloid is seen more often in Negroes than Caucasians. It appears to be due to an injury whereby the healing process is excessive in character. The keloid may be classified between hyperplasia and neoplasia.

Hyperplasia of the skin and mucous membranes is common. A great increase occurs in the hornified layer, which clinically causes the mucous membranes to become white (hyperkeratosis). Hyperplasia of the mucous membranes and skin is the result of an increase in the number of cells. Hyperplasia is an enlargement of tissues associated with inflammation, endocrine disturbances, and pharmacologic agents. Hypertrophy and hyperplasia of the mucous membranes and skin may occur simultaneously so that an increase in the number of cells also indicates an increase in the size of cells. Hyperplasia of ductal epithelium may take place in the excretory ducts of salivary glands. Squamous metaplasia and proliferation of ductal epithelium may be present in excretory ducts. Mucous glands have dilated excretory ducts during hyperplasia. The latter ducts undergo papillomatous hyperplasia and/or squamous metaplasia of ductal epithelium.

Hyperplasia is a common occurrence in the mucous membranes. The redundant hyperplastic tissue may be due to an irritation. Breast hyperplasia is produced by hormonal imbalance, such as excessive estrogenic hormone. The latter cells are governed by estrogenic hormones. Pseudoepitheliomatous hyperplasia is a form of epithelial hyperplasia that may appear histologically similar to the squamous cell carcinoma. However, the epithelium ceases to proliferate. The epithelium is well differentiated and fails to demonstrate dyskeratosis.

Metaplasia of cells is a process whereby one cell type is transformed into another cell type. The transformation involves a change in the form and function of the metaplastic cell. Metaplasia occurs in the excretory ducts of salivary glands transforming the columnar cells into squamous cells. The degenerated columnar cells are replaced by squamous cells, which originate from the undifferentiated reserve cell layer. During vitamin A deficiency, the salivary gland ducts undergo metaplasia of their epithelial lining cells to keratinized squamous epithelium. Osseous metaplasia of muscle tissue may follow trauma. Metaplasia occurs in connective tissue cells with a transformation into cartilage or bone. Chondromatous metaplasia may occur in the mucous membranes following chronic irritation.

INTRODUCTION OF NEOPLASIA

Definitions

Tumor is a symptom of a disease, i.e. a swelling associated with inflammation, neoplasia, and hyperplasia. Hamartoma is an overexpression of tissue, which serves no useful function. Hamartomas consist of normal constituents of the region arranged in an abnormal manner. Choristoma is an overdevelopment of tissue not normally present in the particular tissue. The latter overgrowth of tissue is derived from displaced anlagen.

Neoplasia refers to a specific pathologic process occurring in tissues and organs of the body. Neoplasia refers to a pathologic process whereby cells proliferate above and beyond the normal. Neoplasia is *one* process of unrestricted growth showing aggressiveness, invasion and metastases. The neoplastic process passes through several stages. The first stage is the conditioning of tissue, resulting in dormant cells with neoplastic potential. In the triggering stage, the dormant cells are activated to proliferating neoplastic cells. The final stage includes expansion, infiltration, and metastases of the growing neoplasm. Malignant refers to a clinical behavior pattern elicited by a neoplasm. Benign describe the clinical behavior pattern of a neoplasm.

ETIOLOGY OF NEOPLASIA

While the precise etiology of neoplasia is obscure, extrinsic and intrinsic contributing factors are present.

Extrinsic Factors

In regions where the maximum amount of extrinsic actinic radiation occurs, one finds the highest prevalence of lip and skin neoplasms. Chromium and silica dusts are associated with the production of pulmonary carcinoma (cancer). Workers in the radium dial industry develop neoplasms of the bone marrow. The application of x-rays, coal tar and coal tar derivatives, tobacco, and aniline dyes contribute to the development of neoplasia. Pipe smoking is a contributing factor to carcinoma of the lower lip. Aniline dyes are contributing factors to the development of neoplasms of the bladder. Benzene inhaled as fumes is a contributing factor to leukemia. Excessive smoking is a contributing factor to carcinoma of the lung. Tars, oils, petroleum, oily smegma, chutta (cigar), and khangri (charcoal) are exogenous carcinogens. Inorganic arsenic is carcinogenic to humans. Coal tar pitch is carcinogenic. Hot cutting oils may produce skin (epidermal) neoplasm. Carcinoma may occur in regions of a burn scar, in thermal and chemical burns, roentgen-ray dermatoses, chronic osteomyelitis, chronic sinuses, and in tar and oil dermatoses. Butter yellow dye produces carcinoma of the liver in rats. Pellets of pyrene cause neoplasia at the site of chemical irritation. Radioactive strontium stored in bone tissue and radioactive gold stored in the bone marrow represent contributing factors to neoplasms of bone. Viruses have been implicated as an etiologic agent in human neoplasms. At the present time, the viral theory of neoplasia has gained considerable prominence.

Intrinsic Factors

Heredity or chromosomal defects are intrinsic contributing factors to the development of neoplasms. A high incidence of neoplasia is found in some families. Endocrine disorders and hormonal influences represent intrinsic contributing factors. Age, sex, race, genetic constitution, and alterations in cellular metabolism influence the production of neoplasia. All of the etiologic factors that act selectively on tissues act by repetitive injury, and their effect is accumulative.

CHRONIC IRRITATION AND NEOPLASIA. Chronic irritation may play a contributory role in the production of some neoplasms. The latter irritation factor must represent a specific type of irritation, occurring under very specific conditions. Individuals who have had osteomyelitis of bone tissue for a period of forty to fifty years with multiple sinuses may develop carcinoma at the exit of a draining sinus.

EPITHELIAL NEOPLASMS

The benign epithelial neoplasms utilize the growth form of the neoplasm as the prefix and add the suffix "oma." Malignant epithelial neoplasms are termed *carcinomas*. The *adenoma* is a benign glandular neoplasm of epithelial origin. The *adenocarcinoma* is a malignant glandular neoplasm of epithelial origin.

MESENCHYMAL NEOPLASMS

The *lipoma* is a benign neoplasm of fat tissue, and the *fibroma* is a benign neoplasm of fibrous connective tissue. Malignant neoplasms of mesenchymal origin are termed *sarcomas*.

CHARACTERISTICS OF MALIGNANT NEOPLASMS

Malignant neoplasms grow with unlimited invasion of the adjacent tissue. Malignant neoplasms generally show a rapid rate of growth. The number of chromosomes in neoplastic cells may be double or triple the normal number. Nuclear and cellular pleomorphism are prominent features of malignant cells. Neoplastic cells show low differentiation, bizarre forms, loss of polarity, and anaplasia. The failure of cells to differentiate is terms *anaplasia*. The more anaplastic the neoplasm, the less differentiated the cells comprising the neoplasm and the more malignant is the clinical behavior pattern. Malignant neoplasms have a tendency to recur after removal and following irradiation.

Malignant neoplasms spread to distant organs, producing metastatic neoplasms. Every malignant neoplasm does not produce metastatic lesions. Carcinoma *in situ* does not metastasize. Basal cell carcinomas of the lip or skin do not metastasize.

SPREAD OF MALIGNANT NEOPLASMS

Malignant neoplasms spread by invading the surrounding tissues. Malignant cells may be transported mechanically, following separation from the main neoplastic mass, to the gastrointestinal or respiratory tracts. Malignant neoplasms spread by permeation through the lymphatics. The embolic spread of neoplastic cells is the primary manner of transportation through the lymphatics. Malignant neoplasms may spread by invading the blood vessels. Metastases from neoplasms occur by way of veins to the lungs, the portal circulation to the liver, and the lymphatics to the regional lymph nodes.

CHARACTERISTICS OF BENIGN NEOPLASMS

Benign neoplasms grow by expansion and are generally encapsulated by fibrous connective tissue. Some benign neoplasms show an absence of a connective tissue capsule. A few benign neoplasms locally infiltrate the immediate surrounding tissue. A few benign neoplasms may undergo malignant transformation. Benign neoplasms grow slowly, are self-limiting, and may become arrested in their growth.

REACTION OF BONE TISSUE TO NEOPLASMS

Regardless of the type of primary or metastatic neoplasm, the reaction of bone tissue is always similar. The primary reaction is characterized by resorption of bone due to pressure from proliferating neoplastic cells. The secondary reaction is characterized by apposition of new bone.

CLINICAL DIAGNOSIS OF BENIGN AND MALIGNANT NEOPLASMS

Clinically and roentgenographically, it is difficult to differentiate, with certainty, the benign from the malignant neoplasm. Therefore, all neoplasms should be biopsied and submitted for histopathologic examination. When the lesion is small, it is good judgment to surgically excise it in its entirety (excisional biopsy). When the lesion is large, it is good judgment to do a preliminary incisional biopsy. Biopsy of a neoplasm does not force neoplastic cells into the lymphatics and, therefore, does not speed metastases.

TREATMENT OF NEOPLASIA

The treatment of malignant neoplasms includes surgery, external irradiation, surface radium, interstitial radiation, radium needle implants, radioisotopes, and chemotherapeutic agents. The sensitivity of neoplasms to irradiation depends upon the degree of differentiation of the neoplasm. The more differentiated the neoplastic tissue, the more resistant it becomes to irradiation.

IRRADIATION AND OSTEORADIONECROSIS OF BONE

Irradiation therapy for neoplasms may result in osteoradionecrosis of bone tissue. When the dentition is present in individuals requiring irradiation therapy, preirradiation extractions become a *vital and imperative* matter. The removal of teeth in the path of the irradiation prior to therapy decreases the incidence of postradiation necrosis of the jaws. The opportunities for osteoradionecrosis are decidedly reduced when an intact mucous mucosa is present.

METASTATIC NEOPLASMS TO BONE TISSUE FROM DISTANT PRIMARY SITES

The primary neoplasms most frequently metastasizing to bone tissue result from carcinomas of the breast, thyroid, lung, kidney, testes, uterus, and sigmoid colon. The symptoms most commonly noted are pain, swelling, tenderness, paresthesia, numbness, and neoplastic tissue at the site of metastases.

PATHOLOGY OF INDIVIDUAL NEOPLASMS

Benign Neoplasms of Epithelial Origin

The papilloma is a benign epithelial neoplasm that arises from the stratified squamous epithelium of the mucous membrane. The papilloma consists of projections of squamous epithelium supported by a thin core of connective tissue carrying blood vessels. The adenoma occurs in the glandular structures of the body. The multiplication of glandular elements forms an encapsulated adenoma.

The epithelial cells forming the glandular elements are capable of secreting a fluid leading to distention of the glandular spaces and development of the cystadenoma and the papillary cystadenoma of the salivary glands. The pleomorphic adenoma is a benign neoplasm of the salivary glands. Seventy-five percent of all salivary gland neoplasms are pleomorphic adenomas. The pleomorphic adenoma grows slowly. When the adenoma undergoes malignant transformation, it grows rapidly and causes ulceration of the overlying surface. Histopathologically, the neoplasm is composed of basophilic epithelial cells, which form ducts, acini, chords and nests.

Malignant Neoplasms of Epithelial Origin

Carcinoma is the most common malignant epithelial neoplasm of the skin and mucous membrane. There are several histologic types of carcinomas—squamous cell carcinoma, basal cell carcinoma and adenocarcinoma. The squamous cell carcinoma occurs on the lower and upper lips, oral mucosa, larynx, pharynx, large bronchi, esophagus, and skin. The adenocarcinoma arises from the salivary glands.

The squamous cell carcinoma may be preceded by a thickened and dyskeratotic epithelium. Carcinoma may proliferate in the following gross forms: papillary (exophytic) growth, endophytic bulky mass, and ulcerated (infiltrating) growth. In the infiltrating carcinomas, the margins of the neoplasm are indistinct. Carcinoma cells infiltrate the surrounding tissue spaces, invade the lymphatic channels, and grow along the perineural lymphatics. Tumor cell emboli form in the lymphatics and are carried to regional and distant lymph nodes. Regional lymph node enlargement generally accompanies the carcinoma.

Squamous cell carcinoma occurs in deep fissures, furrows, or thickened epithelium (mucous membrane and skin). If the diagnosis of carcinoma is made when the neoplasm is less than 2 mm in diameter, a relatively good prognosis exists. The epidermoid carcinoma may be extremely difficult to diagnose clinically. The epidermoid carcinoma may appear clinically as an ulcer with an indurated border. Histologically, the epidermoid carcinoma is composed of irregular masses of squamous epithelium, which infiltrate the lamina propria, submucosa, muscle, and bone tissue. The keratin pearls are characteristic of a well-differentiated squamous cell carcinoma. In the undifferentiated squamous cell carcinoma, the cells are characterized by great variation in size and shape and in staining characteristics.

Grading of squamous cell carcinoma indicates the degree of malignancy of the neoplasm. The epidermoid carcinoma may be divided into four grades depending upon the loss of differentiation, the degree of hyperchromatism, and the number and abnormality of mitotic figures. Grade 1 is the most differentiated squamous cell carcinoma and, therefore, the least malignant of the four grades. Grade 1 consists of 75 percent or more of differentiated cells and 25 percent of undifferentiated cells. Grade 2 consists of 50 percent differentiated cells and 50 percent immature cells. Grade 3 consists of 25 percent differentiated cells and 75 percent immature cells. Grade 4 is the least differentiated, most anaplastic and, therefore, the most malignant of the four grades. Grade 4 consists of 75 percent or greater of undifferentiated cells. Grades 3 and 4, the most anaplastic neoplasms, show the best response to irradiation. The prognosis of squamous cell carcinoma is dependent upon location and grading. Squamous cell carcinoma generally has the lowest degree of malignancy when the neoplasm occurs in the lip and skin and the greatest degree of malignancy when it is located in the floor of the mouth and lateral posterior borders of the tongue.

Carcinoma *in situ* appears morphologically and cytologically as a carcinoma. It contains large atypical cells with hyperchromatic nuclei, numerous abnormal mitotic figures, and dyskeratotic epithelium. However, the neoplasm is confined to the epithelium of the mucous membrane and skin and has no invasive characteristics.

Basal cell carcinoma is a common, malignant neoplasm of skin appendages. The basal cell carcinoma occurs on the lips and skin particularly in the nasal and cheek folds. The cure rate for the basal cell carcinoma is 100 percent because the basal cell carcinoma fails to metastasize. The initial manifestation of the basal cell carcinoma is a small, waxy-appearing nodule. The center of the nodule becomes necrotic, and the carcinoma subsequently consists of an ulcer bordered by a rolled, indurated margin. Excessive radiation resulting from prolonged exposure to sunlight and roentgen rays are the most common etiologic factors for the development of the basal cell carcinoma.

The basal cell carcinoma is characterized histologically by masses of cells that have large, deeply basophilic nuclei and minimal cytoplasm. The basal cells generally form solid masses, cysts, or glandlike structures. When epithelial chords composed of basal cells undergo shrinkage with cystic degeneration, the neoplasm is termed *cystic basal cell carcinoma*. The basal cell carcinoma may rarely occur mixed with the epidermoid carcinoma. The latter is termed *basosquamous cell carcinoma* of the mucous membrane.

Adenocarcinoma is a malignant neoplasm that arises from glandular epithelium throughout the body.

Benign Neoplasms of Mesenchymal Origin

The fibroma is a common, benign neoplasm consisting of fibroblasts and collagenous tissue. The fibroma is a well-encapsulated neoplasm, which is firm to palpation. Microscopically, the fibroblasts appear as fusiform cells between interlacing collagenous fiber bundles. A redundant mass of tissue associated with a cause and effect relationship is termed an *irritational fibroma*. Desmoid tumor indicates both benign and malignant fibroblastic neoplasia in muscle tissue and fascial planes. The desmoid tumor consists of well-differentiated fibroblasts and bundles of collagenous connective tissue. The desmoid tumor does not metastasize; however, it may be locally aggressive.

The dermatofibroma protuberans consists of several plaque-like lesions that coalesce and subsequently enlarge, forming a protuberant mass of tissue in the skin. Dermatofibroma occurs in the skin and mucous membranes.

The lipoma is a benign neoplasm composed of mature fat tissue. The lipoma is a soft, yellow, well-circumscribed neoplasm surrounded by a connective tissue capsule. Fibrolipomas are composed predominantly of mature fat and a lesser quantity of fibrous connective tissue. The myxoma is a rare, benign, connective tissue neoplasm, which has a local invasive characteristic. However, the myxoma does not metastasize. The myxoma consists of stellate cells and branching fusiform fibroblasts located in a loose, mucoid matrix. The myxoma is a gelatinous mass, which may attain a considerable size.

The chondroma is a rare, benign neoplasm that produces cartilage following the formation of an intermediary precartilagenous tissue. The chondroma is a hard, gray-colored, lobulated neoplasm surrounded by a connective tissue capsule. When the chondroma occurs in bone tissue, it has the capacity to attain a very large size. Sarcomatous change may occur in the chondroma, a fact that is of the utmost importance to the clinician who is going to treat the chondroma. Chondromas should be considered as potentially malignant neoplasms if they show a tendency to undergo transplantation, regardless of whether or not metastases are present. When chondromas occur in individuals over nineteen years of age, they generally show a tendency toward transplantation and metastases.

True osteoma of bone tissue is a rare neoplasm. Compact osteomas of the maxilla and mandible are termed *torus palatinus* and *torus mandibularis*.

Neoplasms of Myogenic Tissue

The leiomyoma is a benign neoplasm of smooth muscle. Leiomyomas have the capacity to attain a large size. In rare instances, the leiomyoma may undergo malignant transformation. When removed surgically, some leiomyomas show a tendency to recur and undergo transplantation. Histopathologically, the leiomyoma consists of interlacing bundles of smooth muscle separated by minimal amounts of connective tissue. The rhabdomyoma is a benign muscle neoplasm derived from striated or skeletal muscle.

The granular cell myoblastoma is a benign neoplasm of striated muscle that occurs in the tongue, lip, larynx, and esophagus. Histologically, the myoblastoma consists of large polygonal cells with highly granular cytoplasm. The origin of this neoplasm has not been established, i.e. muscular, neurogenic, or fibroblastic. The congenital epulis of the newborn is a rare benign lesion that is morphologically similar to the granular cell myoblastoma. The congenital epulis of the newborn is located only on the gingiva of the newborn and should be classified as a distinct entity.

Benign Angiomatous Neoplasms

Hemangioma represents a new formation of blood vessels, which may be difficult to distinguish from telangiectasia. Telangiectasia is a dilatation of preexisting blood vessels in the skin and mucous membranes. The capillary hemangioma is the most common form of angioma. It is composed of a proliferation of newly-formed capillaries filled with blood. The capillary hemangioma is a frequent cause of macroglossia. The hemangioma may be treated by irradiation, surgery, and sclerosing solutions. Cavernous hemangiomas are less common than capillary hemangiomas. The cavernous hemangioma consists of large, cavernous spaces lined by a single layer of thin endothelial cells. The hemangioma is not encapsulated. Cavernous hemangiomas are common in the lips.

The lymphangioma is a congenital angioma that occurs in both localized and diffuse forms. The lymphangioma consists of small or cavernous spaces lined by a layer of endothelium and filled with lymph. Lymphangioma is frequently the cause of macroglossia. The lymphangioma may be located in the lip, resulting in a diffuse macrocheilia. When the lymphangioma occurs as a diffuse soft swelling in the neck of children, it is termed *hygroma colli cysticum*.

Malignant Neoplasms of Mesenchymal Origin

Sarcomas are malignant neoplasms arising from fibroblasts (fibrosarcoma), osteoblasts (osteosarcoma), and chondroblasts (chondrosarcoma). Sarcomas are not common neoplasms. Sarcomas generallly occur before forty-five years of age. Osteogenic sarcoma occurs in individuals from twelve to thirty-five years of age. The sarcoma is a soft, fleshy mass, that infiltrates the surrounding tissues. Hemorrhage is a common complication. The sarcoma grows by expansion and infiltration. Spread of the sarcoma takes place by way of the blood stream. Tumor cell emboli develop early, and metastases are produced in the lungs and visceral organs. The fibrosarcoma is a well-defined, soft tissue neoplasm consisting of interlacing fascicles of spindle-shaped fibroblasts and frequent mitoses.

The osteogenic sarcoma is composed of the osteoblast type of cell; however, the most predominant portion of the neoplasm is the intercellular tissue. The osteogenic sarcoma produces two types, the osteolytic and sclerotic osteogenic sarcoma. The sclerotic osteosarcoma containing abundant bone tissue has a relatively good prognosis. The osteolytic osteogenic sarcoma containing little or no bone tissue has a relatively poor prognosis. Osteosarcomas of the jaws have a better prognosis than their counterpart in the long bones. Chondrosarcoma is a rare neoplasm that has a rapid growth rate. The chondrosarcoma contains numerous mitotic figures and shows great irregularity in the size and shape of neoplastic cells. The chondrosarcoma involves the sternum and pelvis more commonly than other bones.

Liposarcoma is a rare neoplasm that tends to recur after surgical excision and grows by infiltration. Microscopically, large vacuolated lipoblasts with a signet-ring morphology are arranged around a vascular network. Recurrence is common following surgery. Myxosarcoma is a rare sarcoma undergoing myxomatous change in focal areas. The sarcomatous connective tissue undergoes degenerative changes, resulting in the myxosarcoma. Leiomyosarcoma is a rare neoplasm. The leiomyosarcoma consists of bundles of large, elongated, spindle-shaped cells. The leiomyosarcoma is a dangerous neoplasm when located in the deep tissues of the head and neck. The rhabdomyosarcoma is a rare neoplasm that occurs in voluntary muscle. The clinical behavior pattern of the rhabdomyosarcoma does not follow a highly malignant pattern. Metastases occur to the regional lymph nodes.

Lymphosarcoma is a malignant lymphoma of lymph nodes, spleen, and bone marrow. The lymphosarcoma consists of an uncontrolled proliferation of lymphocytes, resulting in lymphadenopathy. Histopathologically, the lymph node consists of uniform proliferating lymphocytes, which obliterate the nodal architecture. The reticulum cell sarcoma is a malignant neoplasm of lymph nodes. This sarcoma is characterized by an uncontrolled proliferation of reticulum cells in lymph nodes. The reticulum cell sarcoma begins with an insidious onset of localized or generalized enlargement of lymph nodes. Histopathologically, the lymph node consists of masses of proliferating small and large reticulum cells, which obliterate the normal nodal morphology. Ewing's sarcoma is a highly malignant neoplasm of young individuals, which arises from the reticuloendothelial cells of the bone marrow. Ewing's sarcoma of bone tissue may be mistaken for osteomyelitis because it is accompanied by fever, pain, and leukocytosis. Pathologic fracture may occur in the affected bone due to Ewing's sarcoma. Histopathologically, this sarcoma is composed of sheets and masses of undifferentiated, small, round cells located between areas of well-vascularized connective tissue.

Neoplasms of Peripheral Nervous Tissue

The neurofibroma is composed of a mass of tangled nerve bundles and a variable quantity of collagen. The neurofibroma may occur as an independent, benign neoplasm of peripheral nervous tissue or may develop as a generalized neurofibromatosis. Histopathologically, the neurofibroma contains Schwann cells. This neoplasm occurs in the subcutaneous tissue along peripheral nerves as fusiform masses.

Amputation neuromas consist of proliferating nerve fibers, which form bundles surrounded by an epineurium. The amputation neuroma may occur on a branch of the facial nerve or may result following trauma or severance of a peripheral nerve. The mass is movable, grows slowly, and produces pain. Plexiform neuroma consists of a tangled mass of highly differentiated, hypertropic, peripheral nerve bundles. The neoplasm may involve the facial nerve and result in a marked facial deformity. Histopathologically, numerous nerve bundles appear as a tangled mass of fascicles. When the plexiform neuroma is localized to the facial nerve, it is termed *facial gigantism.* Ganglioneuroma is a neoplasm of peripheral nerve cells. It is a slow growing neoplasm, which is composed of ganglion cells in various stages of maturation surrounded by a stoma of Schwann cells.

The neurilemmoma or benign schwannoma is a firm, well-encapsulated, benign neoplasm of peripheral nervous tissue, containing Antoni type A and B tissue. The Antoni type A tissue is a fasciculated or whorled area containing elongated cells and bands or zones of fibrous tissue. The nuclei of the elongated cells are arranged into a palisaded pattern. The palisaded cells surround whorls termed *Verocay bodies.* Antoni type B tissue is composed of minimal collagen fibers and irregularly dispersed cells. Midline lethal granuloma is a nondescriptive, destructive lesion, which involves the palate, nasal chambers, and maxillary sinuses. The granuloma erodes bone, destroying the facial bones, and produces bony sequestrations, a foul odor, and a greatly emaciated patient. It has a relentless clinical behavior pattern and obscure etiology. Histopathologically, the midline lethal granuloma appears as an inflammatory erosive type of lesion.

Neoplasms of Various Embryonic Tissues with a Low-grade Clinical Behavior Pattern

EMBRYOMAS. Embryomas are composed of highly differentiated cells normally present in the part. An example of the embryoma is Wilm's tumor of the kidney of children.

TERATOMAS. The teratoma is composed of cells foreign to a specific area of the body. The cells of the teratoma arise from all germ layers.

Pigmented Malignant Neoplasm

Malignant melanoma occurs in the skin and mucous membrane. It gives rise to widespread metastatic neoplasms. Melanomas may arise from a junctional or compound nevus of the skin. The prognosis of the malignant melanoma is serious. Recurrences result following failure to remove the margins of the neoplasm. Primary malignant melanoma of the mucous membrane is rare. Histopathologically, melanocarcinomatous cells infiltrate the submucosa of the skin.

Cysts and Neoplasms in the Head and Neck

CAROTID BODY TUMOR. The carotid body tumor arises from the carotid bodies located at the bifurcation of the common carotid arteries. Histopathologically, this neoplasm is comprised of alveolar masses of polyhedral-shaped cells. The branchial cleft cyst produces a swelling in the lateral portion of the neck anterior to the sternocleidomastoid muscle. Histopathologically, the branchial cyst is lined by stratified squamous epithelium. Lymphoid tissue and connective tissue are located beneath the epithelial lining.

The epidermoid cyst is lined by several layers of stratified squamous epithelium. It contains sebaceous glands, sweat glands, and hair follicles in the wall of the cyst. The dermoid cyst is a variant of the epidermoid cyst. The connective tissue wall of the cyst may contain hair follicles, sebaceous glands, sweat glands, striated muscle, and mucous glands.

References

Abelev, G.I.: *Cancer Res, 28*:1344, 1968.
Allen, D.W. and Cole, P.: *N Engl J Med, 286*:70, 1972.
Atkin, N.B. and Baker, M.C.: *Br J Cancer, 23*:329, 1969.
Aurelian, L.: *Fed Proc, 31*:1651, 1972.
Baltimore, D.: *Nature (Lond), 226*:1209, 1970.
Bell, J.R., et al.: *Surg Gynecol Obstet, 129*:258, 1969.
Berenblum, I.: In Florey, H.W. (Ed.): *General Pathology*, Philadelphia, Saunders, 1970.
Berg, P.: *Proc R Soc Lond, 177*:65, 1971.
Braun, A.C.: *Am Sci, 58*:307, 1970.
Burnet, F.M.: *Prog Exp Tumor Res, 13*:1, 1970.
Castro, B.C., et al.: *Cancer Res, 33*:819, 1973.
Editorial: E.B. virus, Burkitt's lymphoma and nasopharyngeal carcinoma, *Lancet, 1*:218, 1971.
Epstein, M.A.: *Lancet, 1*:1344, 1971.
Fahmy, O.G. and Fahmy, M.J. *Cancer Res, 30*:195, 1970.
Folkman, J.: *N Engl J Med, 285*:1182, 1971.
Fujimura, S., et al.: *Biochemistry, 11*:3629, 1972.
Gelboin, H.V.: *Cancer Res, 29*:1272, 1969.
Goh, K.: *Arch Intern Med, 122*:241, 1968.
Green, M.: *Fed Proc, 29*:1265, 1970.
Gross, L.: *Cancer, 20*:243, 1970.
Grover, P.L. and Sims, P.: *Biochem Pharmacol, 19*:2251, 1970.
Hellstrom, I., et al.: *Int J Cancer, 7*:1, 1971.
Henle, G., et al.: *J Natl Cancer Inst, 43*:1147, 1969.
Hennings, H. and Boutwell, R.K.: *Cancer Res, 30*:312, 1970.
Hruban, Z., et al.: *Lab Invest, 26*:86, 1972.
Huebner, R.J., et al.: *Proc Natl Acad Sci USA, 67*:366, 1970.
Isselbacher, K.J.: *N Engl J Med, 286*:929, 1972.
Lin, T-Y.: *Scand J Gastroenteral (Suppl), 6*:223, 1970.
MacPherson, I.: *Adv Cancer Res, 13*:169, 1970.
Mazia, D.: *Fed Proc, 29*:1245, 1970.
McNutt, N.S., et al.: *J Cell Biol, 51*:805, 1971.
Miller, J.A.: *Cancer Res, 30*:559, 1970.

Mondal, S. and Heidelberger, C.: *Proc Natl Acad Sci USA, 65:*219, 1970.
Moore, D.H., et al.: *Nature, 229:*611, 1971.
Nahmias, A.J., et al.: *Am J Epidemiol, 91:*547, 1970.
Nowell, P.C. and Morris, H.P.: *Cancer Res, 29:*969, 1969.
Piessens, W.F.: *Cancer, 26:*1212, 1970.
Rawls, W.E., et al.: *Lancet, 2:*1142, 1970.
Ryser, H.J.P.: *N Engl J Med, 285:*721, 1971.
Schlom, J., et al.: *Nature, 231:*97, 1971.
Shabad, L.M.: *Cancer, 27:*51, 1971.
Svoboda, D., et al.: *Cancer Res, 30:*2271, 1970.
Temin, H.M. and Mizutani, S.: *Nature, 226:*1211, 1970.
Warren, S.: *NY Acad Sci, 46:*133, 1970.
Weinstein, I.B., et al.: *Cancer Res, 31:*651, 1971.
Zamcheck, N., et al.: *N Engl J Med, 286:*83, 1972.
ZurHausan, H., et al.: *Nature, 228:*1056, 1970.

CHAPTER 16

HYPERSENSITIVITY (ALLERGY) AND DISEASES OF CONNECTIVE TISSUES

HYPERSENSITIVITY (ALLERGY)

THE RETICULOENDOTHELIAL SYSTEM of the human body provides the cells and fluid that make up the various inflammatory exudates. Opsonins, complement, and properidin are present in the fluid portion of the inflammatory exudate and represent part of the defensive mechanism of the body. Opsonins help during phagocytosis; complement is a bacteriostatic substance and is present in immune reactions along with properidin. When a noxious microorganism (antigen) remains in the tissues for a period of time, an altered serum globulin (antibody) is produced by reticuloendothelial cells. Thus, we have the antigen and antibody mobilized in the injured tissue.

The immune response produces circulating, heat-stable antibodies whose function is to neutralize the effect of the persistent antigen. Acquired immunity is characterized by the following:

1. It develops after a period of seven to fourteen days;

2. It results from the activity of an antigen in cells, causing the cells to elaborate neutralizing serum globulins;

3. The site of antigen-antibody union is intravascular or in the tissue fluids; and

4. The antigen-antibody union has a protective function to reduce or terminate the inflammatory reaction.

Hypersensitivity (allergy) occurs following the union of an antigen and antibody. This union is responsible for producing damage to tissues, and the union either prolongs or exaggerates the inflammatory reaction. Antibodies may circulate in the blood stream and are termed *reagin* or become attached to the tissues or sessile antibodies.

Hypersensitivity (allergy) occurs in man after the individual comes into contact with the antigen (allergen) at least twice. The initial contact with the allergen simply stimulates the immunizing reaction and is called the sensitizing dose. The second contact provokes the hypersensitivity (allergy) phenomenon and is called the shock dose. Seven to twelve days must generally elapse between the initial and shock (second) doses for the hypersensitivity phenomena to occur. Two exceptions occur to the two-dose mechanism at least seven to fourteen days apart. In serum sickness, serum injected only once produces allergic signs and symptoms in seven to twelve days. In the Shwartzman reaction, the sensitizing dose of antigen persists at the local (intradermal) site so that within twenty-four hours of a shock dose of antigen, if given intravenously, thrombosis and vascular necrosis develop at the local (intradermal) site. The mechanism operating in the Shwartzman phenomenon is obscure.

Hypersensitivity (allergy) may be classified into immediate and delayed types. Immediate hypersensitivity is further classified into hereditary and nonhereditary types.

Immediate hereditary hypersensitivity includes hay fever, asthma, urticaria, eczema, migraine, and angioneurotic edema in humans. Anaphylaxis produces the following manifestations in experimental animals, which are important to an understanding of anaphylaxis in man:

1. Reactions are due, in part, to liberation of histamine or H substances by the antigen-antibody union;

2. The reaction is mediated by smooth muscle contraction, increased vascular permeability, spasm, and inflammatory edema.

3. The anaphylactic reaction varies depending upon the individual tissues and their response to the shock dose of antigen; and

4. The hypersensitivity response develops in several minutes following exposure to the shock dose of antigen.

The latter can be correlated with immediate allergy in humans. In humans, antihistamines will, in part, suppress the allergic reactions caused by liberation of histamine and H substances. Constriction and edema of the bronchial wall are present in individuals with asthma. Increased vascular permeability causes hives or urticaria in humans. In asthmatics the bronchi represent the shock organs, and the allergic response is similar regardless of what (food, pollen, dust, etc.) the individual is sensitive to. In humans an immediate allergic response occurs within several minutes after exposure to a shock dose of antigen.

Hypersensitivity (allergy) of the immediate type is present in approximately 10% of individuals in the United States. The latter individuals have a hereditary predisposition to respiratory or skin allergies, which are termed *atopic allergies.* Follow exposures to an antigen, the individuals develop an antibody called *reagin.*

Respiratory allergy occurs as hay fever, chronic allergic rhinitis, and allergic bronchitis (bronchial asthma). Hay fever is a mild, respiratory allergy caused by an airborne antigen or inhalant antigen. The inhalant is generally a pollen but may be dust, inhaled chemicals, etc., which form an antigen by joining with serum proteins. Hay fever has symptoms of a watery secretion from the nose, sneezing, red and itching eyes, and itching nasopharynx. Respiratory mucosa is edematous and may occlude the air passage completely. The tissues contain a perivascular infiltration of eosinophils and a few plasma cells. Chronic allergic rhinitis has the same tissue changes as hay fever. It is, however, nonseasonal and is subject to secondary infection.

Allergic bronchitis (bronchial asthma) is caused by inhalation of pollens, dusts, by ingested foods, or by hypersensitivity to infectious microorganisms present in the respiratory tract. Symptoms are paroxysms of dyspnea, coughing, and wheezing. Wheezing is generally expiratory in nature. However, in severe bronchial asthma, wheezing is both inspiratory and expiratory in nature. Symptoms of bronchial asthma are due to a constriction of the bronchial musculature, edema of the bronchial mucosa, and occlusion of the smaller bronchial passages by a thick, mucoid secretion. The respiratory epithelium and bronchial musculature are hypertrophied due to repeated attacks of asthma. Smaller bronchi become plugged with coiled, inspissated mucus, which contains numerous eosinophils and Charcot-Leyden crystals. Individuals with bronchial asthma have a history of hay fever, eczema, or hives.

Skin hypersensitivity (allergy), urticaria, angioneurotic edema, and eczema are examples of immediate hereditary allergy. Urticaria (hives) is a hypersensitivity to either an ingested antigen or injected antigenic substance. Angioneurotic edema is an inflammatory swelling of the skin, lips, tongue, and rarely, synovial membranes of the joints. The edema develops within thirty minutes in extreme hypersensitivity attacks. Hives are large wheals in the skin, of varying size, number, and distribution, which are accompanied by intense itching. The allergen is in foods or of bacteria in the gastrointestinal tract, or an injection of penicillin or antiserum, all of which reach the skin by way of the blood stream. Endothelium of capillaries of the skin undergoes dilatation and extravasation of plasma and leukocytes, primarily eosinophils. The hives generally begin resolution in twenty-four hours.

Eczema (atopic dermatitis) occurs in infants, children, and adults and is located on the flexor surface of the elbows and knees as well as on the face in infants. Itching (intense) accompanies eczema. Skin becomes red, with minute vesicles located in the epidermis, and appears as moist, crusted areas. Vesicles represent areas of edema or liquefaction necrosis within the epidermis. Edema and dilated capillaries occur with a perivascular infiltration of eosinophils and other leukocytes. Eczema and its allergic manifestations are different from urticaria. In eczema, one or more zones of the skin are chronically involved by an allergic inflammatory response (flexor surface of knees, elbows or on the face and ankles) and a chronic situation endures. In urticaria (hives) the location of the wheal is quite variable, temporary, and the reaction subsidies in twenty-four hours.

During immediate hereditary allergy (atopic allergy), the allergic clinical manifestations may be suppressed by the mechanism of desensitization, i.e. the repeated injections of small amounts of appropriate allergen (antigen). A new blocking antibody (heat stable) circulates and attempts to neutralize the antigen. In order for successful desensitization to take place in an individual with immediate hereditary allergy, the chief antigen must be established.

Immediate, nonhereditary allergies (hypersensitivities) are the transient histamine wheal, the vasospasm, and necrosis without histamine. The latter is termed *Arthus phenomenon.*

The principal effect of the antigen-antibody reaction occurs on endothelium of the blood vessels. Arterioles constrict, and endothelial lining, capillaries, and venules are impaired so that leukocytes and red blood cells stick to the vessel wall. Necrosis and thrombosis follow, and the vascular occlusion of the tissues undergoes ischemic necrosis. The vascular impairment present in the Arthus phenomenon is the result of precipitation of antigen-antibody union since no type of substance similar to histamine has been isolated for the tissues.

The collagen diseases are acute rheumatic fever, rheumatoid arthritis, disseminated lupus erythematosus, and polyarteritis, scleroderma, and dermatomyositis. Therefore, the collagen diseases are believed to be related to the Arthus's phenomenon.

Rheumatic fever, rheumatoid arthritis, and glomerulonephritis are examples of the collagen disease that follow streptococcal infections. For instance, antigens may be elaborated by Type A streptococci. Bacterial antigens acting on human tissues may combine with the tissues to induce an antibody reaction against the injured histologic element. Thus, the bacterial infection may injure the organ and antibodies from the reticuloendothelial system and may be directed against the injured tissue of the organ. In rheumatic fever the heart valves, the myocardium, and pericardium are damaged since mucoid degeneration is present in the stroma, and there is an inflammatory infiltrate of monocytes. The characteristic lesion of the myocardium is the Aschoff body, a sterile granuloma probably produced by the antigen-antibody reaction. In rheumatoid arthritis, multiple joints have painful swellings. The characteristic lesion is the rheumatoid nodule, i.e. a focal fibrinoid degeneration of the synovial tissues of joints.

In other collagen diseases (disseminated lupus erythematosus, polyarteritis, scleroderma, and dermatomyositis), the ground substance of the connective tissue is altered with cementin of the endothelial lining of small blood vessels; in addition, there is thrombonecrosis of blood vessels. Individuals who have asthma and hypersensitivity diseases are more susceptible to collagen diseases. Inherited predisposition to the collagen diseases has not been established. For instance, bronchial asthma may be as high as 25 percent incidence in polyarteritis patients.

DELAYED HYPERSENSITIVITY

Delayed hypersensitivity occurs following repeated exposure to the same antigen plus an interval present between the sensitizing and shock dose. In delayed hypersensitivity, the shock dose causes a response after twenty-four to seventy-two hours. There is an absence of a specific shock organ, but the portal of entry (skin) is generally affected.

Delayed hypersensitivity (allergy) is accompanied by the following:

1. There are no circulating antibodies, and no passive transfer can take place by serum;

2. The appropriate test is the patch test, whereby the suspected antigen is applied to the skin of the allergic individual and allergic inflammation results in the zone of contact in forty-eight hours;

3. Delayed hypersensitivity requires a sensitizing dose and a time interval of seven to twelve days, followed by a shock dose;

4. It differs from immediate hypersensitivity in that everyone can acquire the delayed type, and it shows no hereditary predisposition;

5. The allergic inflammation results directly from the antigen-antibody reaction and no histamine or choline is liberated;

6. There is no specific shock organ;

7. Individuals cannot be desensitized; and

8. Proteins are required for antigens. An example of an antigen for delayed hypersensitivity consists of dead mycobacteria and paraffin oil (vehicle).

Contact dermatitis is a delayed form of hypersensitivity

Hypersensitivity (Allergy) and Diseases of Tissues

(allergy). Contact dermatitis may be caused by plastics, insecticides, weed killers, and new therapeutic agents. The chemical is the allergin, and the body supplies the protein portion of the antigen. The chemical allergins or products make contact with the skin.

There are some common and overlapping areas between immediate and delayed hypersensitivity (allergy). In delayed hypersensitivity caused by bacterial allergy, the leukocytes appear to increase their defensive potential based upon the offender (microorganism).

CONNECTIVE TISSUE DISEASES

Connective tissue diseases or the collagen diseases are characterized by systemic involvement of the connective tissues throughout the body. The diseases of connective tissue reflect a local response of a particular tissue to irritants or injurious agents. In addition to deposition of fibrinoid material, the connective tissue diseases show the following changes: mucoid degeneration, fibrosis, and hyalinization when healing occurs in the fibrinoid material.

SYSTEMIC OR DISSEMINATED LUPUS ERYTHEMATOSUS. Disseminated lupus erythematosus is an acute, subacute, and recurrent febrile disease occurring principally in women. The disease produces widespread involvement of the connective tissue throughout the body. The following features may be present during the course of the disease: erythematous rash on the face; renal, gastrointestinal, and central nervous system involvement; joint pain and swelling; proteinuria; cardiac involvement; lymphadenopathy; fever, anemia, and thrombocytopenia. The most important etiologic factor in systemic lupus erythematosus is hypersensitivity to an antigen. The blood vessels show advanced fibrinoid degeneration in systemic lupus. The thickened basement membrane of glomerular capillary tufts becomes smudgy due to eosinophilic deposits of fibrinoid material, i.e. wire loop lesions.

The lupus erythematosus cells (L.E. cells) appear to be polymorphonuclear neutrophilic leukocytes, which have engulfed large basophilic hematoxylin bodies. The L.E. cell is not pathognomonic for disseminated lupus erythematosus. In the joints, proliferation of the synovial membrane produces arthritis. Disseminated lupus erythematosus is exacerbated by exposure to sunlight. A skin rash is present in approximately 80 percent of affected individuals. The most characteristic skin lesion is an erythematous local maculopapular rash distributed over the bridge of the nose and cheek, producing a butterfly lesion on the face.

CHRONIC DISCOID LUPUS ERYTHEMATOSUS. A form of lupus erythematosus is limited to the skin and is termed *chronic discoid lupus erythematosus.*

SCLERODERMA. Scleroderma is a rare, chronic, systemic connective tissue disease in which the skin and mucous membrane become thickened and stiff due to excessive collagenization. Two forms of scleroderma are recognized—morphea (localized lesion) and diffuse (generalized lesions). The dermatologic and mucous membrane changes constitute the most visible alterations. An indurated skin develops, which is adherent to the atrophic subcutaneous tissue. Induration is followed by atrophic changes in the epithelium, and connective tissue producing a shiny, smooth, and fixed skin containing irregular areas of pigmentation. The main alteration in scleroderma is hyalinization of the connective tissue.

POLYARTERITIS NODOSA. Polyarteritis is a subacute or chronic necrotizing inflammation involving all layers of the walls of medium and small arteries, arterioles, and capillaries. The disease is characterized by a low-grade fever, arthralgia, muscular tenderness, skin eruptions, and central nervous system, renal, and cardiac alterations. The first stage consists of edema, and fibrinoid and mucoid degeneration beginning in the media and extending to the adventitia and intima of medium and small arteries and arterioles. The second stage is characterized by an inflammatory infiltrate of polymorphonuclear leukocytes involving all layers of the vessel wall and perivascular tissues. The third stage is characterized by proliferation of fibroblasts and endothelial cells and formation of granulation tissue. The fourth stage consists of resolution of the inflammatory infiltrate with formation of dense, fibrous, connective tissue.

DERMATOMYOSITIS. Dermatomyositis is a rare, connective

tissue disease involving the skin and skeletal muscles, which is characterized by a sudden onset and acute rapid course. The findings include edema and erythematous rashes involving the face, neck, periorbital region, extremities, and trunk: arthralgia; myalgia; muscle weakness; fever and peripheral neuritis.

SERUM SICKNESS. Serum sickness is a form of hypersensitivity that generally subsides spontaneously. The manifestations of serum sickness may appear without any prior sensitization to an antigen. The manifestations are fever, urticaria, adenopathy, edema, and joint pain. Arthritis commonly accompanies patients with serum sickness. Generalized lymphadenopathy and edema of the eyelids, glottis, hands, and feet are manifestations of serum sickness.

References

Edsall, G.: *J Allergy Clin Immunol, 28*:1, 1957.
Gall, E.A. and Steinberg, A.: *J Lab Clin Med, 32*:508, 1947.
Gore, I. and Isaacson, N.H.: *Am J Pathol, 25*:1029-1043, 1949.
Gutman, A.B.: *Adv Protein Chem, 4*:156, 1948.
Landsteiner, K.: *The Specificity of Serologic Reactions*, rev. ed. Cambridge, Harvard U Pr, 1946.
Landsteiner, K. and Van Der Scheer, J.: *J Exp Med, 57*:633, 1937.
Lawrence, H.S.: The delayed type of allergic inflammatory response. Seminar on Allergy, *Am J Med, 20*:44-63, 1956.
Lepos, I.H.: *J Allergy Clin Immunol, 71*:380, 1953.
Lipton, M.M. and Freund, J.: *J Immunol, 71*:380, 1953.
Lurie, M.B.: *J Exp Med, 69*:579, 1939.
Menkin, V.: *Am J Pathol, 16*:13, 685, 1940.
Miles, A.A.: Some aspects of antibacterial immunity. In *Lectures on the Scientific Basis of Medicine*. London, The Athlone Press, 1953, vol. I, p. 193, 1951-52.
Pillemer, L., et al.: *Science, 120*:279, 1954.
Raffel, S.: *Immunity; Hypersensitivity; Serology.* New York, Appleton-Century-Crofts, 1953.
Rich, A.R.: *The Pathogenesis of Tuberculosis*, 2nd ed. Springfield, Thomas, 1951.
Rosenow, G.: *Acta Haematol (Basel), 5*:1, 1951.
Selye, H.: *Stress*, 1st ed. Montreal, Acta, 1950, pp. 404, 442.
Sternberger, L.A.: *J Allergy Clin Immunol, 28*:40, 1957.
Stoner, R.D. and Hale, W.M.: *J Immunol, 75*:203, 1955.
White, B.V. and Geschicketer, C.F.: *Diagnosis in Daily Practice.* Philadelphia, Lippincott, 1947.

Alarcon-Segovia, D.: *Mayo Clin Proc, 44*:664, 1969.
Amos, D.B.: *Adv Immunol, 10*:251, 1969.
Benacerraf, B. and McDevitt, H.O.: *Science, 175*:273, 1972.
Brent, L.: *N Engl J Med, 284*:499, 1971.
Broder, I.: In Movat, H.Z. (Ed.): *Inflammation, Immunity and Hypersensitivity.* New York, Har-Row, 1971.
Burnet, F.M.: *Cellular Immunology.* London and New York, Cambridge University Press, 1969.
Busch, G.J., et al.: *Hum Pathol, 2*:253, 1971.
Calne, R.Y., et al.: *Nature, 227*:903, 1970.
Cosenza, H. and Nordin, A.A.: *J Immunol, 104*:976, 1970.
Craddock, C.G., et al.: *N Engl J Med, 285*:324, 1971.
Cudkowicz, G. and Bennett, M.: *J Exp Med, 134*:83, 1971.
DeGroot, L.J.: *Med Clin North Am, 54*:1117, 1970.
Fundenberg, H.H., et al.: *N Engl J Med, 283*:656, 1970.
Grumet, F.C., et al.: *N Engl J Med, 285*:193, 1971.
Haas, J.E. and Yunis, E.G.: *Exp Mol Pathol, 12*:257, 1970.
Hobbs, J.R.: *Proc R Soc Med, 62*:773, 1969.
Hood, L.E.: *Fed Proc, 31*:177, 1972.
Klainer, A.S. and Beisel, W.R.: *Am J Med Sci, 258*:431, 1969.
Kleckner, S.S.: *Am J Gastroenterol, 53*:141, 1970.
Lawrence, H.S.: *N Engl J. Med, 283*:411, 1970.
McCluskey, R.T. and Cohen, S.: In Ioachim, H.L. (Ed.): *Pathology Annual 1972.* New York, Appleton-Century-Crofts, 1972.
McDevitt, H.O. and Bodmer, W.F.: *Am J Med, 52*:1, 1972.
Nordin, A.A., et al.: *J Immunol, 105*:154, 1970.
Novack, S.N. and Pearson, C.M.: *N Engl J Med, 284*:938, 1971.
Panayi, G.S.: *Br Med J, 2*:656, 1970.
Pearson, C.M.: In Samter, M. (Ed.): *Immunological Diseases.* Boston, Little, 1971.
Russell, P.S. and Winn, H.J.: *N Engl J Med, 282*:786, 1970.
Sato, T., et al.: *Arch Neurol, 24*:409, 1971.
Schur, P.H.: *N Engl J Med, 282*:1205, 1970.
Sell, S.: *Transplant Rev, 5*:19, 1970.
Sharp, G.C. and Irvin, W.S.: *Am J Med Sci, 259*:365, 1970.
Toth, A. and Alpert, L.I.: *Arch Pathol, 92*:31, 1971.
Whaley, K. and Buchanan, W.W.: *Scott Med J, 15*:261, 1970.
Wigley, R.D.: *NZ Med J, 71*:151, 1970.
Winkelmann, R.K.: *Mayo Clin Proc, 46*:83, 1971.
Yunis, E.J. and Amos, D.B.: *Proc Natl Acad Sci USA, 68*:3031, 1971.

CHAPTER 17

HEART AND BLOOD VESSELS

DEGENERATIVE LESIONS OF THE HEART

Protein Alterations

CLOUDY SWELLING may develop in the heart, producing a swollen and opaque myocardium. The muscle cells undergo enlargement due to an increase in the quantity of water in the muscle cell, but the process is reversible. Cloudy swelling of the heart is due to a high fever or toxemia caused by the breakdown of large protein molecules into small protein molecules that bring fluid into the cell.

Amyloidosis of the heart is due to the accumulation of an abnormal protein-carbohydrate complex in the primary systemic disease. The individual has an enlarged heart with a firm, rubbery myocardium. Muscle cells are separated by pink, homogeneous, amyloid deposits. Amyloidosis of the heart results in chronic congestive heart failure.

Lipid Alterations

Fatty degeneration occurs in the heart due to severe anemia or toxemia. Intracellular lipids appear in muscle cells as red droplets in the cytoplasm (Sudan III or oil red 0 stains). Grossly, minute yellow flecks are visible in the myocardium and are termed *thrush breast* or *tabby cat*. Fatty degeneration of the heart is reversible.

Fatty infiltration of the heart is the intercellular deposition of fat as adipose tissue. Obesity results in accumulation of fat in the epicardial fat and between the muscle fibers of the right ventricle only. The fat deposit disappears as weight is reduced.

Carbohydrate Alterations

Von Gierke's disease (glycogen storage disease) causes glycogen storage in the heart with cardiac enlargement. Cardiac failure, skeletal muscle weakness, and central nervous system involvement result during the first year of life.

Hyalin Alterations

Hyaline forms as a pink, homogeneous material in old scars of the heart where there is an abundance of collagen. Hyalinization of the mitral valve occurs in chronic rheumatic endocarditis. Hyaline material may be deposited in the tricuspid and pulmonic valves in response to carcinoid tumors with metastases.

Pigmentary Alterations

Lipochromes (yellow color of depot fat and adrenal cortex) are related to carotene. Lipochromes may produce a dark brown tinge to the heart of the aging. The heart is generally smaller than normal and is termed *brown atrophy of the heart*.

Hemosiderin is a brown, granular pigment formed by the breakdown of hemoglobin. Hemosiderin may be deposited in the heart muscle cells as red brown granules next to the nuclei. An abundance of hemosiderin pigment granules contributes to cardiac damage and congestive heart failure.

Vitamin Deficiency or Excess

Vitamin B_1 (thiamine) deficiency causes beriberi. The heart is dilated, particularly the right ventricle. Hydropic degeneration of the cardiac fibers and interstitial edema is present in the affected heart.

Vitamin C (ascorbic acid) deficiency causes scurvy. Scurvy is accompanied by hypertrophy of the right ventricle of the heart, but histopathologic changes are present in the heart.

Vitamin D in excess causes focal calcification of the myocardium and arterial walls.

Starvation and Obesity

In starvation, the heart undergoes a reduction in size, first by the loss of epicardial fat and second by atrophy of muscle fibers.

During starvation the fat disappears, and the cells become watery and produce the condition of serous atrophy of the heart. Obesity increases the quantity of adipose tissue present in the epicardial fat and in the interstitial tissue of the heart.

Necrosis and Autolysis

Necrosis occurs in myocardial infarctions. Autolysis is the self-destruction of cardiac cells after death of the individual due to the liberation of enzymes from the lysosomes of the cytoplasm of cardiac cells.

Fragmentation

Myocardial fragmentation is the presence of multiple breaks in the cardiac muscle fibers.

Calcification

Calcium deposition is seen as narrowed coronary arteries, in mitral stenosis or stenosis of aortic valves, and in the dense scar tissue surrounding the heart in chronic constrictive pericarditis. The latter calcification has no metabolic basis and, therefore, is termed *dystrophic calcification*. Focal calcification of the myocardium is also caused by hypercalcemia in hyperparathyroidism and, therefore, is termed *metastatic calcification*.

CONGENITAL LESIONS OF THE HEART AND BLOOD VESSELS

The heart and its blood vessels are susceptible to congenital anomalies during the first three months of fetal life. Mongolism produces developmental defects and congenital cardiac lesions due to chromosomal defects.

Congenital heart disease may be accompanied by cyanosis if the venous to arterial shunts increase the quantity of unoxygenated hemoglobin in the skin capillaries.

Congenital Valve Lesions

Congenital valve lesions include stenosis (abnormally small opening) and atresia (absence of an opening). Stenosis and atresia occur in the aortic valve. Stenosis of a valve produces hypertrophy of the myocardium proximal to the point of stenosis.

Septal Defects: Atrial and Ventricular

Atrial or ventricular septal defects may occur if there is incomplete development of the partitions between the left and right sides of the heart. Intraatrial septal defects may be located near the mitral valve or it may be high due to failure of the foramen ovale to close after birth. Defects in the cardiac septa permit the flow of blood from one side of the heart to the other. An atrial septal defect permits oxygenated blood from the left atrium to mix with unoxygenated blood in the right atrium and cyanosis is present. Intraventricular septal defects are located in the upper portion of the septum below the aortic valve. It is small and well tolerated.

Anomalies of Great Vessels

When the two great arteries leaving the heart are in transposition (interchanged), the systemic venous blood entering the right ventricle is pumped into the aorta and returns by way of systemic veins to the right heart without oxygenation. This condition is not compatible with life unless some oxygenated blood enters the systemic circulation.

Patent ductus arteriosus is the presence of a channel connecting the pulmonary artery to the aorta. A left to right shunt overburdens both the left and right ventricle.

Coarctation of the aorta is a constriction of the distal arch of the aorta. There is an infantile type of anomaly where the entire arch of the aorta is narrowed and the ductus arteriosus remains widely patent so that venous blood from the pulmonary artery enters the aorta and perfuses the abdominal viscera. There is also an adult type of anomaly where the coarctation is localized to a short portion of the aorta distal to or at the entry point of the ductus arteriosus.

The tetralogy of Fallot is a condition in which the septum shifts too far to the right, resulting in a stenosis of the pulmonary artery, an enlarged aorta overriding the right ventricle, an interventricular septal defect, and hypertrophy of the right ventricle.

Arteriosclerosis

Arteriosclerosis is defined as consisting of three different diseases that cause hardening of the arterial wall. The three diseases are atherosclerosis, arteriolosclerosis, and the medial sclerosis of Mönckeberg. Atherosclerosis produces patchy deposits of lipids in the intima of large arteries (aorta) as well as smaller arteries like the coronary, cerebral, mesenteric, popliteal, and femoral arteries. Arteriolosclerosis is the thickening of the intima and media in arterioles associated with hypertension. Medial sclerosis of Mönckeberg is degeneration of medium sized arteries (radial, ulnar) with calcification of the media but without significant reduction in the size of the lumen.

Atherosclerosis

Atherosclerosis is responsible for approximately one-half million deaths due to coronary heart disease per year in the United States. Multiple factors are operating in the production of atherosclerosis. The risk factors in atherosclerosis are diet, serum cholesterol, age and sex, disorders of lipid metabolism, hypertension, cigarette smoking, stress, physical exercise, and overweight. The latter risk factors appear to predispose the individual patient to atherosclerosis.

The pathogenesis of atherosclerosis is still incomplete. Large, cholesterol-containing molecules may be deposited into the intima of arteries in the following ways:

1. By infiltration through the endothelial lining with a breakdown of the macromolecules releasing lipids to the intima;

2. By the accumulation of platelets, fibrin, and constituents of the circulating blood on the vessel lining causing their endothelization and incorporation into the wall; and

3. By hemorrhages from the vasa vasorum that may release blood constituents into the intima.

The normal intima is avascular, but in the late lesions of atherosclerosis the intimal vascularity is significant.

Grossly, the lesions of atherosclerosis are of three types, i.e. the early intimal fatty streak (yellow linear lesion), elevated plaques of lipid (yellow) or fibrous (white) varieties, and the late lesion consisting of necrosis, ulceration, hemorrhage or calcification.

Microscopic findings are characterized by lipid deposition in the intima associated with the collagen and mucopolysaccharide. Lipid deposits begin within the smooth muscle cells of the intima, from which lipid vacuoles enlarge and form foam cells. Cholesterol-laden foam cells become necrotic and release lipid (crystals of cholesterol) forming a mass called the atheroma. As the atheroma (gruel-like mass) expands, the internal elastic lamina becomes fragmented and disappears. Calcium salts deposit on the periphery of the atheromatous deposits. The atherosclerotic lesions have a patchy distribution, and atherosclerosis of the coronary artery produces an eccentric narrowing of the lumen of this blood vessel. Atherosclerosis is most severe in the proximal 3 or 4 centimeters of a coronary artery. It requires many years for atherosclerosis to produce narrowing of a coronary artery and produce myocardial ischemia leading to angina (transient substernal pain relieved by rest), myocardial infarction (persistent substernal pain), or sudden death caused by ventricular fibrillation.

Coronary Occlusion

Thrombosis is the predominate cause of coronary occlusion (incidence is 50 to 80% of fatal coronary occlusion). Thrombosis occurs in a coronary artery when the lumen is severely narrowed as a result of atherosclerosis. The thrombus is attached to cracks in the atheromatous intima of the artery. Coronary occlusion is rarely caused by emboli from thrombi in the left auricle, left ventricle or mitral valve, syphilitic stenosis of coronary ostia, and diseases such as polyarteritis, rheumatic arteritis, and tumors.

Myocardial Infarction

Infarction (ischemic necrosis) results from sudden occlusion of a major coronary artery. The anterior descending branch of the left coronary artery is most common as the site of occlusion resulting in infarction of the anterior portion of the lateral wall of the left ventricle and the anterior one-half of the interventricular septum. Within three or four weeks the periphery of the infarct is replaced by cellular fibrous tissue and contracts to a dense inelastic tissue. Collagenization of the scar continues for two or three months with a tough scar resulting, which is resistant to rupture.

Microscopically, there is necrosis of the myocardium. Within five days, capillaries and fibroblasts migrate into the necrotic zone from the adjacent normal tissue.

The majority of individuals with a myocardial infarction survive their first infarction. Rupture of the heart occurs in 2 to 5 percent of instances of infarction. Complications including ventricular aneurysm, embolism, and chronic congestive heart failure may follow recovery from a very large infarct or from repeated attacks of small infarcts.

Hypertensive Heart Disease

Hypertensive heart disease is defined as the presence of cardiac hypertrophy following a long-standing systemic arterial hypertension. The cause of the elevated blood pressure is obscure, and thus, it is termed *primary* (essential) *hypertension.* Increasing age, female sex, Negro race, high cadmium or salt intake in the diet are predisposing factors to the development of essential hypertension.

Secondary hypertension is defined as hypertension caused by some identifiable disease such as chronic glomerulonephritis, chronic pyelonephritis, polycystic disease, or stenosis of the renal artery, endocrine disorders, and coarctation of the aorta.

Hypertensive heart disease is accompanied by cardiac hypertrophy of the left ventricle caused by a diffuse increased resistance to the blood flow as a result of constriction of the arterioles throughout the body. The heart begins to fail, after many years, from a progressive enlargement due to dilatation with the patient having symptoms of congestive heart failure.

Malignant (accelerated) hypertension generally occurs in an individual with essential hypertension who has a rapid increase in blood pressure at a young age. Blood pressure reaches 300 mmHg or more. Characteristic findings of malignant hypertension are advanced retinal changes including hemorrhages, exudates, and papilledema. Uremia is the cause of death.

Vascular Lesions in Hypertension

The following vascular lesions are associated with hypertension: arteriolosclerosis (arteriolar sclerosis), benign type of essential hypertension, and the malignant or accelerated form of essential hypertension. A third type of arteriosclerosis is Mönckeberg's sclerosis. It fails to produce severe narrowing or occlusion of an artery and is, therefore, not clinically significant.

Rheumatic Heart Disease

Rheumatic fever occurs in children who exhibit manifestations in the heart and joints of the body. The involvement of the joints is transient and undergoes resolution; however, the lesions of the heart may be severe and permanent in character.

Rheumatic fever is a hypersensitivity reaction to an infection with group A beta-hemolytic streptococci. Group A streptococci have antigens that are immunologically similar to antigens of human heart tissue and stimulate the formation of antibodies that are cross-reactive with only the human heart. There is a two– or three-week interval from the initial streptococcal infection in the upper respiratory tract to onset of symptoms of acute rheumatic fever.

Rheumatic heart disease is a pancarditis since it involves the endocardium, myocardium, and pericardium. The initial lesion is a verrucal endocarditis of the endocardium. A row of warty, pink vegetations are present and are firmly attached along the line of contact with the valve cusps. The vegetations consist of platelets and fibrin (which are free of bacteria in uncomplicated cases).

The mitral valve is generally the most commonly affected heart valve, followed by the aortic valve. The tricuspid and pulmonic valves are infrequently affected.

Microscopically, the affected valve(s) becomes edematous and infiltrated throughout with lymphocytes, plasma cells, and monocytes plus scattered Aschoff cells or Anitschkow myocytes. When the acute inflammatory reaction subsides, the vegetations undergo organization by fibroblasts to produce thickening of the valve and adhesions at the commissures. One attack of rheumatic fever is all that is necessary to produce significant damage to the heart valves. Repeated attacks of rheumatic fever produce thickening of the valve and shortening of the chordae tendineae. The latter alterations may produce a stenotic valve or a functionally insufficient valve. If the narrowing of the mitral orifice is very severe, it is described as a fish-mouth mitral valve. At the present time, severely damaged valves are replaced by artificial valves.

Myocarditis is present in acute rheumatic fever and consists of a diffuse inflammatory response in the myocardium plus the formation of focal nodules, i.e. Aschoff bodies. Aschoff bodies are an essential diagnostic feature of acute rheumatic fever. The Aschoff body is characterized by the mobilization of Aschoff cells plus lymphocytes arranged in parallel rows. The Aschoff body develops adjacent to blood vessels. The Aschoff cell has two or three nuclei and arises from the cardiac histiocyte, the Anitschkow myocyte, where the chromatin material of the nucleus is positioned as a serrated bar in the long axis of the nucleus. When healing ensues, the myocarditis and Aschoff nodules are replaced by scar tissue. The scarring contributes to conduction defects and arrhythmias, which occur in the late stages of rheumatic heart disease.

Pericarditis is rather infrequent in acute rheumatic fever and is characterized by a thick fibrinous exudate deposited on the pericardial surfaces of the heart. Healing occurs free of adhesions and compressions of the heart. Rheumatic fever has decreased in frequency due to chemotherapy preventing streptococcal infections in susceptible subjects.

Bacterial Endocarditis

Bacterial endocarditis is defined as a bacterial infection affecting a valve or the endocardium of the heart. Subacute bacterial endocarditis is defined as a bacterial infection of a valve or endocardium of the heart with survival for more than six weeks. Acute bacterial endocarditis has a survival period of less than six weeks.

Subacute bacterial endocarditis has an insidious onset, a low-grade fever, embolic phenomena, and changing heart murmurs. Ninety percent of instances of subacute bacterial endocarditis are caused by nonpyogenic microorganisms *(Streptococcus viridans, Hemophilus influenzae)*. Prophylactic administration of antibiotics will prevent severe risks following dental or surgical procedures.

The majority of instances of bacterial endocarditis develop in hearts where the heart valves have shown previous damage. If the infection begins in a congenital arterial defect (coarctation of the aorta) the disease state is termed *bacterial endarteritis*.

Subacute bacterial endocarditis has an affinity for the mitral and aortic valves, or the aortic valve alone, and only rarely affects the valves of the right side of the heart (same distribution as rheumatic heart disease). Grossly, the lesions of subacute bacterial endocarditis appear as abundant, red brown, friable vegetations located near the line of contact of the cusps of the valve but spreading upward on the atrial surface. Vegetations consist of platelets and fibrin with deeply embedded clumps of bacteria. Fragments of vegetations separate from the main vegetation to produce emboli in the kidneys and spleen. When embolism occurs to the brain, hemiplegia results. Infarcts develop where emboli block the blood supply to an organ. Abscess does not develop since the causative streptococci are not suppurative microorganisms.

Subacute bacterial endocarditis is treated successfully by means of prolonged antibiotic therapy. The chronic infections leave valve deformities; therefore, early diagnosis is essential.

Acute Bacterial Endocarditis

Acute bacterial endocarditis results from either staphylococcus, beta-hemolytic streptococcus, pneumococcus, or other pyogenic virulent organism that infects the endocardium of the heart. The infected valve occurs secondarily to a primary infection in another site in the body after a surgical procedure, and in patients on steroid or antibiotic therapy (organisms are antibiotic resistant).

Normal heart valves are infected more commonly than valves previously damaged by rheumatic disease. Valvular vegetations of acute bacterial endocarditis appear as large, smooth, but lobulated masses, with ulcerations or perforation of the valve a possible feature. Bacterial emboli break off from the vegetations and produce abscesses in the heart, spleen, and kidneys.

Cardiovascular Syphilis

Cardiovascular syphilis represents a minor percentage of cardiovascular deaths. This form of syphilis occurs late in the disease approximately five to fifteen years after the appearance of the chancre. Syphilitic aortitis develops in the ascending portion of the arch of the aorta. Scarring and weakening of the media of the aorta result in aortic insufficiency, aortic aneurysm, and rarely, coronary ostial stenosis.

Aortic insufficiency due to syphilis results from the dilatation of the aortic ring, which permits a separation of the aortic valves at their commissures, and contracture and cordlike thickening of the free margins of the aortic valve cusps. Aortic valvular incompetence leads to dilatation and hypertrophy of the left ventricle of the heart and, subsequently, death due to congestive heart failure.

Stenosis of the coronary ostia occurs in the portion of the coronary artery within the aortic wall. Atherosclerosis of the aorta is more advanced during syphilis. Atherosclerotic lesions (severe) develop in the proximal segment of the aorta during syphilis.

Cor Pulmonale

Cor pulmonale, i.e. hypertrophy and dilatation of the right ventricle, is due to increase resistance in the pulmonary circulation. Tuberculosis, bronchiectasis, embolism, thrombosis, or emphysema leads to cor pulmonale when there is interference with the pulmonary circulation great enough to provoke right ventricular hypertrophy.

Myocarditis

Myocarditis is defined as an inflammatory disease of the myocardium. It produces a dilated flabby heart with areas of pallor. The inflammatory process is interstitial in location and consists of the mobilization of polymorphonuclear leukocytes to mononuclear cells and multinucleated giant cells. The inflammation may be primary in the heart or secondary to the heart due to a variety of infectious agents.

The etiology of myocarditis is generally diphtheria, virus infections (Coxsackie B virus), hypersensitivity reactions (rheumatic fever), and parasitic infections (trichinosis and Chagas' disease). Resolution of myocarditis yields a diffuse interstitial fibrosis.

Cardiomyopathy

Primary myocardial disease (cardiomyopathy) is defined as a variety of cardiac diseases that have in common progressive heart failure without hypertension, cardiac shunts, or significant valvular or coronary disease. The hearts are dilated and hypertrophied with varying degrees of opacity of the endocardium of the left ventricle. Cardiomyopathy is classified into a congenital group, a familial group, a geographical group, and a miscellaneous group.

DISEASES OF THE PERICARDIUM

Acute Pericarditis

Acute suppurative pericarditis follows a bacteremia due to staphylococci, streptococci, pneumococci, and other pyogenic microorganisms. During acute fibrinous pericarditis, the pericardial surfaces become rough due to adherent strands of pink fibrin. Fibrinous pericarditis is generally caused by cardiac infarction, uremia, and rheumatic fever.

Chronic Pericarditis

Chronic constrictive pericarditis (Pick's disease) produces a heart encased in inelastic dense and scarred tissue, which may involve the atria and proximal portion of the great vessels. The scar tissue is a centimeter in thickness and may undergo calcification. The etiology may be obscure or it may be due to a tuberculous infection or secondary to pulmonary, pleural, or lymph node involvement. Chronic constrictive pericarditis alters cardiac function by impairing the filling of the heart during diastole and leads to edema and ascites. Therapy consists of surgical excision of scar tissue.

Hydropericardium

Hydropericardium is defined as an accumulation of more than 10 to 50 mcl of clear fluid in the pericardial sac. The pericardial sac is capable of containing a liter or more of fluid without cardiac compression. Fluid accumulates in the pericardial sac in generalized edema, chronic congestive heart failure, myxedema, and chronic renal disease (nephrosis).

Hemopericardium

Hemopericardium is defined as spontaneous hemorrhage into the pericardial sac commonly resulting from the rupture of a myocardial infarct or the rupture of an aortic aneurysm (dissecting or syphilitic). Three hundred cubic centimeters or more of blood in the pericardial sac is capable of causing cardiac tamponade and death.

Neoplasms (Tumors) of the Heart

Metastatic tumors are more frequent than primary tumors of the heart. Tumors metastasize to the heart from the lungs, breast, lymph nodes, and skin, reaching the heart by way of the blood stream, lymphatic vessels, or by direct extension from an adjacent neoplasm. Small metastatic nodules generally develop in the pericardium, myocardium, or endocardium. The most common primary neoplasm of the heart is the myxoma, a benign tumor generally located in the left atrium. This tumor arises from endocardial cells and does not metastasize; however, they may produce embolism. Primary malignant neoplasms of the heart (rhabdomyosarcoma) are very rare.

Aneurysms of the Aorta

Aneurysm is defined as a localized dilatation of an artery. Aneurysms are classified as true aneurysms if the blood vessel wall forms the actual wall of the aneurysm and false aneurysms if the localized sac is surrounded by connective tissue. Aneurysms are also classified by their morphology as fusiform if the wall is dilated symmetrically or saccular if the localized sac (bulge) involves only one side of the blood vessel wall. An aneurysm may be infected (mycotic aneurysm) or noninfected (bland aneurysm). Aneurysms of the aorta have an incidence of 1 to 3 percent of autopsies. The most frequent aneurysms are the arteriosclerotic, dissecting, and syphilitic aneurysms respectively.

The arteriosclerotic aneurysm is the most common variety of aortic aneurysm. They are fusiform and generally involve the abdominal aorta below the renal arteries since atherosclerosis is extremely severe below the level of the renal arteries. The atherosclerosis is a major contributing factor to atrophy of the media, which is followed by formation of the aneurysm. Rupture is the lethal complication of this aneurysm and occurs in approximately one-third of instances. The small aneurysms measuring less than 4.5 cm in diameter, seldom rupture, however, the larger the aneurysm the greater the possibility of rupture. When the aneurysm enlarges, pain is produced in the abdomen or low back. This pain becomes excruciating in character when the rupture occurs. Mortality rate is 50 percent following a rupture of an aortic aneurysm.

The arteriosclerotic aneurysm generally contains a thrombus in the lumen. Rupture occurs on the lateral wall, producing a massive, left-sided, retroperitoneal hemorrhage. The wall of the aneurysm contains fibrous tissue with the media having disappeared.

Dissecting aneurysm is produced by the penetration of the circulating blood into the wall of an artery (aorta) for some distance. Dissecting aneurysm of the aorta occurs in a male, forty to sixty years of age, who has long-standing hypertension. He suddenly experiences excruciating substernal pain, which extends into the back and abdomen. An untreated dissecting aneurysm has a 75 percent mortality rate in a period of two weeks.

Degeneration of the media of an artery (aorta) is the predisposing factor for dissection. In the hypertensive patient, the lesions consist of defects in the muscle cells of the media. Cystic medionecrosis is a consistent feature of the dissecting aneurysm in cases of arachnodactyly.

Dissection begins in the ascending aorta, just above the aortic valve. An intimal tear occurs, allowing penetration of blood from the lumen of the aorta to the media. From this tear, the dissection proceeds both circumferentially and longitudinally between the middle and outer thirds of the media to involve the entire aorta in approximately one-third of instances of dissecting aneurysm. Death results due to rupture into the pericardial sac, pleural cavities (left), or into the mediastinum.

Syphilitic aneurysm occurs as a late manifestation of syphilis in males from thirty-five to fifty years of age. The aneurysm is more frequently located in the ascending arch and less frequently in the descending thoracic or upper abdominal segment of the aorta. Syphilitic aneurysm is generally saccular with a distinctive ringlike orifice at the site of its origin from the aorta. As the aneurysm enlarges the wall becomes thinner and thinner, ending in a rupture.

Syphilitic aneurysms of the ascending aorta may erode through the sternum and skin to produce massive hemorrhage or extend into the right lung, right main bronchus, or right pulmonary artery. Aneurysm in the descending thoracic or upper abdominal aorta may bulge posteriorly, producing an erosion of the vertebrae while sparing the intervertebral discs due to their lack of vascularity.

Peripheral Vascular Disease

Peripheral vascular disease is defined as the inadequacy of the circulation to an extremity (lower). Early symptoms of arterial insufficiency to the lower extremities are pain in the region of the calf on exertion and relief of pain with rest. This distal aspect of the lower limb may be pale, cold, cyanotic, or develop ulceration and gangrene.

Arteriosclerosis obliterans is the most frequent variety of peripheral vascular disease. It is caused by narrowing of the peripheral arteries due to atherosclerosis in elderly males. Diabetes mellitus is a predisposing factor to the development of this disease. The following blood vessels are involved by arteriosclerosis obliterans: iliac, femoral, popliteal, and tibial arteries. The arteries become thickened, tortuous, and calcified. The vessel lumen is narrowed or obliterated by fibrosis, hyalinization, and by atheroma. The media has disappeared, and calcification replaces this layer.

Raynaud's Disease

Raynaud's disease (syndrome) occurs in young women who complain of an increased sensitivity to cold. Exposure to cold causes blanching, cyanosis, and gangrene of the tips of the fingers. This syndrome is relieved by sympathectomy.

Thromboangiitis Obliterans

Buerger's disease (thromboangiitis obliterans) is a variety of peripheral vascular disease in males (exclusively). This disease is associated with heavy smoking in young Jewish males and is a progressive disease in the smoker.

Symptoms of Buerger's disease include intermittent claudication of one or both legs. The fingers are affected in 50 percent of cases. The lesions of the legs have an affinity for small, peripheral arteries (anterior and posterior tibials) while sparing the large arteries (iliac and femoral arteries). The lesions may be the result of organization of occluding thrombi rather than a primary inflammatory disease of the intima with associated thrombosis.

Temporal Arteritis

Temporal arteritis is defined as an inflammatory disease of obscure causation involving the temporal arteries in elderly females more often than in elderly males. Symptoms begin with malaise, anorexia, body aches, sweats and fever, headache, and extreme tenderness of temporal arteries. Blindness is the most serious complication.

The temporal artery contains a lumen that has nearly been obliterated by fibrous thickening of the intima or occluded completely by thrombosis. Lymphocytes, plasma cells, and giant cells may be present. The media is destroyed and replaced by multinucleated giant cells in the media or outer intima. Cortisone therapy controls the disease.

DISEASES OF VEINS

Phlebothrombosis and Thrombophlebitis

Phlebothrombosis is defined as a noninflammatory process related to alterations in the circulating blood. Thrombi develop in the veins of the lower extremities in over 50 percent of elderly hospitalized patients. These thrombi frequently propagate upward into the pelvic veins and may break loose and result in a fatal pulmonary emboli.

Thrombosis in peripheral veins of the elderly may be associated with an internal neoplasm. Phlebothrombosis occurs in one-third of patients with carcinoma of the body or tail of the pancreas. Thrombi in small pelvic veins undergo organization and subsequently calcify, producing small round opaque bodies (x-ray) termed *phleboliths*.

Thrombophlebitis is defined as a thrombosis occurring as a result of acute inflammation of a vein. Examples of thrombophlebitis are pylephlebitis (portal vein) and cavernous sinus thrombosis.

Varicose veins are defined as venous channels that, have undergone dilatation and become tortuous as a result of increased venous pressure or weakening of the wall of the vein. There is an hereditary weakness to the veins in the lower extremities. Varicose veins are twice as frequent in females as in males. Prolonged standing is a predisposing factor to development of varicose veins. As the veins dilate, their valves become incompetent. Dilated veins of the hemorrhoidal plexus are defined as hemorrhoids that result from chronic constipation or may be due to portal hypertension from cirrhosis of the liver. Esophageal varices also result from portal hypertension and are a common source of fatal hemorrhage in patients with cirrhosis. Varicocele is defined as left-sided dilatation of the pampiniform plexus of the veins in the scrotum. Upon palpation, the dilated vessels produce the sensation that the scrotum is composed of knotted, cordlike anatomic structures.

NEOPLASMS (TUMORS) OF BLOOD VESSELS
Benign Neoplasms of Blood Vessels

Hemangioma, lymphangioma, and the glomus tumor represent the benign neoplasms of blood vessels. Hemangiomas are either capillary or cavernous varieties depending upon the size of the blood vessels. Capillary hemangiomas develop on the skin, lip, and tongue. Cavernous hemangiomas occur in the skin and liver. Microscopically, the hemangioma is composed of large, blood-filled vascular channels lined by endothelial cells. These tumors are asymptomatic but bleed when traumatized.

NEOPLASMS (TUMORS) OF LYMPH VESSELS

Benign Tumors of Lymph Vessels

Lymphangioma is a benign tumor of lymph vessel origin located in the tongue, neck, and a variety of soft tissues. The lymphangioma of the neck or axilla is referred to as a cystic hygroma and is initially noted at birth or shortly thereafter. The lymphangioma is composed of irregular cystic spaces containing a clear fluid and lined by endothelial cells.

Malignant Tumors of Lymph Vessels

Lymphangiosarcoma is a rare malignant tumor of lymphatics, which develops in the lymphedematous arm of a patient following a radical mastectomy five to fifteen years previously. The hemangiopericytoma is a malignant tumor arising from pericytes. It is composed of capillaries surrounded by neoplastic spindle cells. The neoplastic cells are located externally to the vascular sheath of the capillaries.

The glomus tumor (gloangioma) is composed to cells originating from pericytes (cells that lie external to the vascular endothelium). This malignant tumor arises in the myoarterial glomus, a structure that shunts blood from the arterial system into the veins without passing through the capillaries. Pain arises from a tender blue nodule beneath the fingernail.

The hemangioendothelioma is a malignant tumor arising from the endothelium of blood vessels. Proliferation of endothelial cells is the prominent feature that forms capillary-sized channels. This neoplasm occurs during infancy and may be fatal within six months.

References

Angrist, A.A.: *JAMA, 183*:249, 1963.
Armstrong, M.L., et al.: *Circ Res, 27*:59, 1970.
Auerbach, O., et al.: *N Engl J Med, 273*:775-779, 1965.
Barbour, G.H., et al.: *Am J Cardiol, 7*:102, 1961.

Beerman, H., et al.: *Arch Intern Med, 105*:324, 1960.
Bennett, N. McK. and Forbes, J.A.: *Am Heart J, 74*:435. 1967.
Berenson, G.S.: *Hum Pathol, 2*:57, 1971.
Blankenhorn, M.A.: *Ann Intern Med, 23*:398, 1945.
Blount, G.S., et al.: *Circulation, 13*:499, 1956.
Bornstein, P.: *Am J Pathol, 49*:429, 1970.
Bragdon, J.H. and Levine, H.D.: *Am J Pathol, 25*:265, 1949.
Briggs, J.D., et al.: *West J Surg, 61*:499, 1953.
Brill, I.C.: *Mod Concepts Cardiovasc Dis, 26*:425, 1957.
Buerger, L.: *Am J Med Sci, 136*:567, 1908.
Buja, L.M., Khoi, N.B., and Roberts, W.C.: *Am J Cardiol, 26*:394, 1970.
Burch, G.E., et al.: *JAMA, 203*:1, 1968.
Burch, G. and Giles, T.: *J Chronic Dis, 24*:1, 1971.
Burch, G.E., et al.: *Am Heart J, 80*:556, 1970.
Burchell, H.B.: *Circulation, 12*:1068, 1955.
Cabezas-Moya, R. and Dragstedt, L.R.: *Arch Surg, 101*:632, 1970.
Caro, C.G., et al.: *Proc R. Soc Lond, 177*:109, 1971.
Carroll, R.E.: *JAMA, 198*:267, 1966.
Constantinides, P.: *Atherosclerosis, 6*:1, 1966.
Cookson, F.B.: *Br J Exp Pathol, 52*:62, 1971.
Crawford, T., et al.: *Lancet, 1*:181, 1961.
Dahl, L.K.: *N Engl J Med, 258*:1152, 1205, 1958.
Dalldorf, F.G. and Murphy, G.E.: *Am J Pathol, 37*:507, 1960.
Das, S.K.: *Circulation, 44*:612, 1971.
Davies, J.N.P. and Ball, J.D.: *Br Heart J, 17*:337, 1955.
Dayton, S. and Hashimoto, S.: *Exp Mol Pathol, 13*:253, 1970.
DeBakey, M.E. and Crawford, E.S.: *Mod Concepts Cardiovasc Dis, 38*:557, 1959.
Dustan, H.P., Page, I.H., and Poutasse, E.F.: *N Engl J Med, 261*:647-653, 1959.
Economov, S.G., et al.: *Surgery, 27*:21, 1960.
Editorial: Streptococci and rheumatic fever. *Lancet, 1*:485, 1967.
Edmondson, H.A.: *Am J Dis Child, 91*:168, 1956.
Elliot, R.H. and Dunbar, J.M.: *Arch Dis Child, 43*:451, 1968.
Ettinger, M.G., et al.: *Geriatrics, 24*:116, 1969.
Ferrans, V.J. and Roberts, W.C.: *Hum Pathol, 4*:222, 1973.
Finch, S.C. and Finch, C.A.: *Medicine, 34*:381, 1955.
Finland, M. and Barnes, M.W.: *Ann Intern Med, 72*:341, 1970.
Fisher, J.H.: *Can Med Assoc J, 83*:1136, 1960.
Follis, R.H.: *J Pediatr, 20*:347, 1942.
French, J.E.: *Semin Hematol, 8*:84, 1971.
Gore, I.: *Am J Pathol, 29*:613, 1953.
Gore, I and Arons, W.: *Arch Pathol, 48*:1, 1949.
Gore, I. and Barrows, S.: *Am J Clin Pathol, 29*:319, 1958.

Haust, M.D.: *Hum Pathol, 2*:2, 1971.
Heggtueit, H.A.: *Circulation, 29*:346, 1964.
Helfant, R.H., et al.: *N Engl J Med, 284*:1277, 1971.
Hellerstein, H.K. and Santiago-Stevenson, D.: *Circulation, 1*:93, 150.
Hirst, A.E., et al.: *Medicine, 37*:217, 1958.
Hudson, R.E.B.: *Am J Cardiol, 25*:73, 1970.
——: *Med Sci Law, 3*:180, 1968.
Hume, M., et al.: *Venous Thrombosis and Pulmonary Embolism.* Cambridge, Harvard U Pr, 1970.
Hunter, W.C., et al.: *Arch Intern Med, 68*:1, 1941.
Intersociety Commission for Heart Disease Resources: *Circulation, 42*:A55, 1970.
Jackson, B.T.: *N Engl J Med, 279*:80, 1968.
Jones, R.S. and Frazier, D.B.: *Arch Pathol, 50*:366, 1950.
Kagan, A., et al.: *Fed Proc (Suppl 11), 21*:52, 1962.
Kampmeier, R.H.: *Am J Med Sci, 192*:97, 1936.
Kannel, W.B., et al.: *J Occup Med, 9*:611, 1967.
Kannel, W.B.: *Nutr Today, 6*:2, 1971.
——: *Amer J Clin Nutr, 24*:1074, 1971.
——: *Hum Pathol, 2*:109, 1971.
Kaplan, M.H. and Meyeserian, M.: *Lancet, 1*:706, 1962.
Kariv, I., et al.: *Am J Cardiol, 28*:693, 1971.
Keefer, C.E.: *Ann Intern Med, 10*:1085, 1937.
——: *Am Heart J, 19*:352, 1940.
Keys, A.: *Circulation (Suppl 1), 41*:1, 1970.
Korn, D., et al.: *N Engl J Med, 267*:900, 1962.
Klynstra, F.B. and Bottcher, C.J.F.: *Atherosclerosis, 11*:451, 1970.
Larson, R.A. and Smith, F.L.: *Mayo Clin Proc., 18*:400, 1943.
Lehmann, H. and Lynes, J.G.: *Lancet, 1*:557, 1972.
MacDonald, R.A. and Robbins, S.L.: *Ann Intern Med, 46*:255, 1957.
MacMahon, B., et al.: *Br Heart J, 15*:121, 1953.
Mallory, G.K., et al.: *Am Heart J, 18*:647, 1939.
Martin, P. and Pearson, A.C.: *Br J Clin Pract, 10*:161, 1956.
Massumi, R.A., et al.: *Circulation, 31*:19, 1965.
Merkow, L.P., et al.: *Arch Pathol, 88*:390, 1969.
Miettinen, M., et al.: *Lancet, 2*:7782, 1972.
Morales, A.H. and Fine, G.: *Arch Pathol, 82*:9, 1966.
Morfit, J.M.: *Arch Surg, 81*:761, 1960.
Moss, N.S. and Benditt, E.P.: *Lab Invest, 23*:231, 1970.
Neal, R.W., et al.: *Mod Concepts Cardiovasc Dis, 38*:107, 1968.
Nemoto, T., et al.: *Surg Gynecol Obstet, 128*:489, 1969.
Oblath, R.W., et al.: *JAMA, 149*:1276, 1939.
O'Brien, P. and Brasfield, R.D.: *Cancer, 18*:249, 1965.
Osmundson, P.J.: *Postgrad Med, 49*:132, 1971.
Paul, O.: *Hosp Pract, 6*:91, 1971.

Perera, G.A.: *J Chronic Dis, 1*:33, 1955.
Pollack, A.A., et al.: *J Clin Invest, 28*:559, 1949.
Pomerance, A.: *Gerontol Clin, 14*:1, 1972.
Pratt, G.H.: *Am J Surg, 44*:31, 1939.
Price, A.C., et al.: *N Engl J Med, 286*:647, 1972.
Pyun, K.S., et al.: *Arch Pathol, 90*:181, 1970.
Roberts, W.C.: *Am J Med, 49*:151, 1970.
———: *Hosp Pract, 6*:89, 1971.
———: *Am J Med, 49*:151, 1970.
Ronchese, R.: *Am J Surg, 86*:376, 1953.
St. Geme, J.W., et al.: *N Eng J Med, 275*:339, 1966.
Sanders, M.G.: *Q J Stud Alcohol, 31*:324, 1970.
Saphir, O.: *Arch Pathol, 32*:1000, 1941, *33*:88, 1942.
Saphir, O.: *Am J Clin Pathol, 31*:534, 1959.
Saphir, O. and Karsner, H.T.: *J M Research, 44*:539, 1924.
Schatz, I.J., et al.: *Br Heart J, 28*:84, 1964.
Shanoff, H.M.: *Can Med Assoc J, 106*:55, 1972.
Sproul, E.E.: *Am J Cancer, 34*:566, 1938.
Stanbury, J.B., et al.: *The Metabolic Basis of Inherited Disease.* New York, McGraw, 1972, pp. 149-173.
Stamler, J.: *Br Heart J Suppl, 33*:145, 1971.
Stout, A.P.: *Ann Surg, 118*:445, 1943.
Stout, A.P. and Murray, M.R.: *Ann Surg, 116*:26, 1942.
Strehler, B.L., et al.: *J Gerontol, 14*:430, 1959.
Uwaydah, M.M. and Weinberg, A.N.: *N Engl J Med, 273*:1231, 1965.
Wagner, B.M. and Siew, S.: *Hum Pathol, 1*:45, 1970.
Walston, A., et al.: *Am Heart J, 79*:613, 1970.
Watt, H.F.: *Hum Pathol, 2*:31, 1971.
Wessler, S., et al.: *N Engl J Med, 262*:1149, 1960.
Wolf, P.L. and Bing, R.: *JAMA, 194*:674, 1965.
Yarington, C.T.: *JAMA, 173*:506, 1960.

CHAPTER 18

THE RESPIRATORY SYSTEM

PULMONARY EDEMA

WHEN AN obstruction occurs in the alveoli, the air pressure drops; therefore, edema occurs in the alveoli. Anoxia and damage to capillary walls, which take place during shock, are responsible for exudation of edema fluid into the alveoli. Left ventricular heart failure increases the hydrostatic pressure in the pulmonary capillaries, and edema occurs in the alveoli. The latter is the most common cause of pulmonary edema. During pulmonary edema, the alveolar walls are hyperemic and the alveolar spaces are filled with a pink staining, homogeneous fluid. The fluid comprising edema of the lung consists of a rich protein fluid, which is an excellent culture media for microorganisms.

Chronic passive hyperemia of the lung is due to right heart failure. The alveolar walls of the lung are thickened, and macrophages containing hemosiderin (heart failure cells) are present in the alveoli. Although pulmonary emboli are uncommon, they may cause sudden death when an embolus occludes the pulmonary artery.

PULMONARY EMBOLISM AND INFARCTION

A twenty-three-year-old pregnant female succumbed following delivery. At autopsy, an examination of the lungs revealed the presence of an amniotic fluid embolus. During labor, this pregnant female ruptured her membrane. Sudden contractions caused the amniotic fluid to enter a large, open vein. The amniotic fluid embolus terminated in the lung, producing a pulmonary infarction.

ATELECTASIS

Atelectasis is the collapse of a completely expanded lung. Primary atelectasis occurs physiologically in infants and newborns. Secondary atelectasis occurs in adults after a complete (not partial) bronchial obstruction. In an incomplete atelectasis, total collapse of the lung eventually occurs; however, it takes place late in the disease. Extrinsic fluid located in the chest may cause a collapse of the lung. A mechanical collapse of the lungs occurs by opening the chest. The primary atelectatic lung is airless, the lung tissue is not crepitant (crackling) or spongy. Secondary atelectasis consists of a collapsed lung containing black pigmentation (anthracosis).

INFECTIOUS DISEASES OF THE LUNGS

Three types of infectious diseases occur in the lungs, i.e. pulmonary abscesses and the bronchiectatic lung; bacterial pneumonias; and pulmonary infections due to higher forms of bacteria, fungi, viruses, and parasites.

BRONCHIECTASIS. Bronchiectasis is a term meaning the dilatation of bronchi of the lung. Two types of dilatations may occur in the bronchi, i.e. a local cystic or saccular dilated bronchus and a diffuse, fusiform, or cylindrical dilated bronchus. Bronchiectasis may be congenital and appears at birth. Acquired bronchiectasis occurs as a result of infection and overdistention of one bronchus or of a group of bronchi due to a chronic bronchitis. Purulent exudate accumulates in the bronchi. The overdistention of the bronchi results from tearing of the elastic fibers in the bronchial wall. A neoplasm may cause partial obstruction to a bronchus. During inspiration, a slight dilatation occurs in the bronchus as the air passes the partial obstruction. Complete obstruction develops during expiration. The air is trapped by the neoplasm that is obstructing the bronchi. Distal to the obstruction the lung shows emphysema, i.e. a pathologic increase in the air content of the lung, and the bronchi show bronchiectasis.

PNEUMONITIS. Beta-hemolytic streptococci, *Hemophilus influenza*, pneumococcus, and viruses provoke pneumonia. Beta-hemolytic streptococci and *Hemophilus influenza* cause interstitial pneumonia.

An anatomic classification of the pneumonias is the best available classification; however, this classification contains some deficiencies. The anatomic classification includes the following types of pneumonia: bronchopneumonia, lobar pneumonia, influenzal pneumonia, primary atypical pneumonia, interstitial pneumonia, and epidemic pneumonia of the newborn. Pneumonia generally begins as a tracheobronchitis accompanied by a dry cough. The infection extends into the alveolar walls and peribronchial tissue. The respiratory disease begins in the upper respiratory tract extending downward to the tracheobronchial tree.

Bronchopneumonia is an inflammation of the bronchi and peribronchial alveoli due to beta-hemolytic streptococcus in 3 to 5 percent; to staphylococcus in one percent; and to Friedländer's bacillus in one percent of infections of the lung. *Eschericia coli,* pneumococcus, *Hemophilus influenza* and *Nisseria catarrhalis* also produce pneumonia.

Pain is either absent or minimal during bronchopneumonia. The pleura is smooth and irregular nodularity occurs throughout the entire lung. Groups of peribronchial alveoli are affected by the infection and a purulent exudate is present in the bronchi and alveoli.

Lobar pneumonia involves an entire lobe or lobes of the lung, all consolidated as a unit in the same stage of pneumonitis. It is difficult to accurately separate the infection into definite stages; however, lobar pneumonia has four stages. Lobar pneumonia produces a pleuritis, and therefore, pain in the chest is a common finding during the early stages of the infection.

Lobar pneumonia is due to pneumococci, types 1, 2 and 4; and diplococcus or pneumococcus in approximately 90 percent of instances of the infection. The infection spreads from the upper respiratory tract into the terminal bronchi. The organisms spread rapidly from the hilus to the periphery of the lung in a matter of hours. The infection spreads under the pleura, causing an early pleuritis. The initial stage of lobar pneumonia is termed the *congestion stage.* The lung is red and congested or hyperemic. Edema and microorganisms are present in the alveoli along with a fibrinous exudate.

The second stage of lobar pneumonia is termed *red hepatization*. The alveolar walls are hyperemic, and edema, blood, fibrin and polymorphonuclear leukocytes are present in the alveoli. Red hepatization produces a solid lung.

The third stage of lobar pneumonia is termed *gray hepatization*. Pneumococci and fibrin are present; however, leukocytes disappear. Gray hepatization produces adherent lobes with loss of the normal lobar fissures of the lungs. The pleura is thickened during gray hepatization.

The fourth stage of lobar pneumonia is termed *resolution*. All foreign material disappears from the alveoli. Resolution requires several weeks. Organization is a severe complication of lobar pneumonia. However, lobar pneumonia is rarely seen in modern times.

Another epidemic variety of pneumonia is termed *influenzal pneumonia*. In this variety of pneumonitis, the walls of the alveoli undergo necrosis with thrombosis of lymphatics and capillaries.

The clinical syndrome of primary atypical pneumonia includes a cough, cyanosis and a few rales. However, the alveoli are not involved because the inflammation is localized to the alveolar walls. Cold agglutins are high in primary atypical pneumonia.

Interstitial pneumonia is a term describing the pathogenesis of bronchopneumonia. Epidemic interstitial bronchopneumonia is due to beta-hemolytic streptococci. The lungs are congested and edematous with dilated bronchi.

Epidemic pneumonia of the newborn is a viral pneumonia. Cytomegalic viral inclusions are present in the cells of the bronchial epithelium. A thick hyaline membrane lines the alveoli in this viral pneumonia.

LUNG ABSCESS. The formation of abscesses in the lung represents a serious infection because of the lack of resistance of pulmonary tissue. Lung abscesses develop secondarily to bacterial pneumonias and are also due to trauma, atelectasis, and pleura effusions. Aerobic streptococci and staphylococci, and anaerobic fusobacterium, micrococci, streptococci, and bacterioides are present in lung abscesses.

HYALINE MEMBRANE DISEASE OF INFANCY. Hyaline membrane disease of infancy is a fatal disorder producing difficulty in breathing after birth so that retraction of the sternum takes place during inhalation. Obstruction occurs in the trachea and large or small bronchi. The child is cyanotic (blue) and anoxic.

LABORATORY DIAGNOSIS OF THE PNEUMONIAS. Laboratory diagnosis of the pneumonias is made, in part, by sputum studies to determine the predominating organism responsible for the pneumonia. Fresh, single, sputum samples originating in the bronchi are utilized for laboratory diagnosis. A series of single specimens is necessary before a definitive diagnosis is established. Every twenty-four hours a sample of bronchial sputum is obtained for the sputum studies. The sputum is collected in a sterile, wide-mouth bottle, which is well stoppered to prevent contamination by other microorganisms. The sputum is cultured on blood agar. The aerobic organisms are further cultured on broth. Initially, a smear is prepared of the sputum in order to report the tentative diagnosis to the clinician. Within forty-five hours the microbiology laboratory will report the results of the cultured sputum, reporting on the predominate organism. Microbiologic studies are useful in the acute stage of bronchiectasis because the microorganisms present may vary from aerobic to anaerobic types.

In pulmonary infections due to tubercle bacilli, three sputum examinations are generally undertaken, and the smear is prepared using the acid-fast stain. If the organisms on the smear prove to be tubercle bacilli, it still does not provide definite evidence that tuberculosis is present. The tubercle bacilli must first be cultured and then inoculated into guinea pigs. A period of three to eight weeks is required before the guinea pig develops the infection and succumbs to tuberculosis.

BRONCHIAL ASTHMA AND EMPHYSEMA

In bronchial asthma there is an increase in the secretion of mucous into the bronchi, causing dilatation of the bronchial wall. A spasm in the bronchial wall traps air behind a partial obstruction created by the secretion of mucous and accompanying exudate. The obstruction may rupture alveoli and tear the elastic tissue present in the wall of alveoli. Overdistention of the lung may occur in asthma and result in emphysema. The emphysematous lung remains enlarged because the elastic tissue in the wall of alveoli is torn; therefore, the lung cannot collapse.

Emphysema results from chronic bronchitis, pulmonary tuberculosis, whooping cough, and bronchial asthma. The following findings are considered pathognomonic of emphysema: decrease in alveolar depth, increase in alveolar diameter, and flattening of alveolar bases.

PNEUMOCONIOSIS

Any foreign material, animate or inanimate, inhaled into the lungs causes a reaction in the lungs termed *pneumoconiosis*. Anthracosis is due to a foreign material that does not produce a true pneumoconiosis because no tissue reaction is elaborated by the body. Berylliosis is a true pneumoconiosis. Beryllium may be inhaled from either defective or broken fluorescent lights. A transitory pneumonitis results from the inhalation of beryllium. Asbestosis is a pneumoconiosis due to the inhalation of asbestos fibers. A high incidence of carcinoma of the lung appears to be associated with pneumoconiosis due to the inhalation of asbestos.

Silicosis is the most important pneumoconiosis because silica is present in all minerals. Anthracosilicosis (miner's lung) is due to inhalation of coal and silica. The lung contains raised gray nodules, becomes solid, and no longer crepitant. Siderosilicosis is due to inhalation of iron and silica. Silicosis does not develop for approximately three to fifteen years following the initial inhalation of silica. Tuberculosis accounts for 75 percent of deaths in individuals with silicosis. An intense tissue reaction takes place around the silica particles consisting of a proliferation of connective tissue involving an intense proliferation of reticulum.

PULMONARY TUBERCULOSIS

The majority of tuberculosis infections in the lungs are due to the human variety of tubercle bacilli and only rarely to the bovine tubercle bacilli. Racial factors are important in pulmonary tuberculosis. Individuals with pigmented skin are more prone to severe pulmonary tuberculosis. The adult Negro has the same primary reaction as the Negro child because he has a poor immunity to tuberculosis. The degree of hypersensitivity is a most important factor in pulmonary tuberculosis. The balance between immunity and allergy determines the reaction of the pulmonary tissues to the tubercle bacillus.

Polymorphonuclear leukocytes are the initial cells that migrate to the affected area of the lung. The macrophages arrive later in the area of infection and are transformed into epithelioid cells termed *epithelioid histiocytes*. The epithelioid histiocytes fuse to form Langhan's giant cells.

In tuberculosis, large areas of caseation necrosis are present. Langhan's giant cells are centrally located in the early tubercle prior to the development of caseation necrosis. Epithelioid histiocytes contain phagocytized tubercle bacilli in their cytoplasm. Hyaline connective tissue replaces the caseation necrosis in the healed lesion of pulmonary tuberculosis.

Pulmonary tuberculosis may represent a primary and reinfection variety. The pulmonary infection in an adult may appear similar to the primary infection in a child. In the latter instance, the primary pulmonary infection is present in the adult because he has never been previously exposed to tubercle bacilli. The primary infection of tuberculosis is more common in young children than in adults because the degree of immunity is minimal in children and gradually increases with age. Adults undergo a subclinical exposure to tubercle bacilli and, therefore, develop an immunity and hypersensitivity. Caseation necrosis subsequently develops in the lung. The pulmonary infection becomes walled off, calcium is deposited, and ossification occurs in the healed pulmonary lesions of tuberculosis.

In children the situation is different than in adults. The primary pulmonary tubercular infection produces a subpleural lesion located at the extreme outer aspect of any lobe. Bronchopneumonia and pleuritis occur and the infection spreads rapidly by way of the lymphatics to the hilar lymph nodes. Calcification of a pulmonary tubercle does not indicate that healing is complete. Large numbers of viable organisms are present within the calcified tissues as well as within the epithelioid histiocytes.

Reinfection tuberculosis of the lungs is due to endogenous infection from viable tubercle bacilli present in the primary infected area. The liquified necrotic caseous material that develops may be coughed up, leaving a cavity, i.e. cavitation of the lung. The cavity may heal following collapse, provided air is withheld from entering the cavitation. The collapse of a cavitation in the lung is due either to the closure of the bronchus or to stoppage of the oxygen supply. Reinfection tuberculosis occurs in the upper portion of the lungs and spreads to hilar lymph nodes. When the cavitation enlarges, tubercle bacilli grow through the wall of the cavity into viable lung tissue and disseminate throughout the lung. Dissemination also occurs by way of the blood stream, and miliary tuberculosis develops with numerous minute tubercles present throughout the lung. Lymphatic and bronchogenic dissemination are the remaining routes for the spread of pulmonary tuberculosis.

FUNGAL INFECTIONS OF THE LUNGS

Histoplasmosis is the most common fungal disease of the lungs in the Mississippi valley. Fungi enter the respiratory tract and produce a subclinical infection. An atypical pneumonitis results from inhalation of the conidophore of histoplasmosis.

In dry areas of the United States, such as the San Joaquin valley, coccidioidomycosis occurs in the majority of individuals residing in the area. The fungal infection is, therefore, termed *valley fever*. The disease occurs in the form of a subclinical infection of which the individual is not aware. Coccidioidomycosis infection begins in the upper respiratory tract, accompanied by a cough and bronchitis. Five percent of the affected individuals with coccidioidomycosis infection have pleural effusions. Immunity is permanent, and reinfection does not occur in coccidioidomycosis. Subclinical coccidioidomycosis is a disseminated disease. The sedimentation rate drops and the complement fixation test may be useful in the diagnosis of coccidioidomycosis. Individuals with pigmented skin have a predisposition to coccidioidomycosis and are more prone to fatality. Two-tenths of one percent of individuals with valley fever have disseminated coccidioidomycosis. Fifty percent of individuals with disseminated coccidiodomycosis survive the fungal infection.

Monila albicans is an invasive fungus capable of producing pulmonary moniliasis. Monilia infection is found in the lungs of patients with any type of debilitating pulmonary disease.

Actinomycosis is a fungal disease which infects the lungs. *Actinomycosis bovis* is the most common member of this group and is capable of infecting the lung.

NEOPLASMS OF THE LUNG

Carcinoma of the lung is one of the most prevalent carcinomas in humans. Fifteen percent of all carcinomas in the human body are carcinomas of the lung. Lung carcinoma occurs between forty-five and sixty-five years of age. A higher instance of pulmonary carcinoma occurs in the right lung compared to the left lung primarily because the right lung is larger. Males have a higher incidence of carcinoma of the lung than females by a three to one ratio.

Factors to be considered in the production of lung carcinoma include the following carcinogens: (1) arsenic is a carcinogenic agent and is present in cigarette papers, (2) hydrocarbons in the smoke are carcinogens, (3) radium produces a high incidence of lung carcinoma, and (4) asbestos is associated with a high incidence of lung carcinoma.

The initial signs and symptoms of carcinoma of the lung include the following: atypical pneumonitis, atelectasis and bronchiectasis, cough, dyspnea, pain, and enlarged bronchial lymph nodes. The first sign of lung carcinoma may be the presence of hepatic and cerebral metastases. Carcinoma of the lungs is the most widely metastasizing of all carcinomas. Carcinomas of the lung are moderately radioresponsive.

BRONCHIAL ADENOMA. Bronchial adenomas represent the most important benign neoplasm of the bronchi and lung. Bronchial adenomas may undergo malignant transformation and metastasize to the regional lymph nodes. The mean age for the occurrence of bronchial adenomas is twenty-eight years.

BRONCHOGENIC CARCINOMA. Primary lung carcinoma is principally bronchogenic in origin and develops from the bronchial mucosa. There are three basic types of bronchogenic carcinomas of the lung, i.e. the squamous cell carcinoma, the adenocarcinoma and the anaplastic carcinoma (oat cell carcinoma).

Squamous cell carcinoma of the lung is the most common bronchogenic carcinoma. It represents 40 to 60 percent of all pulmonary carcinomas. Over 90 percent of squamous cell carcinomas of the lung occur in male cigarette smokers. There is strong evidence that lung carcinoma is due to heavy cigarette smoking. Squamous cell carcinoma generally arises from the bronchi adjacent to the hilus of the lung. Metastatic squamous cell carcinomas from the pharynx, larynx, and oral cavity may metastasize to the lungs and, therefore, may be readily confused with primary bronchogenic carcinoma of the lungs. The development of the squamous cell carcinoma may be preceded by metaplasia of the cylindrical bronchial epithelium to squamous epithelium.

The adenocarcinoma is the rarest of the bronchogenic carcinomas. Thirty-five percent of bronchogenic carcinomas in females are adenocarcinomas. The adenocarcinoma may occur as an undifferentiated (anaplastic) bronchogenic carcinoma arising from the mucous-secreting glands of the bronchi.

The anaplastic carcinoma or oat cell carcinoma arises from the bronchial epithelium of the main stem bronchi. It comprises approximately 40 percent of the bronchogenic carcinomas. The anaplastic carcinoma spreads by the lymphatics and blood stream. Metastases are present in approximately 90 percent of instances due to the explosive spread of neoplastic oat cells.

Bronchiolar carcinoma represents a fourth type of carcinoma of the lung. The bronchiolar carcinoma (alveolar cell carcinoma) develops from the cells of the terminal bronchioles or cells lining the alveoli of the lung. The bronchiolar carcinoma generally arises from the mucous-secreting epithelium of the terminal bronchioles. Bronchiolar carcinoma represents less than 4 percent of all forms of lung carcinoma.

Bronchogenic carcinomas spread far and wide. Metastatic neoplasms may be the initial evidence that a primary carcinoma of the lung is present. Bronchogenic carcinomas spread throughout the lungs by way of the lymphatics and bronchioles. The neoplasm spreads to lymph nodes by way of the lymphatics and to distant organs by way of the blood stream and lymphatics.

References

Auerbach, O., et al.: *Arch Environ Health, 21*:754, 1970.
Azzopardi, J.G. and Williams, E.D.: *Cancer, 222*:274, 1968.
Bignall, J.R. and Martin, M.: *Lancet, 2*:60, 1972.
Burrows, B. and Kettel, L.J.: *Geriatrics, 24*:72, 1969.
Carrington, C.B.: *N Engl J Med, 280*:787, 1969.
Falk, J.A. and Briscoe, W.A.: *Ann Intern Med, 72*:595, 1970.
Farber, S.M. and Wilson, R.H.L.: *Ciba Found Symp, 20*:35, 1968.
Farr, G.H., et al.: *Am J Pathol, 60*:347, 1970.
Grieco, M.C.: *Bull NY Acad Med, 46*:597, 1970.
Hagadorn, J.E.: *Am J Pathol, 57*:17, 1969.
Hammond, E.C., et al.: *Arch Environ Health, 21*:748, 1970.
Henle, W., et al.: *J Natl Cancer Inst, 44*:225, 1970.
Hume, M., et al.: *Venous Thrombosis and Pulmonary Embolism*, Cambridge, Harvard U, Pr, 1970.
Koffler, D., et al.: *Am J Pathol, 54*:293, 1969.
Kueppers, F.: *Science, 165*:899, 1969.
Larson, R.K., et al.: *Ann Intern Med, 72*:627, 1970.
Laurenzi, G.A.: *Advances Cardiopulm Dis, 4*:198, 1969.
Lieberman, J.: *N Engl J Med, 281*:279, 1969.
Mittman, C., et al.: *Chest, 60*:214, 1971.
Pollak, V.E. and Mendoza, N.: *Med Clin North Am, 55*:1397, 1971.
Poskitt, T.R.: *Am J Med, 49*:250, 1970.
Pratt, P.C. and Kilburn, K.H.: *Hum Pathol, 1*:443, 1970.
Sanerkin, N.G.: *Ann Allergy, 28*:528, 1970.
Sevitt, S. and Gallagher, N.G.: *Br J Surg, 55*:481, 1968.
Szentivanyi, A.: *J Allergy Clin Immunol, 42*:203, 1968.
Walcott, G., et al.: *Am J Med, 49*:70, 1970.
Willoughby, W.F. and Dixon, F.J.: *J Immunol, 104*:28, 1970.
Wynder, E.L. and Hoffman, D.: *Med Clin North Am, 50*:631, 1966.
Ziskind, M. and Saunders, M.: *Am J Med Sci, 222*:81, 1953.

CHAPTER 19

KIDNEYS AND LOWER URINARY TRACT

CONGENITAL ABNORMALITIES OF THE KIDNEYS

AGENESIS OF THE KIDNEY. Renal agenesis may be unilateral or bilateral (incompatible with life). The newborn presents the following external features at birth, which indicate agenesis of the kidneys: complete absence or diminished amniotic fluid, long and low placed ear lobes, receding chin, prominent intercantus of the eye, increased spacing between the eyes, and flattened tip of the nose.

CONGENITAL HYPOPLASIA AND DYSPLASIA OF THE KIDNEY. The true hypoplastic kidney is a small organ regardless of the age of the individual. In the hypoplastic kidney a reduction is present in both the nephrons and glomeruli. Unilateral hypoplasia is more common than the bilateral form. If one kidney is not functioning, the other kidney becomes enlarged due to compensatory hypertrophy.

Abnormality of position may result in the fusion of two kidneys producing the horseshoe kidney. In the horseshoe kidney an isthmus is present in the caudal portion joining the two kidneys. The kidney may migrate and become fused with the kidney on the opposite side, forming either a double kidney or a fused single kidney. Ectopic kidneys occur when they move downward from their normal site.

Congenital polycystic disease of the kidney is generally bilateral; rarely is it unilateral. Congenital polycystic kidney is divided into two types, i.e. the congenital infantile and the congenital adult types. The congenital infantile polycystic kidney is initiated *in utero* and undergoes a prenatal increase in size so that the combined weight of the kidneys is 600 gm. The fetus lives *in utero* with the polycystic kidney because it is not dependent on renal filtration. However, the newborn may succumb several days or weeks following delivery due to renal failure. Cysts may occupy the majority of the renal substance, therefore only a few nephrons are left to operate. Adult congenital polycystic disease of the kidney begins *in utero* and is found in late infancy, childhood, young adults, and adults from forty to sixty years of age. The disease is present throughout the life of the individual.

DISEASES OF THE KIDNEYS THAT TERMINATE IN UREMIA

UREMIA. Uremia is of unknown etiology and represents the terminal phase of renal insufficiency. Uremia is due to the retension of metabolic nitrogenous products, which are generally excreted by the kidney. The complex findings consist of the following: acidosis, high concentration of urea, nitrogen, uric acid, and acid creatinine in the blood. The calcium/phosphorus ratio is abnormal with a great increase in phosphorus and decrease in calcium. The kidneys are unable to concentrate urine or to function under increased demands. Uremia may be accompanied by bone changes and hypoplasia of the parathyroid glands, uremic pericarditis, edematous lungs, edematous brain, gastrointestinal tract hemorrhage, necrosis of the spleen, termed *spotted spleen,* inspissation of secretions in the pancreas, and hemorrhages in the skin and mucous membranes. A frost forms over the skin termed *uremic frost.*

The tissue alterations in uremia due to renal failure start in the glomeruli as a glomerulonephritis. Renal failure is preceded by vascular lesions, which cause destruction of glomeruli and nephrons, and by bacterial infection and inflammation, which destroy the glomeruli.

GLOMERULONEPHRITIS. Glomerulonephritis is an inflammation of the glomerular tufts. The inflammation may result in proliferation or exudation in the glomeruli. The etiology of the disease is obscure; however, it is related to infection probably with streptococci. The disease may be the result of an allergic phenomena of renal tissue to microorganisms or their products.

There are three stages of glomerulonephritis, i.e. acute, subacute, and chronic. The three stages are not distinct entities but rather blend together into one disease entity.

Acute glomerulonephritis may be initiated by group A hemolytic streptococcus—type 12 in young individuals. The surface of the kidneys is smooth and is studded with numerous petechial hemorrhages (flea-bitten kidney). The enlarged glomeruli are highly cellular due to the proliferation of capillary endothelium, exudation of polymorphonuclear leukocytes in the glomerular tufts, and thrombi in the capillaries. The flow of blood through the glomeruli is slowed, resulting in decreased output of urine, and leakage of red blood cells and albumin into the urine. Diffuse involvement of glomeruli during acute glomerulonephritis may result in death.

Subacute glomerulonephritis may be accompanied by uremia in a matter of months. The kidneys are enlarged, mottled yellow, and there is involvement of practically all of the glomeruli. The most prominent alteration in the glomeruli consists of proliferation of the epithelium of the capsule of the glomeruli to form "glomerular crescents." The glomerular tufts are, however, separated from the glomerular crescents, and hyalinized tufts are generally absent. The tubules become atrophic and contain red cell casts. The urinary output is normal or decreased, and large amounts of protein are excreted in the urine. The plasma proteins are diminished, and A/G ratio is reversed to 1/1. Subacute glomerulonephritis may be unilateral; however, this phase is generally a bilateral diffuse form of the disease.

Chronic glomerulonephritis may follow the acute and subacute forms of the disease by a progressive failure of renal function. The disease slowly progresses for many years with minimal clinical symptoms. However, there is a decrease of renal function. The terminal phase of the disease is always the development of uremia and an inability to concentrate urine. The unconcentrated urine is, therefore, excreted in large quantities, producing nocturia and polyuria.

Grossly, depressed zones are present on the surface of the kidney. These zones represent scars located beneath the capsule. The elevated portion of the surface of the kidney represents areas of viable nephrons. The kidneys are small and contracted during chronic glomerulonephritis.

Numerous glomeruli are converted into partial hyaline areas or a complete hyalinization takes place in the capillary tufts. The renal tubules undergo atrophic changes, and there is an increase in the interstitial connective tissue around the glomeruli and between the tubules. The tubules contain hyaline casts. Some glomeruli show capsular adhesions and are highly cellular. Hypertension develops in the terminal phase of chronic glomerulonephritis as a result of loss of the glomerular nephrons, scarring, and vascular sclerosis. It may be difficult to distinguish between nephrosclerosis and chronic glomerulonephritis. A secondarily contracted kidney indicates that it has passed through the stages of acute and subacute glomerulonephritis.

VASCULAR DISEASE OF THE KIDNEY

Thrombosis of the renal artery, arteriosclerosis, and renal venous thrombosis may result in infarction of the kidney. Changes in the small vessels of the kidney are almost invariably associated with an elevated blood pressure.

Glomerulonephritis is associated with hypertension. A small change is readily produced in the vessels of the kidney during hypertension. Diffuse changes occur in the arterioles throughout the body as well as in the kidney during hypertension. Essential hypertension occurs when the systolic pressure is over 200 and the diastolic pressure is 130. Alterations in the nephrons are due to narrowing of the interlobular artery, which results from atrophic changes. Glomeruli shrink into hyalinized balls due to a deficient blood supply to the glomeruli. Nephrons in the area undergo atrophic changes. However, not all nephrons undergo hyalinization, and some nephrons are retained in a normal state. The contracted kidney does not have a normal blood supply and is poorly vascularized. It is possible for some nephrons to survive because they obtain blood by means of anastomosis. Grossly, due to essential hypertension, the contracted kidney has an adherent capsule and a granular surface.

Essential hypertension is due to nephrosclerosis, fibrosis, and the contracted kidney. Seven to ten percent of individuals with essential hypertension die of uremia. Essential hypertension may be complicated by malignant hypertension. Malignant nephrosclerosis may be superimposed on early or late essential hypertension.

Malignant nephrosclerosis produces alterations in arterioles termed *necrotizing arteriolitis*. The necrotizing change is superimposed on hyaline arteriolar changes which occur in the less affected arterioles. No structures are recognized in malignant nephrosclerosis. The afferent arterioles, glomeruli and capillary tufts undergo fibrinoid necrosis. In malignant nephrosclerosis the patient generally dies of uremia and cardiovascular changes.

PYELONEPHRITIS

Pyelonephritis is another renal disease leading to a contracted kidney. Glomerulonephritis, arteriolar nephrosclerosis, malignant nephrosclerosis, and pyelonephritis all terminate in the contracted kidney and uremia. The hypertension that accompanies unilateral pyelonephritis is curable. However, the hypertension that accompanies bilateral pyelonephritis in incurable. Enterococci, *Proteus vulgaris, Escherichia coli, Pseudomonas aeruginosa* and *Aerobacter aerogenes* are responsible for the development of pyelonephritis. The disease generally reaches the kidneys by the ascending route and is commonly due to an obstructive phenomenon, causing stasis of fluid. In pyelonephritis the infection may be of the uncommon descending type, in which instance it spreads downward to involve the kidney.

Grossly, the pyelonephritic kidney is enlarged with multiple abscesses located on the surface of the organ. Perinephritic abscesses occur since the infection spreads through the adherent capsule to the perirenal tissue. The individual may die of a suppurative pyelonephritis with renal failure, uremia, and sepsis. The pyelonephritis may, however, subside or undergo acute exacerbations.

In the chronic stages of pyelonephritis, the kidney becomes small and contracted, weighing approximately 100 gm. The surface contains irregular retracted areas with either smooth or granular parenchyma.

The kidney in acute glomerulonephritis is large, red, and

hemorrhagic. In subacute glomerulonephritis the kidney is large and pale. In chronic glomerulonephritis the kidney is small, pale, and granular, representing a secondary contracted kidney. In arteriolonephrosclerosis a red, contracted kidney is present, containing finely uniform granularity. In chronic pyelonephritis the kidney is contracted, irregularly scarred, and granular.

TUBERCULOSIS OF THE KIDNEY

Tuberculosis of the kidneys may be unilateral or bilateral. The initial tubercular focus spreads to the calyces, infundibulum, pelvis, and ureters. Tuberculosis of the mucous membrane of the pelvis has the gross appearance of a nonspecific ulcer. The infection starts in the renal pelvis, which initially undergoes enlargement. Tubercle bacilli spread into a static urine, and the bacilli ascend into the kidney proper, resulting in infection of renal substance. Tubercles are studded irregularly over the surface of the thickened ureter and occur irregularly and conglomerantly throughout the substance of the kidney.

In tuberculous pyelonephritis the ureteral stricture is involved by ulceration, dilatation occurs in the pelvis, and the calcyes are ulcerated. Two factors are responsible for enlargement of the pelvis and calyces, i.e. obstruction and retention of urine, and the progress of tuberculous ulcers with erosion of pyramids. If obstruction of the ureter occurs, the rate of progression of the tuberculosis is enhanced. The entire kidney may be replaced by caseation necrosis, leaving a shell of viable renal tissue.

HYDRONEPHROSIS

Nephritis means inflammation of the kidney. Nephrosis means a degenerative change in the kidney. Hydronephrosis means a dilated renal pelvis and dilated infundibulum and calyces accompanied by degeneration of renal parenchyma due to pressure atrophy. Hydronephrosis is brought about either by a disturbance in the flow of urine from the renal pelvis or by a congenital abnormal nerve supply to the ureter.

In hydronephrosis the obstructive phenomenon produces a dilatation of the ureters and the renal pelvis. The pelvis enlarges as a result of the obstruction, and hydronephrosis develops. A stricture may occur at the ureter-pelvic junction or stones may be present, giving rise to hydronephrosis in the proximal or distal ureter. In hydronephrosis the pelvis and infundibulum are enlarged and the calyces become hollowed out. Hydronephrosis may occur accompanied by an acute infection of the kidney. The fluid that is present in hydronephrosis has a clear watery consistency. When suppuration is superimposed upon the hydronephrosis the clear fluid changes its character and a pyelonephrosis results, i.e. pyelonephritis plus hydronephrosis.

Expansion of the kidney and atrophy of the renal parenchyma occur in pyelonephrosis. The kidney increases from three to five times its normal size during hydronephrosis.

Renal calculi are renal stones that form in the kidney and may be found in the bladder. The calculi may be small in size and therefore are capable of migrating down the ureter, resulting in ureteral cholic. The smaller calculi are generally passed by the patient. A spasm may occur in the ureter containing the renal calculi with resultant pain. Hydronephrosis may occur as a consequence or complication of the renal calculi. Large calculi occur in the renal pelvis and have the morphology of fingerlike projections termed *staghorn renal calculi*.

NEOPLASMS OF THE KIDNEY

BENIGN NEOPLASMS OF THE KIDNEY. Benign neoplasms are frequently located in the kidney. *Fibromas* occur as nodules in the pyramids of the kidney. Occasionally, smooth muscle combines with a fibrous connective tissue proliferation to form a leiomyofibroma of the kidney. Small lipomas are located in the cortex more frequently than in the medulla. Leiomyomas may occur on the renal parenchyma not associated with the fibroma. Adenomas occur in the scarred areas of the kidney as small well-circumscribed masses.

Papillomas occur in the renal pelvis and resemble papillomas of the bladder. The papilloma of the bladder has certain inherent dangers. The papilloma of the renal pelvis may have a benign architecture and still tend to spread down the ureter. The pelvic papilloma may become a frankly invasive neoplasm.

MALIGNANT NEOPLASMS OF THE KIDNEY. Wilms' tumor is a

rare neoplasm of the kidney in children, generally prior to seven years of age. Wilms' tumor is responsible for one-fifth of all of the malignant neoplasms of children. This neoplasm is a mixed tumor containing glandular elements and sarcomatous tissue both arising from misplaced mesodermal tissue, which retains the ability to form both epithelial and connective tissues. Wilms' tumor grows rapidly, invades the surrounding tissue, and metastasizes by way of the blood stream to the brain, lymph nodes, and liver.

Hypernephroma or renal cell carcinoma is a common malignant tumor of the kidneys of adults. Small foci of adrenal cells may be displaced to the kidney. It is hypothesized that the latter adrenal cells give rise to the hypernephroma. However, the latter observation is inconclusive. The hypernephroma is fundamentally an adenocarcinoma of the kidney, which develops more frequently in males over forty years of age. This neoplasm consists of large, clear cells in sheets and cords with minimal connective tissue stroma. The neoplasm grows, causing atrophy of the kidney. In advanced stages there is widespread invasion of renal tissue. Metastases follow renal invasion to the bones, liver, and lungs. The early stage of this neoplasm may be difficult to diagnose because clinical symptoms are minimal.

PELVIS AND URETER

ABNORMALITIES OF THE PELVIS AND URETER. A double pelvis or two ureters are examples of abnormalities arising in the pelvis and ureters. The ureters either unite and fuse into a single structure, or they have separate openings into the bladder.

URETERITIS AND PYELITIS. Inflammation of a ureter is termed *ureteritis* and inflammation of the pelvis of the kidney is termed *pyelitis*. Calculi may be associated with both ureteritis and pyelitis.

NEOPLASMS OF THE PELVIS AND URETER. Papillomas of the pelvis and ureter are benign neoplasms; however, they show a great tendency to recur. Malignant neoplasms of the pelvis and ureter include the papillary carcinoma, transitional cell carcinoma, and infiltrating squamous cell carcinoma.

URINARY BLADDER

INFLAMMATORY CYSTITIS. Inflammation of the urinary bladder is termed *cystitis*. Inflammatory cystitis is generally secondary to infection in the surrounding organs and tissues and may follow the placement of a catheter or use of the cystoscope. The inflammation causes increased urination accompanied by burning and painful micturition. The urine contains pus, bacteria, and albumin.

NEOPLASMS OF THE URINARY BLADDER. Benign neoplasms (rare) of the urinary bladder have a tendency to recur following excision. The transitional papilloma is a histopathologically benign lesion, which recurs and is considered a grade one transitional cell carcinoma. The malignant neoplasms of the urinary bladder include the papillary transitional cell carcinoma, epidermoid carcinoma and the adenocarcinoma. Papillary carcinoma is the most common neoplasm of epithelial origin occurring in the bladder. Hematuria, dysuria, and secondary infection are clinical and are laboratory findings associated with papillary carcinoma of the urinary bladder. Epidermoid carcinoma is less common than the papillary carcinoma.

References

Angell, M.E., et al.: *N Engl J Med, 278:*1303, 1968.
Aoki, S., et al.: *N Engl J Med, 281:*1375, 1969.
Arakawa, M.: *Lab Invest, 23:*489, 1970.
Bailey, G.L., et al.: *Circulation, 38:*582, 1968.
Berger, J.: *Transplant Proc, 1:*939, 1969.
Black, D.A.K., et al.: *Br Med J, 3:*421, 1970.
Bokisch, V.A., et al.: *J Exp Med, 129:*1109, 1969.
Boyce, W.H.: *Am J Med, 45:*673, 1968.
Bryant, R.E., et al.: *J Infect Dis, 126:*1, 1972.
Burkholder, P.M., et al.: *Lab Invest, 23:*459, 1970.
Cameron, J.S.: *Br Med J, 4:*285, 1970.
Cameron, J.S., et al.: *Br Med J, 4:*7, 1970.
Churg, J., et al.: *Lancet, 1:*1299, 1970.
Combes, B., et al.: *Lancet, 2:*234, 1971.
Cotran, R.S.: *J Infect Dis, 120:*109, 1969.
Dodge, W.F., et al.: *N Engl J Med, 286:*273, 1972.
Eknoyan, G., et al.: *N Engl J Med, 280:*677, 1969.
Feldman, B.H.: *Invest Urol, 8:*575, 1971.

Franklin, W.A., et al.: *Arch Pathol, 94*:230, 1972.
Gault, M.H., et al.: *Ann Intern Med, 68*:906, 1968.
Habib, R. and Kleinknecht, C. In Sommers, S.C. (Ed.): *Pathology Annual*, New York, Appleton-Century-Crofts, 1971, p. 414.
Hand, W.L., et al.: *J Lab Clin Med, 77*:605, 1971.
Hodson, C.J.: *J Infect Dis, 120*:54, 1969.
Hollenberg, N.K., et al.: *N Engl J Med, 286*:877, 1972.
Hopper, J., et al.: *Medicine, 49*:321, 1970.
Hoyer, J.R., et al.: *Lancet, 2*:773, 1972.
Kaufman, D.B., et al.: *J Pediatr, 77*:37, 1970.
Koffler, D., et al.: *Am J Pathol, 54*:293, 1969.
Kondo, y., et al.: *Lab Invest, 27*:620, 1972.
Kunin, C.M.: *J Infect Dis, 120*:1, 1969.
Leonard, C.D., et al.: *Ann Intern Med, 73*:703, 1970.
Lewis, E.J. and Couser, W.G.: *Pediatr Clin North Am, 18*:467, 1971.
Lewis, E.J., et al.: *J Clin Invest, 49*:1103, 1970.
Lewis, E.J., et al.: *Hum Pathol, 2*:185, 1971.
Lewis, E.J., et al.: *Ann Intern Med, 75*:555, 1971.
Mattern, W.D.: *Am J Med, 52*:187, 1972.
McCluskey, R.T.: *Bull NY Acad Med, 46*:769, 1970.
McIntosh, R.M., et al.: *J Chronic Dis, 24*:787, 1971.
Merrill, J.T. and Hampers, C.L.: *N Engl J Med, 282*:953, 1970.
Mond, N.C., et al.: *Br Med J, 1*:602, 1970.
Pollak, V.E. and Pirani, C.L.: *Mayo Clin Proc, 44*:630, 1969.
Proskey, A.J., et al.: *Am J Med, 48*:162, 1970.
Rastogi, S.P., et al.: *Q J Med, 38*:335, 1969.
Relman, A.S.: *Am J Med, 44*:706, 1968.
Richardson, J.A., et al.: *Lancet, 2*:180, 1970.
Rosen, S.: *Hum Pathol, 2*:209, 1971.
Schainuck, L.I., et al.: *Hum Pathol, 1*:631, 1970.
Seymour, A.E., et al.: *Am J Pathol, 65*:550, 1971.
Siegel, R.R.: *Am J Med Sci, 259*:201, 1970.
Treser, G., et al.: *Clin Invest, 49*:762, 1970.
Tu, W.H., et al.: *Ann Intern Med, 71*:335, 1969.
West, C.D. and McAdams, A.J.: *Nephron, 7*:193, 1970.
White, R.H.R., et al.: *Lancet, 1*:1353, 1970.

CHAPTER 20

THE GASTROINTESTINAL TRACT

DISEASES OF THE ESOPHAGUS

CONGENITAL ANOMALIES. Agenesis is complete absence or imperfect development of the esophagus. In atresia, the upper portion of the esophagus ends blindly.

Diverticuli (acquired) may occur in the esophagus. In older individuals, the diverticuli may become very large and contain a volume of 300 cc of fluid. If the mouth of the diverticulum is small, infection will result due to stagnation, and a diverticulitis occurs. Diverticulitis may lead to perforation.

CIRCULATORY DISTURBANCES OF THE ESOPHAGUS. Submucosal and subserosal esophageal varices are due to distention of blood vessels. The esophageal varices may rupture, with hemorrhage occurring from the point of rupture. Clinically, the diagnosis of esophageal varices is made by utilizing balloons.

In cardiac patients or terminally in patients with debilitated disease a poor circulation occurs in the esophagus, and an acute esophagitis with or without esophagomalacia (soft esophagus) develops.

INFECTIONS OF THE ESOPHAGUS. Infections of the esophagus are not common. Esophagitis may be due to monilia infection in infants. Acute and subacute esophagitis produces erosion and inflammation in the esophageal wall with desquamation of epithelial cells.

SCLERODERMA OF THE ESOPHAGUS. Scleroderma results in a firm, immovable (stiff) esophagus due to collagen degeneration in the wall.

PLUMMER-VINSON SYNDROME. This syndrome produces the

following symptoms in females between forty and fifty years of age: dysphagia, soreness and atrophy of the esophageal mucosa, achlorhydria, and hypochromic anemia. The dysphagia is caused either by a thin membranous web passing across the lumen of the esophagus or by narrow, constricting bands that encircle the lumen of the esophagus. It has been hypothesized that the neoplasia associated with Plummer-Vinson syndrome arises in the atrophic esophageal mucosa.

NEOPLASMS OF THE ESOPHAGUS. Malignant neoplasms occur in the esophagus. The esophageal carcinoma is the only common neoplasm. It develops in males over fifty years of age. Fifty percent of esophageal carcinomas develop in the middle third of the esophagus, 25 percent in the lower third, and 25 percent in the upper third. The squamous cell carcinoma is the predominant esophageal carcinoma. It invades the adjacent tissues and metastasizes to the lymph nodes, liver, and lungs.

DISEASES OF THE STOMACH

ANOMALIES OF THE STOMACH. Gastric malrotation accompanied by intestinal malrotation is an anomaly occurring in the stomach. Diverticuli may be present in the fundus of the stomach. Atresia of the pylorus or cardiac regions of the stomach is a rare anomaly. Diaphragmatic hernia is the most common hernia that occurs in the chest.

CIRCULATORY DISTURBANCES OF THE STOMACH. Circulatory disturbances occur in the stomach during congestive heart failure, due to focal obstruction, congestion of the stomach, and terminally in cardiac patients. Gastromalacia may occur terminally in cardiac patients.

INFLAMMATORY LESIONS OF THE STOMACH. Acute gastritis is an inflammation of the stomach caused by irritating substances, foods, alcohol, and the ingestion of poisons. Prior to the advent of the antibiotics, a purulent gastritis (acute) occurred secondary to osteomyelitis, pneumonia, and scarlet fever.

Chronic gastritis occurs in atrophic and hypertrophic forms. Chronic atrophic gastritis occurs during vitamin D deficiency, pernicious anemia, chronic alcoholism, and chronic pellagra. The lining of the stomach contains flattened rugae, and there is a reduction in the surface area of the gastric mucosa. The mucosal glands are decreased in number, and leukocytes infiltrate the mucosa and submucosa. Metaplasia may occur in the gastric mucosa during chronic gastritis. The metaplasia is commonly present during carcinoma of the stomach. However, it has not been established whether the gastric metaplasia leads to the development of gastric carcinoma.

Chronic hypertrophic gastritis produces a lining mucosa, which contains large rugae and a hypertrophic polypoid lining. The gastric mucosa is hyperplastic, and lymphocytes and eosinophiles are infiltrated throughout the lamina propria.

PEPTIC ULCER OF THE STOMACH. Peptic ulcer is an erosion of the stomach caused by the action of acidic gastric juice upon the gastric mucosa. Acute peptic ulcers are small, common, superficial erosions produced by injuries (hot foods, coarse foods), blood stream infections, and skin burns. They generally heal rapidly in the gastric mucosa but occasionally may become chronic peptic ulcers.

Chronic peptic ulcers of the stomach are more common in males and Caucasians. Chronic peptic ulcers occur only in areas of the gastric mucosa that are exposed to the acidic gastric juice. Excessive acidity is commonly associated with the peptic ulcer of the stomach.

A circulatory theory for formation of the peptic ulcer states that an alteration occurs in the vascular supply of the gastric mucosa as a result of thrombosis. Local infections may produce the peptic ulcer. The neurogenic theory states that disturbances in the nervous system provoke the peptic ulcer. The gastric peptic ulcer generally develops proximal to the pyloric ring and in the pyloric portion of the stomach (posterior wall near lesser curvature). The gastric peptic ulcer is a single small ulcer, which remains small. Chronic peptic ulcers of the stomach are punched-out, indurated areas with hyperemia surrounding the ulcerations. The ulcer involves the mucosa, submucosa, and muscular layers. The base of the ulcer consists of fibrous tissue, and over the fibrous base are granulation tissue, necrotic tissue, and an exudate of inflammatory cells. Healing of the peptic ulcer occurs by organization and fibrosis. The gastric mucosa grows over the fibrosis from the edges of the ulcer. Malignant transformation may occur in the chronic gastric peptic ulcer in less than five percent of peptic ulcerations.

NEOPLASMS OF THE STOMACH. Benign neoplasms are not common and are of minor clinical significance. The common benign neoplasms of the stomach are the fibroma, lipoma, leiomyoma, gastric adenomatous polyps, and neurofibroma. The gastric mucosa may be the site of development of a single polypoid adenoma or of multiple polyps. The adenomatous polyps may rarely undergo malignant transformation.

The adenocarcinoma of the stomach is the most common and significant gastric malignant neoplasm. Gastric malignant neoplasms are responsible for approximately 10 percent of all deaths from neoplasia in the United States. Gastric carcinoma is more common in males after fifty years of age. Gastric carcinoma has a high incidence in Icelanders and Japanese. This neoplasm appears to have an hereditary susceptibility. Gastric adenocarcinoma may develop at any site in the stomach but more commonly arises from glandular cells located in the lesser curvature.

The adenocarcinoma of the stomach arises from the glandular and mucous cells of the stomach. The adenocarcinoma of the stomach appears as a large polypoid or cauliflower mass, which extends into the lumen of the stomach. The adenocarcinoma spreads by direct expansion and invasion of adjacent and surrounding tissues as well as by the lymphatics and blood vessels. Gastric carcinomas metastasize to the liver, lungs, bones, and regional lymph nodes.

Sarcomas represent only a small number of malignancies of the stomach. The lymphosarcoma, leiomyosarcoma, and fibrosarcoma may rarely develop in the stomach.

DISEASES OF THE SMALL INTESTINES

CONGENITAL ANOMALIES. The order of frequency of congenital anomalies is greatest in the duodenum, followed by the ileum, colon, and jejunum. The duodenum, ileum, jejunum, and colon may be the site of either congenital atresia or stenosis. Atresia is the closing down of the lumen of the bowel.

Meckel's diverticulum is an outgrowth or outpouching of the

intestines located in the left abdomen and has been referred to as left-sided appendicitis. Meckel's diverticulum may become infected with the development of an acute Meckel's diverticulitis. Thirty percent of individuals with diverticuli in the small bowel show the presence of heterotrophic gastric mucosa, which may cause a peptic ulcer complication. Meckel's diverticulum may, therefore, be the site of a bleeding peptic ulcer.

VASCULAR DISTURBANCES. Hyperemia, edema, and hemorrhage may occur in the small intestines. Infarction of the small intestines is due to occlusion of the superior or inferior mesenteric arteries by emboli or thrombi. The extent of an infarction of the small intestines is directly related to the size of the occluded vessel. The bowel proximal to the infarction becomes distended due to ileus. Chronic passive congestion of the small bowel occurs in males more commonly than females (3:2 ratio). This vascular disturbance has a sudden onset with acute paroxysmal abdominal pain. Chronic passive congestion of the small intestines is rarely localized and may be associated with reflex vomiting.

INFLAMMATION. Duodenal peptic ulcer is a chronic peptic ulcer of the duodenum and probably has a similar etiology to the peptic ulcer located in the stomach and esophagus. Duodenal stasis, related to mesenteric occlusion at the duodenal-jejunal junction, may play a role in the etiology and pathogenesis of the duodenal peptic ulcer. The duodenal peptic ulcer is characterized clinically by pain, vomiting, and hematemesis. The duodenal peptic ulcer may perforate, bleed, undergo scarring, and produce stenosis. The ratio of gastric to duodenal peptic ulcer is 1:2 respectively. The duodenal peptic ulcer occurs most frequently between the ages of twenty and fifty years. Seventy-five percent of duodenal peptic ulcers occur in males. The duodenal peptic ulcer is generally located 2 to 3 cm below the pylorus along the posterior wall of the duodenum or lesser turn against the head of the pancreas. Microscopically, the duodenal peptic ulcer exhibits the following layers: the layer of exudation, the layer of necrosis, layer of granulation tissue, and the layer of scarring. An acute perforation (complication) may lead to generalized peritonitis. Massive hemorrhage or slow bleeding and stenosis are complications of the duodenal peptic ulcer.

Regional ileitis is an acute or chronic inflammatory disease of the bowel of obscure etiology. The inflammation occurs in the ileum in 60 percent of affected individuals, in the ileum and colon in 35 percent, and in the jejunum in 3.5 percent of the instances of regional ileitis. The disease is characterized by inflammation of all layers of the wall of the bowel. Clinical features include pain and formation of a mass or swelling.

A diffuse or circumscribed inflammation is evident accompanied by hyperplasia, hypertrophy, and granular polypoid proliferation. Multiple ulcerations, perienteritis and pericolitis, stenosis, chronic perforation, fistula, peritonitis, thickened mesentery, and a tumorlike mass are associated with regional ileitis.

INTESTINAL OBSTRUCTION. Obstruction of the intestines indicates that a disturbance is present involving the intestinal contents, which prevents their movement onward through the bowel lumen. Actual physical closure of the lumen, i.e. dynamic ileus, may be responsible for the obstruction. A disturbance may be present in muscular contraction, resulting in cessation of intestinal motor activity, i.e. paralytic ileus.

The pathologic effects of intestinal obstruction are fluid and elctrolyte loss, distention, changes in the wall of the bowel, absorption from obstructed bowel, strangulation, and mechanisms by which the obstruction causes death. Obstructions of the bowel may develop at a high or low level. If the obstruction is high, vomiting and loss of hydrochloric acid result. If the obstruction is low, abdominal distention and acidosis result.

NEOPLASMS OF THE SMALL INTESTINES. Benign neoplasms are rare in the small intestines. The lipoma, fibroma, leiomyoma, and benign polyps may involve the small intestines. Carcinoma of the small intestines is rare. Malignancies of the small bowel are more common in males between fity and sixty years of age. Adenocarcinoma causes obstruction and jaundice.

DISEASES OF THE APPENDIX

CONGENITAL ANOMALIES. The congenital anomalies of the appendix include atresia, absence, reduplication, and diverticulae.

INFLAMMATORY DISEASE. Acute appendicitis is the most common disease of the abdomen, necessitating surgical intervention. Appendicitis occurs equally in males and females. Fifty percent of instances of appendicitis occur in individuals under twenty years of age. The inflammation is rare in children. Appendicitis occurs in individuals living in highly civilized regions of the world. Clinically, the findings are abdominal pain, nausea, vomiting, leukocytosis, fever, rigidity at McBurney's point, and tenderness. Chronic appendicitis results from the acute inflammatory process. Fecaliths (stones) may cause stasis or obstruction in the distal one-third of the appendix. Foreign bodies are important factors in causing obstruction and appendiceal stasis. Lymphoid hyperplasia frequently occurs in teenagers, and the resulting hyperplasia may obstruct the lumen of the appendix. Bacterial infection and obstruction are the two most important etiologic agents in the production of appendicitis.

Bacteriological investigations reveal that *Bacillus coli* was present in 57 percent, *Bacillus coli* and streptococci in 19 percent, and streptococci only in 9 percent of instances of appendicitis. Anaerobic microorganisms have been isolated in less than 50 percent, nonhemolytic streptococci and pneumococci in 100 percent, enterococci in 65 percent, gram-positive rods and coliform group in 50 percent, gram-negative rods of the influenzal form in 25 percent, and bacterium coli mucosum in 14 percent of instances of appendicitis.

The gross appearance of the appendix is dependent upon the type of inflammation, i.e. acute, suppurative, hemorrhagic, and gangrenous appendicitis. Histopathologically, the mucosa is edematous, hyperemic, and may be ulcerated. Polymorphonuclear leukocytes infiltrate the wall of the appendix.

Obliterative appendicitis occurs when the distal end of the lumen of the appendix is plugged by lymphoid tissue containing no mucosal covering. Chronic lymphoid appendicitis occurs in children and is usually accompanied by lymphadenitis.

MUCOCELE OF THE APPENDIX. Mucocele of the appendix occurs in the distal end. The mucocele of the appendix is due to obstruction. The lumen of the appendix becomes filled with mucin, which arises from the glands of the mucosa and produces a morbidly distended appendix. Mucin fills the entire lumen of the appendix.

CARCINOID OF THE APPENDIX. Carcinoid (neoplasm) of the appendix commonly arises from theca cells located in the wall of the appendix. The benign carcinoid neoplasm initially involves the submucosa; however, it subsequently invades the remainder of the wall of the appendix.

DISEASES OF THE LARGE INTESTINES

CONGENITAL ANOMALIES. Anomalies of length and size, i.e. congenital megacolon or Hirschsprung disease, occurs in the large bowel. Megacolon means the presence of a markedly dilated descending or sigmoid colon. The marked intestinal dilatation is due to the congenital absence of neural elements in the segment of large bowel below the dilatation.

Diverticuli are common in the colon. Diverticuli develop in the weakened bowel wall at the site of entry of blood vessels. Herniation of the lining mucosa occurs into the wall of the colon and the muscle layer is pushed aside. Diverticuli are commonly located in the descending and sigmoid colon. Approximately 10 percent of the population over sixty years of age develop diverticuli. Left-sided acute appendicitis is actually acute diverticulitis.

VASCULAR DISTURBANCES. Infarction, hemorrhage, and hemorrhoids represent the major vascular disturbances in the colon.

INFLAMMATORY DISEASES. Tuberculosis of the intestines is the most common secondary lesion of this granulomatous disease. Intestinal tuberculosis occurs as a result of dissemination of pulmonary tuberculosis. The iliocecal region is the most common intestinal site for the development of tuberculosis.

Typhoid fever involves the terminal ileum. The lesions of typhoid fever are located in the iliocecal region of the intestines. The lymph nodes, spleen, liver, and reticuloendothelial system are involved during typhoid fever. Swelling and congestion of Peyer's patches of the terminal ileum are the principal alterations. Stuffing and ulceration develop in the intestinal mucosa at the sites of Peyer's patches.

Bacillary dysentery produces lesions in the sigmoid colon and rectum. The intestinal lesion appears as a superficial ulceration with a pseudomembrane covering the ulceration.

Endamoebic dysentery involves the cecum and rectum. Minimal inflammation is present; however, small, superficial ulcerations develop in the mucosa of the cecum and rectum. Endamoeba histolyticus enters the wall of the cecum producing a deep, flask-shaped ulceration.

Regional ileitis or enteritis is a disease of unknown origin. The disease may involve any portion of the ileum; however, the terminal portion of the ileum is most commonly involved. Approximately 20 to 30 centimeters of the terminal ileum are generally involved in regional ileitis. The alteration that occurs is well demarcated at both ends of the inflammatory zone. The gross lesion of an ileitis has the appearance of a carcinoma.

Ulcerative colitis is an inflammatory disease of the colon of obscure eitology. Chronic ulcerative colitis is a specific inflammatory disease of the colon occurring in middle adult life. Proposed etiologic factors are allergy, infection, neurogenic disturbances, and enzymatic necrosis of the colon. The disease is accompanied by remissions and exacerbations over an extended period of time. An edematous large intestine, rectum and sigmoid colon undergoes necrosis and ulceration. The ulcerations are small; however, coalescence of individual ulcerations may result in formation of large and very irregular ulcerations. The wall of the bowel undergoes fibrosis and thickening and the ulcerations undergo resolution by fibrosis and scarring. Perforation, hemorrhage and peritonitis are severe complications. Multiple polypoid masses may be associated with chronic ulcerative colitis.

Malignant transformation may occur in the polypoid proliferations associated with chronic ulcerative colitis. Carcinoma has a greater instance in the colon affected with chronic ulcerative colitis when compared to the unaffected colon.

Uremia causes superficial nonspecific ulcers in the colon.

BENIGN NEOPLASMS. Benign neoplasms are rare in the large bowel. Benign adenomas or adenomatous polyps develop in the colon as polypoid, sessile, or ulcerated benign gross neoplasms. The adenomatous polyp may have a predisposition to undergo malignant change. However, this change is currently debatable. Multiple adenoma or benign polyposis of the colon and rectum is a definite premalignant lesion in the descending colon, sigmoid colon, and rectum. Polyposis of the colon and rectum may occur as a diffuse disease (polyposis) or as a solitary disease (polyposis). The solitary polyposis consists of a few adenomatous polyps whereas the diffuse polyposis consists of a large number of polyps throughout the entire colon and rectum.

MALIGNANT NEOPLASMS. Carcinoma of the large intestines is a very important neoplasm. Ninety-five percent of all malignant neoplasms of the intestines occur in the colon. One percent of all carcinomas (human) occur in the colon. Carcinoma of the large intestines is more common in males than females. It is rare in individuals under forty years of age. Fifty percent of carcinomas of the colon occur in the rectosigmoid region. Two-thirds occur in the left colon and one-third in the right colon. Twenty-five percent of carcinomas of the large intestines occur in the sigmoid colon. Two predisposing factors to malignancies of the large bowel are polyps and ulcerative colitis. Adenocarcinoma of the colon and rectum develops as a polypoid or annular constrictive neoplasm. The annular adenocarcinoma proliferates and grows around the colon and rectum, causing a decrease in the size of the lumen. The polypoid adenocarcinoma projects as a cauliflower-like mass into the lumen of the colon and rectum, producing obstruction. The colon above the obstruction becomes dilated. Chronic obstruction develops in the advanced stage of carcinoma of the colon.

Metastases from adenocarcinoma of the large intestines commonly occur to the regional lymph nodes and liver. Malignant neoplasms of the abdomen spread by way of the circulation, resulting in metastatic liver involvement. Metastases from the large bowel also occur to the lung, adrenal gland, and brain.

DISEASES OF THE PERITONEUM

INFLAMMATION. Acute peritonitis is an inflammation of all or part of the peritoneum. Bacteria or chemical agents are generally the etiology of acute peritonitis; however, multiple initiating extrinsic and intrinsic factors may be present. Bile and gastric juice are chemicals that are capable of producing peritonitis. The organisms responsible for provoking peritonitis are *Bacillus coli*, nonhemolytic streptococci, diphtheroid bacillus, *Bacillus lactis aerogenes, Bacillus melanogenicum,* pneumococcus, and hemolytic streptococcus. There are four possible routes of entry of bacteria into the peritoneum, i.e. by way of the blood stream, vagina and fallopian tube, wall of the gastrointestinal tract, and transdiaphragmatic as a complication of pulmonary diseases.

Grossly, there is generally some type of peritoneal exudate, which ranges from a serous to a purulent and fibrinous exudate. Peritonitis produces chills, fever, and leukocytosis, stimulation of nerve endings leading to pain, pain resulting in muscle spasm in the abdominal wall and rigidity, the presence of the exudate in the peritoneal cavity, which helps to distend the abdomen, inhibited intestinal motility, and nausea and vomiting.

MISCELLANEOUS DISTURBANCES OF THE GASTROINTESTINAL TRACT

HERNIA. Hernia is the protrusion of an entire viscus or its wall through the enclosing wall. An abdominal hernia can be reduced. A hernia may be internal or external, and acquired or congenital.

INTERSUSSCEPTION. Intersussception is an invagination of one loop into another loop of the bowel. In children, intersussception is due to the enlargement of a lymph follicle or to local persistence of peristalsis. In adults, intersussception occurs secondary to pedunculated neoplasms and thickened bowel walls.

VOLVULUS. Volvulus is a twisting of the sigmoid colon or small intestines. The mesenteric vessels are compressed, resulting in infarction and gangrene. The prognosis and mortality depend upon the length of time that the volvulus has been present.

INTESTINAL POLYPOSIS (PEUTZ-JEGHERS SYNDROME). Peutz-Jeghers syndrome is an inherited syndrome consisting of multiple fibromas, polyposis of the small bowel, and focal melanin pigmentation of the oral mucosa and lips. The polyposis associated with the Peutz-Jeghers syndrome are benign lesions that only rarely become malignant.

References

Asquith, P., et al.: *Lancet, 2*:129, 1969.
Baeza, M.: *Dis Colon Rectum, 12*:147, 1969.
Black, B.M.: *Surg Clin North Am, 51*:955, 1971.
Burdette, W.J.: *Cancer, 28*:51, 1971.
Burkitt, D.P.: *Cancer, 28*:3, 1971.
Castle, W.B.: *Am J Med, 48*:541, 1970.
Chapman, B.L. and Duggan, J.M.: *Gut, 10*:443, 1969.
DeDombal, F., et al.: *Gut, 10*:270, 1969.
Devroede, G.J.: *N Engl J Med, 285*:17, 1971.
Djar, T., et al.: *JAMA, 221*:31, 1972.
Eisenman, B. and Heyman, R.L.: *N Engl J Med, 282*:372, 1970
Goldman, H., et al.: *Arch Pathol, 89*:349, 1970.
Haenzel, W. and Correa, P.: *Cancer, 28*:14, 1971.
Horn, R.C.: *Cancer, 28*:146, 1971.
Hornsby, L.G.: *Dis Nerv Syst, 31*:338, 1970.
Ivey, K.J.: *Gut, 12*:750, 1971.
Joyal, R.K., et al.: *N Engl J Med, 282*:1298, 1970.
Kraft, S.C. and Kirsner, J.B.: *Gastroenterology, 60*:922, 1971.
Kraft, S.C., et al.: *Gastroenterology, 54*:1251, 1968.
Kronman, B.S.: *Cancer, 28*:82, 1971.
McCusick, V.A.: *JAMA, 182*:271, 1962.
Mann, J.G.: *Am J Med, 48*:357, 1970.
Max, M. and Menguy, R.: *Gastroenterology, 58*:329, 1970.
Menguy, R.: *Am J Surg, 120*:282, 1970.
Mitchell, D.N. and Rees, R.J.W.: *Lancet, 2*:168, 1970.
Mitchell, D.N., et al.: *Lancet, 2*:496, 1970.
Myren, J., et al.: *Scand J Gastroenterol, 6*:511, 1971.
Painter, N.S.: *Lancet, 2*:586, 1969.
Palmer, E.D.: *Am J Med, 44*:566, 1968.
Parks, T.G.: *Br Med J, 4*:639, 1969.
Robinson, D., et al.: *Gut, 12*:789, 1971.
Shiner, M. and Ballard, J.: *Lancet, 1*:1202, 1972.
Spratt, J.S. and Watson, F.R.: *Cancer, 28*:153, 1971.
Stokes, P.L., et al.: *Lancet, 2*:162, 1972.
Thayer, W.R.: *Scand J Gastroenterol, Suppl 6, 5*:164, 1970.
Tizes, R.: *N Engl J Med, 282*:1273, 1970.
Watson, D.W.: *Gastroenterology, 56*:944, 1969.
Watson, D.W.: *Gastroenterology, 56*:385, 1969.
Zamcheck, N., et al.: *N Engl J Med, 286*:83, 1972.
Zamcheck, N., et al.: *N Engl J Med, 252*:1103, 1955.

CHAPTER 21

THE LIVER AND BILIARY TRACT

THE LIVER FUNCTIONS as a chemical laboratory and performs the following functions: (1) bile production and excretion; (2) metabolism of fats, carbohydrates, vitamins, and minerals; (3) storage of vitamins A, C, and D; (4) chemical detoxification by hepatic cells; (5) reticuloendothelial participation in detoxification by means of phagocytosis by Kupffer cells; and (6) hematopoiesis and coagulation by means of storage of vitamin B_{12} and vitamin K.

Bile is produced by the liver and passes into the duodenum. Bile aids in the emulsification of fat along with the action of lipase, which prepares the fat for absorption. Vitamins A and K are fat soluble vitamins, therefore, when fat is decreased or absent, vitamins A and K are not absorbed. Bile contains bilirubin, bile salts, and cholesterol. The bile salts are formed in the liver. Cholesterol is produced and eliminated by the liver. Bilirubin is derived from the breakdown of hemoglobin.

DEGENERATIVE CHANGES IN THE LIVER

FATTY CHANGE. Fatty change produces a greasy, yellow-colored liver. Microscopically, the liver cord cells contain large, clear vacuoles located in the cytoplasm. The fat vacuole pushes the centrally located nucleus to the periphery of the cell.

CHRONIC PASSIVE CONGESTION. During chronic passive congestion, the liver is hyperemic in the area of the central veins. Compression of liver cords occurs with atrophy of hepatic cells. Central lobular necrosis is the result of chronic passive congestion.

INFARCTION. Infarction is rare but may occur in the liver

when complete obstruction is present in the portal vein or hepatic artery located in the portal triad. Complete necrosis does not occur in the liver because of the double circulation to this organ. Partial necrosis occurs when an obstruction is present in either the portal vein or hepatic artery. If an obstruction occurs to the portal vein before it enters the liver, no infarction results because the hepatic artery provides the blood supply. However, if the obstruction develops suddenly, infarction will occur in an organ (liver) with a double blood supply.

Infarction of the liver is, therefore, rare for the following reasons: (1) double blood supply; (2) 65 percent of the blood supply occurs by way of the portal vein; (3) the liver is resistant to relative anoxia; (4) collateral vessels pass from the diaphragm to the liver; and (5) the hepatic artery does not arise directly from the aorta. The liver has a limited ability to regenerate parenchymal cells.

AMYLOIDOSIS. Amyloidosis of the liver produces stiff margins and overall increase in the size of the organ.

NECROSIS. Five types of liver necrosis may be identified, i.e. central zonal, midzonal, peripheral zonal, focal and diffuse necrosis. Central zonal necrosis of the liver is due to anoxia, chronic passive hyperemia, chemical poisons, and acute viral hepatitis.

The most common necrosis occurs around the central vein. Midzonal necrosis of the liver is due to yellow fever, infectious diseases, burns, and tannic acid. The rare peripheral zonal necrosis is due to eclampsia and phosphorus poisoning. Focal necrosis of the liver is due to typhoid fever and other infectious diseases. Diffuse necrosis of the liver is due to syphilis, Weil's disease, viral hepatitis, and acute yellow atrophy.

When a large quantity of poison is consumed, or if liver disease or congestive heart failure is present, acute yellow atrophy of the liver occurs rather than the zonal type of necrosis. Chemicals and drugs that are directly toxic to the liver may provoke a hypersensitivity reaction, i.e. a focal type of liver necrosis. Bacterial toxins accompanied by a generalized septicemia result in focal areas of necrosis in the liver.

Cholangitis is produced when organisms reach the liver through the portal vein resulting in infection of the biliary tract and bile ducts. The infection spreads through the liver, producing abscesses in the parenchyma.

INFECTIONS OF THE LIVER

Infectious agents may reach the liver by direct extension in the event of trauma or from an infection in the peritoneal cavity. Rarely do infectious agents reach the liver by way of the portal vein or hepatic artery. Any infection in the spleen and gastrointestinal tract (rarely, intestinal infection) may lead to liver damage by means of bacterial or septic emboli. The liver is a fairly resistant organ, which contains phagocytic cells of the reticuloendothelial system. When infection takes place in the liver, the microorganisms generally follow the mesenteric and portal veins with abscess formation in the right lobe of the liver. Bacteria present in the gall bladder may enter the liver through the bile ducts. Bacteria enter the liver following either partial or complete obstruction of the bile ducts due to bile stones, carcinoma, or after extensive surgical procedures.

ABSCESSES OF THE LIVER. Abscesses of the liver are more commonly located in the right lobe. Multiple abscesses of the liver are due to *Eschericia coli* or gram-negative intestinal microorganisms. The liver abscess contains green pus because of the presence of bile in the exudate. The abscess spreads and involves adjacent liver parenchyma. Recent abscesses of the liver consist of focal areas of tissue necrosis and dead and dying polymorphonuclear leukocytes. Older liver abscesses are walled off by organization of tissue at the periphery. Empyema, lung abscess, or pancarditis may occur following rupture of the liver abscess through the diaphragm.

GRANULOMATOUS INFLAMMATIONS OF THE LIVER. Rarely, syphilis involves the liver by production of either a diffuse type of liver involvement, termed *syphilitic cirrhosis,* or gumma of the liver with fibrosis and scarring. Congenital syphilis produces a diffuse fibrosis or hyperplasia of the connective tissue of the liver. In adults with congenital syphilis, the gummas and fibrosis produce an acute syphilitic hepatitis.

Acquired syphilis is responsible for production of diffuse hepatitis or gumma of the liver. The areas of gummatous necrosis heal by fibrosis and produce a large, nodular, and deformed liver divided by deep fissures termed *hepar lobatum*.

Tuberculosis produces an enlarged liver, i.e. hepatomegaly. Miliary tuberculosis of the liver generally results from a hematogenous spread of tubercle bacilli from the lungs. Tubercles are located in the portal triads. Brucellosis infection of the liver gives rise to hepatitis and produces small granulomata in the portal and intralobular areas of the liver.

SPIROCHETAL INFECTIONS OF THE LIVER. Leptospirohemorrhagica or Weil's disease is an occupational hazard in stockyard workers and butchers. Rats excrete the spirochetal organisms, which enter the water and propagate. The spirochetes pass through the skin of the workers and enter the circulating blood. The symptoms of Weil's disease are painful, enlarged liver, jaundice, and fever.

VIRAL INFECTIONS OF THE LIVER. Infectious hepatitis is a mild viral infection of the liver, which may occur in epidemic fashion or following administration of human blood or serum containing the filterable virus. The resistant filterable virus provokes a hepatitis and hepatic necrosis. Jaundice accompanies infectious hepatitis due to obstruction of the intralobular bile canaliculi with plugs of bile. Following resolution, there may be full restoration of hepatic cells because these cells have the ability to regenerate so long as the framework and vasculature of the liver are still present. Histopathologically, the advanced hepatic lesion shows degeneration and necrosis of hepatic cells and mononuclear inflammatory cells. In most instances, scarring is absent; however, chronic hepatitis may be accompanied by scarring and occasional cirrhosis of the liver.

Yellow fever is a viral disease transmitted by the *Aedes aegypti* mosquito. Liver damage results from the viral infection, and the liver may be enlarged or normal in size. Midzonal necrosis is present; however, the peripheral cells of the liver lobule are preserved. Gastrointestinal symptoms, severe jaundice, hepatocellular damage, and plugged bile canaliculi are the principal findings in yellow fever. The infection provides a good immunity. Vaccines are available against the virus of yellow fever.

FUNGAL AND PARASITIC INFECTIONS OF THE LIVER. The most

common fungal infections of the liver include actinomycosis and histoplasmosis. Actinomycosis produces sulfur granules in the liver, surrounded by polymorphonuclear leukocytes. *Histoplasma capsulatum* microorganisms are located in the Kupffer cells following infection of the liver. The entire reticuloendothelial system is invaded by the *Histoplasma capsulatum,* yeastlike fungi.

Malaria produces alterations in the liver due primarily to the presence of the malarial parasite and secondarily to severe anemia and anoxia. Excessive malarial pigment (hematin pigment) is deposited in the liver. The malarial pigment, high fever, and antimalarial drugs produce degenerative changes in the liver.

The liver is enlarged in malaria. Microscopically, the Kupffer cells are enlarged and are actively phagocytic to the malarial parasite, malarial pigment (hematin), and red blood cells. Hyaline necrosis is present, and central lobular necrosis develops. The necrosis is due to anoxia resulting from blockage of the blood supply. Portal cirrhosis develops in the late stages of malaria.

JAUNDICE

Jaundice (icterus) is a term indicating the presence of bile pigment in the tissues of the body, plus a high concentration of bilirubin in the blood. The bile pigment is normally produced in the reticuloendothelial cells of the spleen and bone marrow from the breakdown of hemoglobin. Two types of jaundice are recognized, i.e. retention jaundice and regurgitation jaundice. During retention jaundice, the hepatic cells are incapable of removing all of the bilirubin from the blood; therefore, the pigment is not excreted by the kidneys. During regurgitation jaundice, bilirubin passes back into the blood after the pigment has been acted upon by hepatic cells. Bilirubin is excreted by the kidney and is present in the urine. Retention jaundice results from anoxemia, febrile disease, and hepatic malfunction. Regurgitation jaundice results from necrosis of hepatic cells, obstruction of the biliary tree, and from idiopathic causes. Clinically, retention jaundice reveals pigmentation of the tissues and organs of the body. Clinical findings in regurgitation jaundice are pruritis, bleeding tendencies, and renal and central nervous system involvement.

CIRRHOSIS OF THE LIVER

Cirrhosis of the liver refers to the development of fibrosis, i.e. scarring of the liver. Cirrhosis is a chronic disease process that is progressive and dynamic rather than static. The fibrosis is diffuse and may involve every lobule of the liver by connective tissue, which causes disruption of the normal architecture of the liver. There are three forms of cirrhosis based on morphologic characteristics, i.e. portal (Laennac's) cirrhosis, postnecrotic cirrhosis, and biliary cirrhosis. The most common portal atrophy (Laennac's cirrhosis) is related to protein, sulfur containing amino acid, choline, cystine, and methionine nutritional deficiencies. A choline deficient diet and a methionine deficient diet result in a fatty liver and cirrhosis.

PORTAL CIRRHOSIS (LAENNEC'S CIRRHOSIS). Portal cirrhosis occurs in approximately 2 to 3 percent of the population of the United States. The age distribution in the United States is from forty to sixty years. Portal cirrhosis is more common in males than females. Portal cirrhosis shows a higher incidence in the Negro than in the Caucasian. The etiology of portal cirrhosis is obscure. Fifty percent of patients with portal cirrhosis give a history of alcoholism. However, many alcoholics never have portal cirrhosis. Protein, carbohydrate, and vitamin deficiencies (malnutrition), and infectious diseases are etiologic factors.

During portal cirrhosis, the liver is generally smaller than normal and is firm, nodular, and yellow in color. The cut section of the liver reveals fine nodules with a yellow color to both the cut and capsular surfaces. The liver has a tough consistency and cuts with increased resistance.

The clinical features of portal cirrhosis include the following: dyspepsia, anorexia, lower abdominal pain, constipation, tenderness in right hypergastric region (upper gastric region), amenorrhea, sterility in males, gynecomastia, and terminal edema and jaundice. The most important clinical feature of portal cirrhosis is ascites. The liver is palpable in 80 percent and the spleen is palpable in 50 percent of patients with portal cirrhosis.

Diffuse fibrosis is present; however, it is more conspicuous in the portal areas which become attached to one another. Regenerative activity is evident, and binucleated cells are present with darkly stained nuclei. Ten to fifteen times the normal number of small bile ducts are present in the portal areas during portal cirrhosis. New bile ducts proliferate in all forms of cirrhosis.

Bile stasis may be present in portal cirrhosis. Bile plugs occur in canaliculi, bilirubin is located in liver cells, and there is destruction of blood and bile circulation. Jaundice occurs in approximately 10 to 20 percent of individuals with portal cirrhosis.

Ascites develops early in portal cirrhosis. Portal hypertension occurs due to the anastomosis between the portal vein and hepatic artery with an increase in pressure. The damaged liver fails in its function of detoxification. Hyperestrogen, gynecomastia and increased intra-abdominal pressure accompany the failure of detoxification and an increase in hormones.

BILIARY CIRRHOSIS. Biliary cirrhosis is not as common as portal cirrhosis. Biliary cirrhosis is due to obstruction of the bile duct system and alterations in the biliary system. The biliary obstruction may be intrahepatic or result from an obstruction outside of the liver (posthepatic biliary cirrhosis).

Posthepatic biliary cirrhosis is due to a pancreatic carcinoma, gallstone, or stricture. In posthepatic biliary cirrhosis, the liver is enlarged terminally. In postnecrotic biliary cirrhosis, the obstruction causes stasis in the large bile ducts (polystasis). Inflammation ocurs secondarily to the polystasis.

Hypertrophic biliary cirrhosis is due to a primary cholangitis of the small branches of bile ducts. The portal areas contain a proliferation of connective tissue, a prominent inflammatory exudate, and proliferation of bile capillaries. Hepatic cell atrophy is a result of the pressure exerted by the fibrosis, interference with the circulation, and anoxia. The normal architecture of the liver is subsequently replaced by pseudolobular formation due to the periportal cirrhosis.

Differentiation of intrahepatic from the extrahepatic type of biliary cirrhosis is possible since the large bile ducts contain bile thrombi in the extrahepatic type. When the etiology of the biliary cirrhosis is intrahepatic in origin, bile thrombi are present in the small bile ducts.

When biliary cirrhosis is due to hyperlipemia and hypercholesterolemia, yellow xanthomas develop on the lower extremities and eyelids.

POSTNECROTIC CIRRHOSIS. Postnecrotic cirrhosis follows necrosis of hepatic cells. Infectious agents, toxins, poisons, and malnutrition may lead to massive necrosis. Alcoholism plus portal cirrhosis predispose the liver to development of large areas of necrosis. Grossly, the liver is reduced in size. Large, irregular nodules are present, which represent regenerated liver cells. Irregular, broad areas or bands of fibrosis extend into the liver lobule due to the postnecrotic changes.

CARDIAC CIRRHOSIS. Cardiac cirrhosis is associated with pericarditis and rheumatic heart disease. Central lobular dilatation and chronic passive congestion lead to central lobular necrosis. The reticulum collapses, and periportal fibrosis results. A fine, regular nodularity occurs in cardiac cirrhosis. Less bile duct proliferation takes place, and the fibrosis is not marked in cardiac cirrhosis as compared to portal cirrhosis.

CIRRHOSIS WITH HEMOCHROMATOSIS. Cirrhosis of the liver accompanied by hemochromatosis is a metabolic disorder resulting in increased absorption of iron and deposition of iron in the liver, pancreas, lymph nodes, skin, and other organs. Severe fibrosis occurs in the pancreas, which is responsible for producing diabetes mellitus. The skin is pigmented, and the alteration is termed *bronzed diabetes*. The liver is enlarged and brown colored, due to the tremendous deposition of iron pigment, hemosiderin, and hemofuscin. Fibrosis occurs predominantly in the portal region and is multilobular in distribution.

PARASITIC CIRRHOSIS. Parasitic cirrhosis is due to hepatic infection by the liver fluke *(Clonorchis sinensis)* or schistosomiasis. The parasites obstruct the blood stream, producing portal cirrhosis, and/or the bile ducts, producing biliary cirrhosis. Malarial parasites produce portal cirrhosis.

WILSON'S DISEASE. Wilson's disease is a chronic disease due to hepatolenticular degeneration. Three basic findings are present in Wilson's disease, i.e. portal cirrhosis, degeneration of basal ganglion in the brain, and green pigmentation at the outer edge of the cornea.

NEOPLASMS OF THE LIVER

Benign neoplasms of the liver are uncommon. The most important benign neoplasms of the liver are the hemangioma and the adenoma. The adenoma is a cholangioma derived from bile ducts.

Primary carcinoma may occur in the liver. The primary carcinoma of the liver occurs in individuals from fifty to sixty years of age and is more common in males than females. Cirrhosis of the liver is an etiologic factor in primary carcinoma of the liver. The primary carcinoma of the liver occurs in two histologic types, i.e. the hepatocarcinoma and cholangiocarcinoma. The hepatocarcinoma causes an enlarged liver, which may be multinodular or diffusely infiltrated with neoplastic cells. The hepatocarcinoma is the most frequent carcinoma of the liver and consists of neoplastic cells situated in columns similar to hepatic cords and abnormal lobule formation. The clinical features of primary carcinoma of the liver are pain, dyspepsia, weight loss, enlarged liver, enlarged pigmented spleen, and jaundice (80% of patients).

DISEASES OF THE BILIARY TRACT

Inflammation, neoplasia, and lithiasis are the principal pathologic processes that involve the biliary tract. The hepatic duct passes downward from the liver to join the cystic duct in forming the common bile duct (common hepatic duct). The common bile duct joins the pancreatic duct, forming the ampulla of Vater, just proximal to their site of entrance into the duodenum. Bile is secreted by the liver and concentrated in the gall bladder. Bile contains bile salts, bile pigments (bilirubin and biliverdin), alkali carbonates, cholesterol, mucin, and water. If equilibrium of bile constituents is not maintained, a deposition of elements takes palce, providing a nidus for the formation of stones.

INFLAMMATION OF THE GALL BLADDER. Bacteria may enter the gall bladder by way of the blood stream or biliary system. Microorganisms grow in the biliary system if there is stasis of bile or if an obstruction is present. Acute cholecystitis may occur due to bacterial infection with streptococci, staphylococci, *Eschericia coli* and typhi. Acute cholecystitis may occur as a nonbacterial inflammation due to increased retention of bile salts. The infection starts in the mucosa and extends into the wall of the gall bladder.

CHRONIC CHOLECYSTITIS. Chronic cholecystitis may occur as chronic inflammation from the start or the acute disease may become chronic. A thick, fibrosed gall bladder with adhesions and areas of inflammation and necrosis occurs in chronic cholecystitis. Cholecystitis is responsible for the formation of gallstones.

Cholesterolosis is a strawberry gall bladder containing seedlike spots on the surface. The yellow areas are due to masses of cholesterol esters, which are deposited in the mucosal lining and in deeper areas of the wall of the gall bladder.

EMPYEMA OF GALL BLADDER. Empyema is the accumulation of pus in the gall bladder due to a severe infection and obstruction. The lumen is distended, mucosal folds are obliterated, and an exudate covers and mucosa.

HYDROPS OF THE GALL BLADDER. When obstruction occurs to the passage of bile from the gall bladder, in the absence of infection, the gall bladder becomes distended with mucin. The mucin plugs the ducts and the gall bladder becomes distended with white bile (mucin), i.e. hydrops of the gall bladder.

CHOLELITHIASIS. Cholelithiasis is the formation and presence of gallstones in the gall bladder and bile passages including the bile ducts of the liver. Pure cholesterol gallstones develop as solitary stones termed *metabolic stones.* Pure calcium bilirubinate gallstones develop in hemolytic jaundice as multiple stones due to increased hemolysis. Calcium bilirubinate stones are black, friable, multiple small stones. Ten percent of patients with hemolytic jaundice develop calcium bilirubinate stones. Pure calcium carbonate gallstones form rare, solitary, gray, amorphous stones. Mixed cholelithiasis form as faceted multiple stones. Ten percent of all cholelithiases are pure stones and 90 percent are mixed, faceted, multiple stones associated with infection.

The etiologic factors in the formation of cholelithiasis include the following: infection, stasis of bile, high serum cholesterol, and high bile cholesterol. The most common complications of cholelithiasis include obstruction, perforation of the ileum or colon, ulceration, and formation of a fistula.

NEOPLASMS OF THE GALL BLADDER. Papillomas occur in the

neck of the gall bladder. Adenomas and adenomyomas occur in the fundus of the gall bladder. Malignant neoplasms of the gall bladder are associated with long-standing cholelithiasis and are more common in females than in males. Carcinoma occurs in the neck or fundus of the gall bladder. The neoplastic cells infiltrate the wall of the gall bladder and are responsible for ulceration of areas of mucosa.

The adenocarcinoma is the predominant carcinoma of the gall bladder. Metastasis takes place to the liver and to the area surrounding the gall bladder. Obstructive jaundice and biliary cirrhosis occur following metastases. Squamous cell carcinoma of the gall bladder is rare. It is due to metaplasia of the epithelium due to long-standing irritation from cholelithiasis.

References

Alpert, M.E. and Davidson, C.S.: *Am J Med, 46:*325, 1969.
Alpert, M.E., et al.: *Lancet, 1:*1265, 1968.
Black, M. and Billing, B.H.: *N Engl J Med, 280:*1266, 1969.
Blumberg, B.S., et al.: *N Engl J Med, 283:*349, 1970.
Blumberg, B.S., et al.: *Am J Med, 48:*1, 1970.
Boyer, J.L. and Klatskin, G.: *N Engl J Med, 283:*1063, 1970.
Brewin, A.W.: *J Am Coll Health Assoc, 20:*328, 1972.
Callahan, E.W. and Schmid, R.: *Gastroenterology, 57:*134, 1969.
Carey, C.M. and Small, D.M.: *Arch Intern Med, 130:*506, 1972.
Dane, D.S., et al.: *Lancet, 1:*695, 1970.
Dienstag, J.L., et al.: *Lancet, 1:*765, 1975.
Doniach, D., et al.: *N Engl J Med, 282:*86, 1970.
Dudley, F.J., et al.: *Lancet, 2:*2, 1971.
Feizi, T.: *Gut, 9:*193, 1968.
Fleischner, G. and Arias, I.M.: *Am J Med, 49:*576, 1970.
Fox, R.A., et al.: *Lancet, 1:*959, 1969.
Fox, R.A., et al.: *Gut, 12:*574, 1971.
Gitnick, G.L., et al.: *Lancet, 2:*285, 1969.
Giustino, V., et al.: *Lancet, 2:*850, 1972.
Havens, W.P.: *Med Clin North Am, 54:*455, 1970.
Iseri, O. and Gottlieb, L.S.: *Gastroenterology, 60:*1027, 1971.
Krugman, S. and Giles, J.P.: *JAMA, 212:*1019, 1970.
Lieber, C.S.: *Ann Rev Med, 18:*35, 1969.
Lieber, C.S., and Rubin, E.: *N Engl J Med, 280:*705, 1969.
Liebowitz, H.R.: *NY J Med, 69:*2012, 1969.
Lin, T.Y.: *Scand J Gastroenterol, (Suppl), 6:*223, 1970.
London, W.T., et al.: In Ioachim, H.L. (Ed.): *Pathology Annual,* New

York, Appleton-Century-Crofts, 1972, p. 207.
MacKay, I.R. and Morris, P.J.: *Lancet, 2*:793, 1972.
Mistilus, S.P. and Blackburn, R.B.: *Am J Med, 48*:484, 1970.
Moertel, C.G., et al.: *Am J Dig Dis, 15*:983, 1970.
Mosley, J.W.: *Can Med Assoc J, (Suppl), 196*:427, 1972.
Mosley, J.W., et al.: *Nature, 225*:953, 1970.
Paronetto, F. and Popper, H.: *N Engl J Med, 282*:277, 1970.
Poland, R.L. and Odell, G.B.: *N Engl J Med, 284*:1, 1971.
Popper, H.: *Can Med Assoc J, (Suppl), 106*:447, 1972.
Popper, H. and Orr, W.: *Scand J Gastroenterol, (Suppl), 6*:203, 1970.
Popper, H., et al.: *N Engl J Med, 281*:1455, 1969.
Porta, E.A., et al.: *Exp Mol Pathol, 12*:104, 1970.
Prince, A.M., et al.: *N Engl J Med, 282*:988, 1970.
Reynolds, T.B., et al.: *Ann Intern Med, 70*:497, 1969.
Rubin, E., et al.: *Hum Pathol, 2*:343, 1971.
Schweitzer, I.L. and Spears, R.L.: *N Engl J Med, 283*:510, 1970.
Sherlock, S.: *Gut, 13*:297, 1972.
Shulman, N.R.: *Am J Med, 49*:669, 1970.
Skikne, M.I. and Talbot, J.H.: *Lab Invest, 31*:246, 1974.
Small, D.M.: *Adv Intern Med, 16*:243, 1970.
Small, D.M.: *N Engl J Med, 279*:588, 1968.
Smith, J.B.: *Med Clin North Am, 54*:797, 1970.
Sutnick, A.I., et al.: *Am J Dis Child, 123*:392, 1972.
Tartakow, I.J.: *Am J Med, 50*:313, 1971.
Taswell, H.F., et al.: *JAMA, 214*:142, 1970.
Trey, C., et al.: *New Engl J Med, 279*:798, 1968.
Vischer, T.L.: *Br Med J, 2*:695, 1970.
Vogel, C.L., et al., *Lancet, 2*:621, 1970.

CHAPTER 22

THE LYMPH NODES AND SPLEEN

DISEASES OF THE LYMPH NODES

INFLAMMATORY DISEASES OF THE LYMPH NODES. Lymph nodes contain reticuloendothelial cells, which act as a filtering system to remove irritants that pass to the lymph node by way of the lymphatics. Acute lymphadenitis is the most common alteration of lymph nodes.

Lymphadenitis may develop in those lymph nodes draining any region of acute inflammation. The lymph nodes become enlarged and tender or painful. The enlargement of lymph nodes during acute lymphadenitis is due to hyperplasia of the cellular elements and infiltration of acute inflammatory cells. Diphtheria, pharyngitis, measles, scarlet fever, gastroenteritis, vaginitis, pyogenic infection and abscess, cellulitis, and mononucleosis are representative of the wide range of pathologic processes associated with localized and generalized acute lymphadenitis.

The enlarged lymph nodes due to acute lymphadenitis may persist for several weeks, and in children the enlargement is commonly accompanied by fever, fluctuations, convulsions, and meningitis.

Chronic lymphadenitis occurs in lymph nodes draining areas of low-grade inflammation. The nodes show proliferation of mononuclear cells. The lymph nodes do not reach a large size during chronic lymphadenitis.

Chronic granulomatous lymphadenitis is due to tuberculosis, sarcoidosis, cat-scratch disease, lymphopathia venereum, brucellosis and tularemia. The lymph nodes show areas of necrosis and proliferation of epithelioid histiocytic cells and hyperplasia of reticulum cells.

Infectious mononucleosis is a contagious disease affecting the cervical lymph nodes. During infectious mononucleosis, immature white blood cells, probably lymphoblasts, are present in the circulating blood.

NEOPLASMS OF LYMPH NODES. The malignant lymphomas comprise neoplastic pathologic processes involving the lymph nodes of the body. The giant follicle lymphosarcoma is a malignant lymphoma of lymph nodes and lymphoid tissues. The neoplasm produces a prominent follicular pattern. The large follicles are closely packed together, and a condensation of reticulum fibers is present at the periphery of follicles. The enlarged follicles are located in the peripheral area as well as in the central zone of the lymph nodes. In the advanced stage of this lymphoma, the follicular pattern disappears.

Lymphosarcoma is a malignant lymphoma of the lymph nodes, which arises from lymphoid tissue at a mean age of forty-five years. Lymphadenopathy occurs early in this lymphoma, with the cervical lymph nodes most commonly involved. Extension to other lymph nodes occurs in the early stage of this neoplasm. Metastasis takes place later by way of the blood stream to affect various organs throughout the body. The lymphosarcoma arises from the undifferentiated mesenchymal cell of the lymph node. Lymphosarcoma has been classified into the following: lymphocytic variety composed of well-differentiated, small lymphocytes; lymphoblastic variety composed of undifferentiated, large lymphocytes; mixed variety composed of lymphocytes and reticulum cells; and reticulum cell variety (reticulum cell sarcoma).

Reticulum cell sarcoma is a malignant lymphoma of lymph nodes of obscure etiology. The sarcoma may be localized or generalized, and the affected individual loses weight, and develops fever and anemia. The reticulum cell sarcoma is commonly present in the visceral lymph nodes, causing displacement of the kidney, stomach, and intestines. The affected lymph nodes become matted together into one syncytium.

The lymphosarcoma destroys the normal architecture of the lymph node due to proliferation of neoplastic cells. Lymphoblasts proliferate and destroy the sinuses of the affected lymph nodes.

The neoplastic cells are similar in morphology, penetrate the capsule of the node, and invade the adjacent structures.

Lymphatic leukemia is a form of malignant lymphoma involving the lymph nodes. Lymphatic leukemia is accompanied by fever, anemia, and lymph node enlargement. Lymphatic leukemia has a similar morphologic appearance to the lymphosarcoma. The architecture of the lymph nodes is destroyed by small lymphocytes and some large and young neoplastic cells.

Hodgkin's disease is a form of malignant lymphoma involving the lymph nodes or lymphoid tissue in the spleen, gastrointestinal tract, and bone marrow. The etiology of Hodgkin's disease is obscure; however, it has been considered a viral infection, a neoplasm of lymphoid tissue, and a chronic granuloma. Hodgkin's disease is two to three times more common in males than females. It occurs more commonly in individuals between twenty and forty years of age but may occur at any age. Hodgkin's disease is twice as common in young adults as the lymphosarcoma. However, Hodgkin's disease has the same frequency in children as the lymphosarcoma. Hodgkin's disease begins as an enlargement of the cervical lymph nodes in the neck. The enlarged cervical nodes are initially discrete. However, during the late stages of the disease the individual nodes become fused together. Splenomegaly, hepatomegaly, and anemia are present. In early Hodgkin's disease, the lymph nodes are affected by a lymphoblastic hyperplasia. In late Hodgkin's disease, a reticulum cell hyperplasia with eosinophils and giant cells is the dominant histopathologic feature. In still a later stage of Hodgkin's disease, there is a replacement of the cellular structure of lymph nodes by fibrous connective tissue, producing a hard and contracted lymph node. The architecture of the affected lymph node is obliterated in all instances of Hodgkin's disease. The lymphoblastic proliferation of early Hodgkin's disease may be confused with the lymphosarcoma. The pleomorphism of reticulum cells suggests that Hodgkin's disease may be an infective granuloma. Large, pale reticuloendothelial cells (epithelioid cells), Reed-Sternberg multinucleated giant cells, and fibrosis in the late stage constitute the histologic features of Hodgkin's disease (Hodgkin's granuloma).

Hodgkin's disease has been classified into the following types on the basis of histopathology: Hodgkin's paragranuloma, Hodgkin's granuloma, and Hodgkin's sarcoma. Hodgkin's paragranuloma is a benign disease of the cervical lymph nodes, producing cervical lymphadenopathy as the main symptom. Hodgkin's paragranuloma may undergo transformation into Hodgkin's granuloma, which is probably the most common variety of Hodgkin's disease. Hodgkin's granuloma is synonymous with Hodgkin's disease. Hodgkin's sarcoma is the most anaplastic variety of the disease. This neoplasm runs a highly malignant course and has the same incidence in males and females between fifty and seventy years of age. Pleomorphic lymphocytic and reticulum cells, mitoses, fibrosis, and the presence of Reed-Sternberg cells are the principal histopathologic findings.

METASTATIC NEOPLASMS TO THE LYMPH NODES. The metastatic neoplasms to the lymph nodes are much more common than the primary lymphomas. The majority of metastatic neoplasms to lymph nodes are epithelial in origin. The metastatic cells in the lymph nodes may be either the same degree of differentiation or less differentiated than the cells of the primary neoplasm.

DISEASES OF THE SPLEEN

The spleen is a vascular organ that represents the largest single collection of lymphoid and reticuloendothelial tissues in the body. The spleen has the function of detaining and altering the blood as it passes through the organ. The spleen is a filter for bacteria and hemolyzed red blood cells. The spleen is capable of production of blood cells (extramedullary hematopoesis).

ANOMALIES OF THE SPLEEN. An accessory spleen is an anomaly of principal interest to surgeons since it may be overlooked during splenectomy in the treatment of primary splenic disease.

RETROGRADE CHANGES IN THE SPLEEN. Amyloidosis is a degenerative, irreversible change in the spleen, characterized by deposition of amyloid either locally or diffusely, causing splenomegaly. Focal necrosis, atrophy, and pigmentation may occur in the spleen. Rupture of the spleen may occur spontaneously or result from trauma. Splenic rupture is characterized by a possible history of splenomegaly or injury followed by a sudden onset of abdominal pain, nonshifting paravertebral dullness, increasing anemia, decrease in hematocrit, and leukocytosis. A ruptured spleen may be associated with typhoid fever, malaria, and infectious mononucleosis.

CIRCULATORY DISTURBANCES IN THE SPLEEN. Chronic passive hyperemia produces a congested and enlarged spleen as a result of mitral valve disease or in following portal obstruction. Infarction of the spleen is caused by embolic occlusion of a branch of the splenic artery. Infarction of the spleen is usually associated with subacute bacterial endocarditis and leukemia.

Banti's syndrome (splenic anemia) includes enlargement of the spleen, nonhemolytic anemia, leukopenia, and possible portal cirrhosis. The enlarged spleen is congested and fibrotic. Hemorrhages develop and precede the fibrosis. Dilated splenic sinusoids are present with thick, collagenous walls. The original lesion in Banti's syndrome may be cirrhosis of the liver.

Felty's syndrome is a symptom complex consisting of enlargement of the spleen in adults, chronic arthritis with leukopenia, and lymphadenopathy.

Hemolytic jaundice is an inherited and congenital disease transmitted as a Mendelian dominant characteristic. Hemolytic jaundice is characterized by an enlarged spleen, jaundice, fever, and spheroid-shaped erythrocytes with increased fragility (spherocytic anemia). The splenic enlargement is the result of hypertrophy of phagocytic cells and the accumulation of blood in the splenic pulp.

Pernicious anemia is accompanied by an enlarged spleen with hemosiderin pigment deposited in the splenic pulp. Polycythemia vera is accompanied by vascular thrombosis and excessive red blood cells in the enlarged spleen. The thrombosis may cause splenic infarcts, producing abdominal pain.

INFLAMMATION OF THE SPLEEN. Acute splenitis (acute splenic tumor) is characterized by an enlarged and tender spleen, which accompanies bacteremias or septicemias. The softest spleen occurs during septicemia and pyemia. The enlarged spleen results from a proliferation of mononuclear cells, blood, and hyperplastic follicles.

Myeloid metaplasia of the spleen is characterized clinically by anemia, pallor, slight icterus, splenomegaly, hepatomegaly, and bone pain. The affected individual has a history of polycythemia vera or diseases of bone tissue. The bone marrow is acellular and fibrotic. The splenomegaly may be due to the development of active hematopoietic tissue in the spleen.

NEOPLASMS OF THE SPLEEN. Hodgkin's disease causes an enlarged spleen since it represents a disease of the reticuloendothelial system. All forms of leukemia produce splenomegaly. The lymphoid reticuloendothelial cells proliferate, and the sinuses of the spleen are filled with leukemia cells. Lymphosarcoma results in infiltration of the splenic parenchyma with neoplastic lymphoid cells and prolymphocytes.

LIPIDOSIS OF THE RETICULOENDOTHELIAL SYSTEM. The lipidosis are rare lipid storage diseases and are characterized by an accumulation of lipids in varying quantities in reticuloendothelial cells, i.e. Gaucher's disease and Niemann-Pick disease. A nonlipid reticuloendotheliosis or osseous xanthomatosis termed *Hand-Schüller-Christian syndrome* also affects the spleen.

Gaucher's disease is a chronic, familial, cerebroside lipoidosis in which kerasin accumulates abnormally in the reticulum cells of the spleen, lymph nodes, liver, and bone marrow. The disease is initiated during childhood and continues for many years into adulthood. Massive enlargement of the spleen occurs. The lymph nodes are only moderately enlarged. The spleen contains collections of large, mononuclear cells filled with kerasin. The large, pale, mononuclear cells are termed *Gaucher cells*. The latter cells accumulate and cause the excessive enlargement of the spleen.

NIEMANN-PICK DISEASE. Niemann-Pick disease is a lipidosis due to the abnormal accumulation of sphingomyelin in reticuloendothelial cells and histiocytic cells of tissues and organs. The disease occurs in young infants and is fatal by two years of age. Lipid-filled cells are present in the spleen, lymph nodes, liver, and bone marrow. However, the sphingomyelin-containing cells may be present in the lung, adrenal, thyroid, brain, pancreas, and glomeruli of the kidney. Deposition of sphingomyelin in the ganglion cells of the brain may result in idiocy.

Hand-Schüller-Christian Syndrome is basically an osseous xanthomatosis in children and adults. The symptom complex includes defects of membranous bones, diabetes insipidus, and exophthalmos. Defects are common in the skeleton, particularly in the skull. The latter defects consist of collections of xanthoma cells, which contain cholesterol. The cholesterol accumulates in phagocytic cells of the reticuloendothelial system.

References

Banfi, A., et al.: *Eur J Cancer, 4*:319, 1968.
Bennett, J.M., et al.: *Bull WHO, 40*:601, 1969.
Butler, J.J.: In *14th Annual Clinical Conference on Cancer, 1969*. Chicago, Year Bk Med, 1970, p. 135.
Cole, P. and MacMahon, B.: *Lancet, 2*:1371, 1968.
Davies, J.N.P.: *Hum Pathol, 3*:297, 1972.
Dmochowski, L.: In *14th Annual Clinical Conference on Cancer, 1969*. Chicago, Year Bk Med, 1970, p. 37.
Editorial: Further in the Hodgkin maze. *Lancet, 1*:1053, 1971.
Fudenberg, H.H.: *Am J Med, 51*:295, 1971.
Goldman, J.M. and Aisenberg, A.C.: *Cancer, 26*:327, 1970.
Henle, W., et al.: *J Natl Cancer Inst, 44*:225, 1970.
Hoover, R. and Fraumeni, J.F.: *Lancet, 2*:55, 1973.
Johansson, B., et al.: *Int J Cancer, 8*:475, 1971.
Klein, G., et al.: *J Exp Med, 129*:697, 1969.
Lukes, R.J. and Parker, J.W.: In Brunson, J.G. and Gall, E.A. (Eds.): *Concepts of Disease*. New York, MacMillan, 1971, p. 924.
Lukes, R.J., et al.: *Lancet, 2*:1003, 1969.
MacMahon, B.: *Cancer Res, 27*:416, 1971.
Newell, G.R.: *J Natl Cancer Inst, 45*:311, 1970.
Order, S.E. and Hellman, S.: *Lancet, 1*:571, 1972.
Penn, W., et al.: *Transplant Proc, 1*:106, 1969.
Rappaport, H., et al.: *Cancer Res, 31*:1864, 1971.
Strum, S.B. and Rappaport, H.: *Arch Pathol, 91*:127, 1971.
Strum, S.B., et al.: *Cancer, 26*:176, 1970.
Vianna, N.J., et al.: *Lancet, 1*:1209, 1971.
Vianna, N.J., et al.: *Lancet, 1*:431, 1971.
Weiss, L.: *J Biophys Biochem Cytol, 3*:599, 1957.

CHAPTER 23

BLOOD AND BONE MARROW

INTRODUCTION TO DISEASES OF THE BLOOD AND BONE MARROW

BLOOD FORMATION starts in the liver after the second month of intrauterine life and continues for a period following birth. The spleen participates in blood formation after the second month of intrauterine life and continues until the seventh month of fetal life. Eventually, the marrow takes over the function of hematopoiesis. All of the bone marrow throughout the body is red or hematopoietic bone marrow until puberty. At puberty there is a regression of active bone marrow. Hematopoietic bone is located in the ribs, vertebrate, distal portion of the femur, humerus, sternum, and innominate bones. All blood cells are formed in the bone marrow. The entire circulating red blood cells and their precursors originate in the bone marrow. Oxygen is carried by the hemoglobin. Approximately fifteen different chemical types of hemoglobin have been described.

ALTERATIONS IN RED BLOOD CELLS

Loss of hemoglobin and decrease in the number of red blood cells results in anemia. The general morphology of the organs of the body during anemia depends upon the severity and duration of the disease.

ANEMIAS DUE TO BLOOD LOSS. Anemias may be due to loss of blood from the body. Chronic hemorrhage leads to chronic anemia. In chronic anemia, the nails are brittle and spoon shaped. Cardiac cells, epithelial cells of renal tubules, hepatic cells, and ganglion cells of the central nervous system show fatty degeneration.

Hemolytic anemias are due to extrinsic factors, i.e. bacterial toxins, antigens, or hematologic injury to red blood cells. Intrinsic factors also produce hemolytic anemias due to anoxia. When rapid hemolysis occurs, the result is acute tubular necrosis, hemosiderosis, and hyperplastic normoblastic bone marrow.

Spherocytic anemia (congenital hemolytic anemia) is a congenital, familial, Mendelian dominant disease, which becomes clinically evident early in life. There is an inherent defect in the red blood cells, which affects individuals of any race and in both sexes. The disease is characterized by prolonged or recurrent attacks of jaundice accompanied by varying degrees of anemia and splenomegaly. The red blood cells are biconvex discs (spherocytes) and show excessive fragility and decreased resistance.

The spleen is enlarged, congested, and contains enlarged sinusoids. Foci of extramedullary hematopoiesis develop in the liver, and excessive hemosiderin pigment is present in the bone marrow and parenchymal organs. Proliferative changes occur in the outer plate of the skull, producing the tower skull. The clinical finding of spherocytic anemia include mild jaundice, high incidence of gall stones, chronic leg ulcers, and hemorrhage that may occur into the intestines.

Sickle cell anemia is a congenital, hemolytic anemia transmitted as a Mendelian dominant hereditary characteristic. Sickle cell anemia is present in approximately 7 to 10 percent of Negroes in the United States. The disease occurs in young adults of either sex. The sickle cell trait produces sickled red blood cells, i.e. the formation of bizarre-shaped cells when exposed to low oxygen tension. The sickling of red blood cells is due to the presence of hemoglobin S in individuals with sickle cell anemia. Hemoglobin S is less soluble and crystallizes as compared to normal hemoglobin. In the individuals with sickle cell anemia there is less oxygen, more sickling in the venous blood, and the hemoglobin is all hemoglobin S. In the latter individuals, the fetal hemoglobin is replaced by hemoglobin S instead of by normal adult hemoglobin A. During a hemolytic crisis, the patient will have some fetal hemoglobin, jaundice, leukocytosis, and decreased platelets. The spleen is congested and enlarged. There are recurrent attacks of weakness, fatigue, and anemia. Pain occurs in the gastrointestinal tract, and nausea and vomiting are present.

Cooley's Mediterranean anemia or thalassemia is a form of erythroblastic anemia. The disease is congenital and familial and occurs among children of the Mediterranean races. The disease is due to the persistence of fetal hemoglobin. The disease follows a severe course, and death occurs in childhood. The clinical features are thickening of the skull and long bones, Mongoloid facies, enlarged spleen, pallor, and enlarged abdomen due to hepatomegaly and splenomegaly. There is reduced destruction of blood and less hemosiderosis; however, hemosiderin may be found in the parenchymal organs. Hyperplasia of the bone marrow is present in the porous long bones with thickened cortex.

Erythroblastosis fetalis or hemolytic disease of the newborn is a congenital disease of the newborn in which an excessive quantity of immature red blood cells is present in the peripheral blood. Excessive hemolysis and destruction of red blood cells occur in the peripheral blood. Extramedullary hematopoiesis is present in the spleen and liver. Red blood cells are present in various tissues of the body. The acute disease of the newborn is characterized by hydrops fetalis, i.e. edema and ascites, icterus gravis neonatorum (intense jaundice), and kernicterus (bile pigmentation of basal ganglia of the brain, which accompanies erythroblastic anemia of the newborn).

The Rh factor is important in erythroblastosis fetalis. The child born from an Rh-negative mother and Rh-positive father has a good chance of inheriting the Rh factor. When the Rh factor is inherited, the fetus produces anti-Rh agglutinins in the maternal blood stream. The anti-Rh agglutinins pass through the placenta, causing destruction of the red blood cells of the fetus.

Hemoglobinuria is caused by syphilis and exposure to cold. Hemoglobinuria is the result of hemolysis of red blood cells intravenously. Moderate splenomegaly and heptomegaly are present and the urine has a clear, port wine color and contains hemolyzed red blood cells. The intravascular release of hemoglobin produces methemoglobin which colors the plasma pink.

ANEMIAS DUE TO DECREASED RED BLOOD CELL PRODUCTION. Hypochromic anemias result from a deficiency of iron caused by acute or chronic hemorrhage, chronic infections, parasitic infections, pregnancy, neoplasms, diseases of the gastrointestinal tract, and lead poisoning. When acute hemorrhage occurs in a patient with hypochromic anemia the findings include leukocytosis, increased reticulocyte count, and hyperplasia of the normoblasts of bone marrow. The red blood cells are smaller than normal, and the hemoglobin concentration is less than 30 percent of normal. The parenchymal organs show degenerative changes.

Idiopathic hypochromic anemia occurs in Caucasians, generally females between forty and fifty years of age. The disease has an occasional familial incidence. The findings include normal to slightly reduced red blood cell count, markedly decreased hemoglobin, decreased color index, decreased hematocrit, microcytosis, normal leukocytes, achlorhydria, atrophy of mucous membrane and dysphagia. The anemia is progressive with no spontaneous remissions. Administration of iron is the recommended therapy.

Pernicious anemia is due to a deficiency of the extrinsic factor, i.e. vitamin B_{12} and of the intrinsic factor (unknown substance) produced by cells of the stomach. The gastric deficiency produces gastric achlorhydria and variable gastrointestinal and neurological disturbances. The intrinsic factor is necessary for absorption of vitamin B_{12} from the small intestines.

Pernicious anemia affects both sexes but is more common in males. It occurs in individuals from forty to sixty years of age. Pernicious anemia is chiefly a disease of the Caucasian race (Nordic types). The disease is insidious and progresses slowly. The anemia has remissions and exacerbations. The clinical triad of pernicious anemia is weakness, sore tongue, and numbness or tingling. The pernicious anemia patient has a lemon-yellow pallor, no free hydrochloric acid in the stomach, and gastrointestinal and central nervous system symptoms. The blood picture in pernicious anemia is a macrocytic hypochromic anemia. There is a variation in the size of the red blood cells, and the abnormal red blood cells do not have a normal survival time. The white blood cells are also affected in pernicious anemia (lymphocytosis and abnormal granulocytes).

The stomach is affected by an atrophic gastritis. Gastric analysis reveals an achylia following histamine stimulation. The central nervous system changes include atrophy and degeneration of the dorsal and lateral columns of the spinal cord, degeneration of ganglion cells, and demyelination. There is also degeneration of peripheral nerves. Patients with pernicious anemia have a predisposition to carcinoma of the stomach, cirrhosis of the liver, sprue and celiac disease, pellagra, and intestinal disorders. Diarrhea, loss of weight, paresthesia, glossitis and sore tongue, and achlorhydria are the principal findings. Treatment with vitamin B_{12} produces a proliferation of normoblastic tissue, which replaces the megaloblastic tissue in the bone marrow. Erythropoietic tissue is converted to normaloblastic tissue in twenty-four hours following initiation of therapy.

Aplastic anemia results from failure of blood cells to undergo maturation at an early phase. A severe anemia, leukopenia, and thrombocytopenia develop. Individuals with aplastic anemia show weakness, fatigue, dyspnea, sepsis and fever, and purpuric manifestations. The anemia is common in young adult females.

Myelophthisic anemia is an anemia characterized by replacement of the bone marrow and blood-forming elements by proliferating neoplastic tissue, fibrosis of the marrow, or due to storage disease.

DISEASES DUE TO INCREASED RED BLOOD CELLS. Polycythemia (Erythemia) is an increase in the number of red blood cells (7 to 10 million RBC per cubic millimeter of blood). There is excessive erythroblastic activity in the bone marrow which produces a persistent polycythemia and splenomegaly.

A mild polycythemia is due to poor oxygenation. A second kind of polycythemia is of unknown etiology, i.e. polycythemia rubra. The latter occurs in middle-aged individuals and is due to a proliferation of leukopoietic (granulopoietic and erythropoietic) tissue. The red blood cells may increase to 13.5 million per cubic millimeter of blood due to overproduction rather than to increased longevity. The bone marrow is engorged and hyperplastic. Splenomegaly and hepatomegaly, ecchymoses in the skin and mucous membranes, and thrombosis are the main findings. All of the parenchymal organs are engorged, and the capillaries are hyperemic. Polycythemia may be associated with a long survival period. The individual has a cyanotic appearance. Complications are due to hemorrhage and thrombosis.

ALTERATIONS IN WHITE BLOOD CELLS

LEUKOCYTOSIS AND LEUKOPENIA. Leukocytosis is an increase in the number of circulating leukocytes. The number of immature, neutrophilic leukocytes is increased in the circulating blood. Leukocytosis is present in most pyogenic infections. Leukopenia is a reduction in the number of circulating leukocytes. It may result from chemicals, drugs, radiation, aplasia of the bone marrow, infections, redistribution of white blood cells within the vascular channels, and increased destruction of white blood cells.

INFECTIOUS MONONUCLEOSIS. Infectious mononucleosis is an acute, benign, infectious disease of obscure etiology characterized by the following clinical findings: irregular fever, sore throat, lymphadenopathy, splenomegaly, hepatomegaly, purpura, and jaundice. Infectious mononucleosis is characterized by a leukocytosis with atypical lymphocytes, lymphocytosis, and anemia. Infectious mononucleosis is generally self-limiting in approximately three weeks; however, the disease has been reported to exist for weeks to as long as months.

The clinical laboratory findings concerning infectious mononucleosis include the following: leukocytosis (10,000 to 25,000), lymphocytosis (50% to 90%), atypical lymphocytes, normal erythrocytes, possible decreased platelets, normal bone marrow, serum heterophile agglutinin titre above 1:120, which is diagnostic, and bone marrow eosinophilia.

The lymph nodes are enlarged and show extreme hyperplasia of lymphocytes and reticulum, with atypical lymphocytes present in the sinuses.

Agranulocytosis is a marked depression in the formation of leukocytes accompanied by a decrease in the number of granulocytes in the circulating blood. Agranulocytosis is associated with infections, chemicals, and drugs. There is an absence of anemia.

CYCLICAL NEUTROPENIA. Cyclical neutropenia is a rare, periodic decrease in circulating polymorphonuclear leukocytes. The disorder affects both males and females and persists without remissions. The neutropenia generally follows a rhythmical pattern of three-week periodicity. Every three weeks the following symptoms appear: anorexia, malaise, and lymphadenitis.

LEUKEMIA. Leukemia is a neoplasm of white blood cells, which terminates fatally. Widespread proliferation of leukocytes and their precursors infiltrates the blood and tissues of the body with numerous immature and abnormal cell forms. The bone marrow is stimulated by some obscure etiologic factor(s) into producing leukocytes or their precursors at the expense of the normal erythroblastic tissue.

The leukemias are classified according to the type of white blood cells produced by the leukocyte-forming tissue present in the bone marrow, i.e. myeloid, lymphatic, and monocytic. The latter three types may be acute or chronic. Acute leukemias develop during the first decade of life; chronic myeloid leukemia develops between twenty-five and forty-five years of age, and chronic lymphoid leukemia develops between forty-five and sixty years of age.

Acute leukemia develops insidiously, and the neoplasm follows a rapid course with high white blood counts, anemia, and thrombocytopenia. The bone marrow throughout the body is densely infiltrated with primitive, undifferentiated white blood cells.

Chronic myeloid leukemia results from a hyperplasia of the bone marrow with a tremendous increase in granular leukocytes in the circulating blood, and numerous immature myeloblasts and myelocytes are readily visible in blood smears. The white blood cell count is extremely elevated and may reach 500,000 or more per cubic millimeter. Normocytic anemia and increased platelets, and decreased erythropoiesis occur as the bone marrow is displaced by proliferating, immature leukocytes. The leukemia follows a chronic course and may last for one to five years, terminating fatally. Chronic myeloid leukemia has the most rapid course of all chronic leukemias. The bone marrow contains predominantly myelocytes, and myeloid infiltration causes an enlarged spleen and liver. Myeloid cells infiltrate the kidney, lymph nodes, heart, and viscera.

Chronic lymphatic leukemia is accompanied by a white blood cell count under 100,000 lymphoid cells per cubic millimeter.

Anemia results from a reduction of red blood cells. The spleen, lymph nodes, and liver are infiltrated with lymphoid cells. The bone marrow is replaced by an infiltrate of mainly lymphocytes with minimal numbers of lymphoblasts. The skin contains infiltrations of lymphocytes. This leukemia has an insidious onset with weight loss, fatigue, lymphadenopathy, and bone tenderness.

Monocytic leukemia occurs in the chronic form in 10 to 11 percent of instances of this leukemia. Acute monocytic leukemia is the most common form of this leukemia. Mature and immature monocytes are present in the circulating blood but in greatly increased numbers. Monocytic leukemia occurs in two types, i.e. the Naegeli type and the Schilling type. The Naegeli type consists of immature monocytes intermediate between monocytes and myeloblasts. The Schilling type consists of immature cells in the blood resembling monocytes and reticuloendothelial cells. Skin and oral mucosal infiltrations plus hyperplasia are common as well as hemorrhage from the oral and mucous membranes.

Plasma cell leukemia is more correctly termed *multiple myeloma*, i.e. abnormal plasma cells are present in the circulating blood. Multiple myeloma is a primary neoplasm of the elements of the bone marrow.

Aleukemic leukemia is characterized by splenomegaly in individuals of middle age or older. The peripheral blood may contain immature red blood cells and there is a leukocytosis with or without features of leukemia. The bone marrow may be filled with abnormal white blood cells. This reaction may represent a form of myeloid leukemia or a response of hematopoietic cells to a nonspecific stimulus and, therefore, may not be associated with anemia.

DISEASES ASSOCIATED WITH ELEVATED WHITE BLOOD CELL COUNTS. Lymphocytosis is present in viral diseases, bacterial infections, tuberculosis, syphilis, brucellosis, infectious mononucleosis, and in convalescent patients. Elevated basophiles occur in chronic granulocytic leukemia, smallpox (variola), irradiation, and polycythemia. Elevated eosinophiles are present in familial eosinophilia, allergic diseases, recovery phase of infections, parasitic infections, collagen diseases, dermatologic diseases, reticuloendotheliosis, hypoadrenal-corticism and metastatic neoplasms. Elevated neutrophiles occur in pyogenic infections, physiological neutrophilia, necrosis, neoplasms, intoxication, abnormal metabolism, and polycythemia.

DISEASES ASSOCIATED WITH LOWERED WHITE BLOOD CELL COUNTS. Leukopenia is caused by irradiation, typhoid fever, chemotherapy with cytotoxic drugs, sulfonamides, thiouracil, and amidopyrine. Leukopenia may be due to lymphopenia or neutropenia.

PURPURA

THROMBOCYTOPENIC PURPURA. Purpura is the presence of an extravasation of blood (petechiae and ecchymosis) beneath the skin and mucous membranes of the body. Purpura accompanies various pathologic processes, i.e. leukemias, advanced anemia, and certain severe infectious diseases. Thrombocytopenic purpura is a specific form of purpura that is associated with a decrease in the number of blood platelets (thrombocytes) in children and young adults. The blood vessel walls undergo an alteration so that spontaneous hemorrhages occur into the mucous membranes, skin, and joints. Thrombocytopenic purpura occurs secondarily to systemic diseases, i.e. severe infections and septic states, meningococcus septicemia, chemicals, poisons, and drugs. The disease is common in Caucasian females.

The bone marrow is normal and, therefore, platelet formation is not affected. The spleen may or may not be palpated. Females with thrombocytopenic purpura have a prolonged and heavy menstruation. Small hemorrhages occur in the central nervous system. In rare instances, platelet agglutination occurs. The latter patients are destroying their own platelets. The cause of platelet agglutination is unknown.

THROMBOTIC THROMBOCYTOPENIC PURPURA. This rare condition is a disease of the arterioles and capillaries characterized by platelet thromboses, hemolytic anemia, thrombocytopenic purpura, fever, and neurological disturbances. The arterioles and capillaries are occluded by hyaline or eosinophilic (fibrinoid) material. The spleen is congested and enlarged, and there is a reduction in blood platelets to less than 50,000 per cubic millimeter. This purpura is fatal in a matter of weeks. The etiology is currently obscure; however, the disease has similarities to the collagen diseases.

HEMOPHILIAS

Hemophilia is an inherited disease transmitted as a recessive sex-linked Mendelian factor. Females carry the gene, but the disease appears only in males.

Classic hemophilia A is due to deficiency of antihemophilic globulin (AHG). Blood coagulation is prolonged; however, the following hematologic tests are normal: bleeding time, clot retraction, prothrombin concentration, and the tourniquet test. The platelets fail to release thromboplastin. Prolonged hemorrhage results from trauma. Hemarthroses produces painful and deformed joints.

Christmas disease or hemophilia B is due to a deficiency of plasma thromboplastic component (PTC). The deficiency is a sex-linked Mendelian recessive disease. The findings are petechiae and ecchymoses in the mucous membrane and skin, epistaxis, and hemarthrosis, which are all of a lesser severity than the manifestations of hemophilia A.

Hemophilia C is due to a rare deficiency of plasma thromboplastic antecedent (PTA) or factor XI. The disease affects both males and females. The genetic nature of this disease is obscure; however, it is not a sex-linked Mendelian recessive disease. The clinical manifestations of hemophilia C are milder than those of hemophilia A.

Von Willebrand's disease is a hereditary hematologic disorder of obscure etiology, which affects both males and females. The platelet count is normal, the bleeding time is prolonged, the clotting time and clot retraction are normal; however, there is increased capillary fragility. Females with this disorder bleed heavily during menstruation.

References

Awano, I., et al.: *Tohoku J Exp Med, 102*:233, 1970.
Brain, M.C.: *Ann Rev Med, 21*:133, 1970.

Brodsky, I. and Siegel, N.H.: *Med Clin North Am, 54*:555, 1970.
Castle, W.B.: *Am J Med, 48*:541, 1970.
Colman, R.W. and Rodriguez-Erdmann, F.: *N Engl J Med, 282*:99, 1970.
Deykin, D.: *N Engl J Med, 283*:636, 1970.
Edson, J.R.: *Hum Pathol, 1*:387, 1970.
Fialkow, P.J., et al.: *Lancet, 1*:251, 1971.
Gabuzda, T.G.: *Del Med J, 43*:124, 1971.
Gallo, R.C., et al.: *Nature (Lond), 228*:927, 1970.
Gardikas, C., et al.: *Acta Haematol, 46*:201, 1971.
Greenberg, P.L., et al.: *N Engl J Med, 284*:1225, 1971.
Harrington, W.J.: *Med Times, 99*:53, 1971.
Ichikawa, Y.: *J Cell Physiol, 76*:175, 1970.
Kahn, S.B.: *Med Clin North Am, 54*:631, 1970.
Keitt, A.S.: *Mod Treat, 8*:402, 1971.
Kwaan, H.C.: *Med Clin North Am, 46*:177, 1972.
Marks, P.A. and Bank, A.: *Fed Proc, 30*:977, 1971.
Nalbandian, R.M. and Evans, T.N.: *Mich Med, 70*:411, 1971.
Nalbandian, R.M., et al.: *Hum Pathol, 2*:377, 1971.
Nathan, D.G.: *N Engl J Med, 286*:586, 1972.
Pauling, L.: In Nalbandian, R.M. (Ed.): *Molecular Aspects of Sickle Cell Hemoglobin. Clinical Applications.* Springfield, Thomas, 1971.
Pederson, B. and Hayhoe, F.G.J.: *Br J Haematol, 21*:251, 1971.
Sandberg, A.A., et al.: *Cancer, 27*:176, 1971.
Schumacher, H.R., et al.: *Cancer, 26*:895, 1970.
Spiegelman, S., et al.: *Nature (Lond), 227*:1029, 1970.
Sullivan, L.W.: *Am J Med, 48*:609, 1970.
Szippin, C., et al.: *Blood, 37*:59, 1971.
Valentine, W.N.: *Adv Intern Med, 16*:303, 1970.
White, J.G. and Heagan, B.: *Am J Pathol, 58*:1, 1970.
Wiernik, P.H. and Serpick, A.A.: *Medicine, 49*:505, 1970.

CHAPTER 24

THE ENDOCRINE SYSTEM

Introduction

ALL OF THE endocrine glands of the body are interrelated and interdependent. Each endocrine gland represents one unit of the total endocrine system. For example, the body requires more insulin during hyperthyroidism and less insulin during atrophy or total absence of the pituitary gland.

The cortices of the pituitary and adrenal glands have a special and intimate relationship. Stress, i.e. the presence of internal lacerations, produces adrenocortical hypertrophy only if ACTH is present. When the entire pituitary gland is excised, the adrenal gland also becomes defective. The adrenal gland is the only endocrine gland vital to life. The adrenal gland exhibits self-regulation. Hypertrophy of the adrenal gland is not possible if the connection with the hypothalamus is severed. If one adrenal gland is surgically excised, the remaining gland undergoes compensatory hypertrophy.

Neural relationships are intimately associated with the anterior pituitary gland. The hypothalamus and the posterior pituitary influence the release of ACTH by two mechanisms. Epinephrine released from the medulla, and direct neural connection and the central nervous system neurohumorals all impinge upon the hypothalamus and posterior pituitary. The portal circulation carries the humoral agents from the hypothalamus and posterior pituitary to the anterior pituitary. The adrenal cortex secretes steroid compounds (17-oxycorticosteroid or 17-hydroxycorticosteroid), which take part in the feedback or servomechanism by acting upon the anterior pituitary and possibly upon the hypothalamus. The feedback mechanism, therefore, reacts upon the anterior and posterior pituitary and hypothalamus. The central nervous system is stimulated during stress. This nervous system reaction is mediated by the hypothalamus.

The adrenal glands consist of a cortex and a medulla. The adrenal cortex secretes aldosterone, hydrocortisone, androgens, and three to eight steroids. Only two steroids have a physiological effect. Approximately 10 percent of the functional adrenal cortical cells is all that is required to maintain cortical function.

The thyroid gland is under the control of the anterior pituitary gland, which produces and releases the thyroid stimulating hormone (TSH) into the blood stream. The TSH acts directly on the cells of the thyroid gland. Thyroid cells take up iodine under the control of the thyroid stimulating hormone in the blood. Thyroglobulin is secreted by the thyroid gland. Thyroxine is a true hormone produced by the thyroid gland. Thyroxine is liberated from the thyroglobulin and directly enters the blood stream. The active hormones of the thyroid gland are thyronine, thyroxine, and diiodotyrosine. The highest potency is present in thyronine and the lowest potency in diiodotyrosine. Thyroxine regulates hormone production by the pituitary gland through production and secretion of thyrotropic hormone or TSH. The thyroid gland is itself influenced by the adrenal cortex; whereas, the thyroid gland influences the function of the gonads and the islets of Langerhans in the pancreas.

Iodine enters the gastrointestinal tract and circulating blood and is taken up by the thyroid gland. If excessive thyrotropic hormone is produced, there is a greater uptake of iodine and thyroxine. The thyroid gland contains storage epithelium and secreting epithelial cells. All of the different cells of the thyroid gland secrete iodine into the blood stream.

Hyperplasia of the thyroid gland is generally treated with therapeutic doses of iodone. Iodine therapy causes the thyroid acini to return to their original position, and the acinic cells undergo flattening. Colloid accumulates in the thyroid acini, which has undergone enlargement, i.e. involution of the thyroid gland.

The function of the parathyroid glands is to control and

regulate the blood serum levels of calcium and phosphorus. The parathyroid glands produce parathormone (parathyroid hormone) and calcitonin (humoral agent). Parathormone elevates and maintains the normal level of blood calcium. Parathormone controls the liberation of calcium from bones and increases the urinary excretion of phosphates. The parathyroid glands are part of the endocrine system and are a biologic catalyst controlling calcium and phosphates.

DISEASES OF THE PITUITARY GLAND

Congenital Anomalies of the Pituitary Gland

Displaced squamous epithelial cells from Rathke's pouch may be present in the pituitary gland as a congenital anomaly. Epithelial rests from neural tissue are also present in the pituitary but are of no significance. The craniopharyngioma (tumor) of the pituitary gland has its origin in the epithelial rests from Rathke's pouch.

Syndromes of the Pituitary Gland

Destruction of the pituitary gland (anterior pituitary) includes the following syndromes: Simmond's disease; and Sheehan's, Fröhlich's, and Cushing's syndromes. Simmond's disease is caused by infarction and necrosis plus fibrosis and atrophy of the anterior pituitary. Extreme hypofunction of the anterior pituitary produces pituitary cachexia (Simmond's disease). The adult develops the following symptoms due to hypofunction of the anterior pituitary: premature old age; wrinkled, thick skin; myxedema; hypogonads; diminished blood pressure; drop in body temperature; very low basal metabolic rate; marked loss of weight or cachexia; weakness; atrophy of viscera; atrophy of thyroid, adrenals, and gonads; negative nitrogen balance; and osteoporosis of bone tissue.

Sheehan's syndrome is a variety of Simmond's disease that is related to pregnancy, i.e. pituitary cachexia associated with pregnancy and with severe intrapartum or postpartum hemorrhage.

Fröhlich's syndrome is caused by a chromophobe adenoma or more commonly by a craniopharyngioma. This syndrome is related to a peculiar distribution of body fat. Pelvic obesity occurs accompanied by hypogonadism, diabetes insipidus, loss of hair, thin soft skin, and polyuria. When the craniopharyngioma expands in a superior direction, blindness results.

Cushing's syndrome is due to the basophil adenoma of the pituitary gland. In this syndrome the face, neck, and trunk are obese, purple striae are present on the skin, and hypertension and sexual disturbances are present. The clinical findings in this syndrome are generally but not always associated with degenerated changes in the basophils of the pituitary gland.

Diabetes Insipidus

Hypofunction of the posterior pituitary leads to diabetes insipidus. This diabetes is accompanied by polyuria and increased thirst (polydipsia). Hypofunction of the posterior pituitary results from a failure of the hypothalamic-pituitary system, which results in a deficiency of the antidiuretic hormone (ADH). Decreased ADH causes the distal convoluted tubules to lose their ability to concentrate urine. Polyuria results, and the urine has a very low specific gravity.

Functional Hyperplasia of the Pituitary Gland

Gigantism and acromegaly are functional hyperplasias of the pituitary gland. The result of excessive growth hormone depends upon the age of the affected individual. When the individual is young and open epiphyseal plates are present, the excess growth hormone produces gigantism. The bones become long, and the individual may grow to 7 feet 8 inches. Generalized hyperplasia occurs in the viscera since there is an increase in connective tissue in the viscera and bones.

Functional hyperplasia of the eosinophil cells of the anterior pituitary begins after twenty years of age with the development of acromegaly. In the adult who has a functional adenoma of the pituitary gland, the epiphysial plate is closed, and growth of bones occurs only at sites where it normally forms after maturity is reached. Therefore, there is no increase in height in acromegaly. Bone apposition takes place beneath the periosteum and leads to widening and enlargement of specific bones. The hands, feet, skull, nose, and jaws become enlarged. Scoliosis develops with a curvature of the spine. Acromegaly may be associated with secondary disorders such as hypogonadism. Headache and visual disturbances develop in acromegaly and are due to the presence of a tumor occupying the entire sella turcica and adjacent region. Alterations in acromegaly are the result of excessive function of the pituitary gland. Excessive sweating, hypertrophied laryngeal tissues, and deepening of the voice are additional clinical findings of acromegaly.

Neoplasms of the Pituitary Gland

Pituitary tumors produce headache, visual alterations, and diplopia. The presence of a nonfunctional tumor may destroy all of the functional tissue in the pituitary gland. The common chromophobe adenoma of the pituitary causes partial or total destruction of the basophil and eosinophil cells, resulting in pituitary insufficiency. The chromophobe adenoma is capable of destroying the entire pituitary gland, sella turcica, and adjacent neural tissue plus hypothalamus, resulting in hypopituitarism.

The craniopharyngioma is a benign tumor of the pituitary gland, which is capable of destroying the pituitary when it enlarges by means of expansion, resulting in pituitary hypofunction. Cysts may develop in the pituitary gland following either hemorrhage or from the epithelial rests of Rathke's pouch. Cysts slowly expand and produce pituitary insufficiency.

When the hypothalamus is involved by a tumor or other pathology, obesity develops. The fat metabolic center of the body is located in the hypothalamus. The obesity has a specific distribution throughout the body, involving the trunk and neck but sparing the extremities. Carcinoma of the pituitary gland is a destructive tumor causing hypopituitarism.

Mongolism is a developmental disturbance that is accompanied by pituitary gland changes as well as secondary alterations in the gonads, thyroid, and adrenal glands. The mongoloid has characteristic features. The head is smaller than normal, the musculature is hypotonic, and an enlarged tongue (macroglossia) may or may not develop. The etiology of the Mongoloid features and the enlarged tongue is unknown. The jaws are abnormal in size.

The upper jaw is small and the lower jaw is protruded. There is an underdevelopment or absence of the nasal bones, and alterations are present in the shape of the head, i.e. brachycephalic or hyperbrachycephalic Mongoloid head.

DISEASES OF THE ADRENAL GLAND

Retrograde Changes in the Adrenal Gland

Hypertrophy of the adrenal gland with focal necrosis is due to ACTH. One form of local infection of the adrenal gland is tuberculosis, which has the capacity to destroy the adrenal. Bilateral confluent tuberculosis with a caseous necrotic mass causes destruction of the adrenal gland, resulting in a small sac filled with caseous necrosis. Amyloidosis results in partial destruction of the adrenal gland. However, life is compatible with adrenal amyloidosis, and primary or secondary amyloidosis rarely leads to adrenal insufficiency. Metastatic tumors to the adrenal gland or primary tumors of the adrenal cause retrograde changes in the gland. The total destruction of the adrenal gland leads to Addison's disease and adrenal insufficiency. Atrophy of the adrenal gland is due to arteriosclerosis of adrenal arteries.

Hemorrhage occurs in the adrenal gland, accompanying severe infections, i.e. meningococcus infection with toxemia. A fulminant meningococcal toxemia, streptococcal or staphylococcal septicemia accompanied by cyanosis, hypertension, and purpura is termed *Waterhouse Friderichsen syndrome*. The adrenal glands in this latter syndrome undergo bilateral cortical necrosis and hemorrhage, indicating that a hemorrhagic infarct has taken place. Petechiae occur in the skin and mucous membranes in the Waterhouse-Friderichsen syndrome.

Chronic Adrenal Insufficiency

Addison's disease is a clinical manifestation of adrenal cortical insufficiency. Tuberculosis of the adrenal is the cause of 60 to 70 percent of instances of Addison's disease, the most common cause of adrenal insufficiency in the United States. Addison's disease is also caused by histoplasmosis, sarcoidosis, and secondary amyloidosis. Atrophy of the adrenal glands is another cause of chronic adrenal cortical insufficiency of Addison's disease.

Addison's disease represents a syndrome characterized by lowered blood pressure, profound loss of weight, weakness, pigmented skin, and pigmentation of mucous membranes. The following metabolic disturbances are present during Addison's disease: low blood sodium and low chloride, high blood potassium, and slightly elevated blood urea nitrogen. There is a conservation of water by the body and diminished metabolites occur and 17-ketosteroids and 17-hydroxysteroids are diminished in the urine. Addison's disease is accompanied by loss of weight, anorexia, and asthenia.

Hyperplasia of the Adrenal Gland

Cushing's syndrome, adrenal hyperplasia, and pseudohermaphroditism are associated with adrenal hyperplasia and adenoma or carcinoma of the cortex of the adrenal. Hyperplasia occurs in patients with renal disease and hypertension. An enlarged adrenal is evident in the latter diseases. Acromegaly produces an enlarged adrenal gland. Only a small percentage of adenomas or hyperplasia of the adrenal gland produce clinically detectable symptoms of endocrine disturbances.

Cushing's syndrome is the opposite of Addison's disease since it represents hyperplasia of the adrenals. The individual with Cushing's syndrome is obese, with fat located in the neck, face, and trunk. The obese face is termed *moon face*. Hypertension, polycythemia altered androgen metabolism, altered cortisone metabolism, and decreased glucose tolerance are present in Cushing's syndrome. Estrogen and androgen production are disturbed and hypogenitalism develops in Cushing's syndrome. The bones are osteoporotic, weak, and may fracture easily. The skin develops purplish striae in patients with Cushing's syndrome. There is increased retention of sodium and chloride and a decrease in serum potassium. The blood urea nitrogen is unaltered. Uric acid is increased in the blood. Alterations develop in the formed elements of the blood, producing an eosinophilia, increase in neutrophils, and leukopenia during Cushing's syndrome.

The adrenogenital syndrome is a rare variant of Cushing's syndrome in which hypermasculinization is present. The individual undergoes precocious development, and preadolescent boys develop pubic hair and a large glans penis. Girls and adult females show masculinization. Individuals with the adrenogenital syndrome are sterile. There is a large production of androgens in individuals with this syndrome. The defect occurs in the adrenal glands. The defect in this syndrome is in the production of C_{11} oxysteroids.

Neoplasms of the Adrenal Gland

The adrenal cortex gives rise to the adenoma and carcinoma (rare). Functional carcinoma of the adrenal gland produces an endocrine disturbance due to excessive production of androgen and estrogen. The majority of instances of primary carcinoma of the adrenal cortex are nonfunctional and are associated with disturbances of androgen and estrogen metabolism. Metastatic tumors to the adrenal glands are generally from primary bronchogenic carcinomas. Metastatic tumors are commonly bilateral.

Pheochromocytoma is a benign tumor of the adrenal gland, which arises from the medulla of the adrenal. This tumor is formed by large cells similar to mature adrenal medullary cells. Cells of the pheochromocytoma produce an epinephrinelike substance; therefore, hypertension develops in the form of paroxysmal crisis due to the large release of adrenaline. Surgery for removal of the pheochromocytoma is curative. This adrenal tumor is generally unilateral with about 5 percent of neoplasms showing a bilateral distribution. This tumor occurs in young adults who experience palpitation of the heart, rapid pulse, sweating, nausea, headache, crisis, and hypertension, which is increased when the patient changes positions.

Neoplasms of the adrenal medulla also include the neuroblastoma, sympathicoblastoma, and ganglioneuroma. Neuroblastoma is one of the most common malignancies of infancy and childhood up to five years of age. The sympathicoblastoma is practically identical to the neuroblastoma. The ganglioneuroma from the medulla is a more benign tumor than the neuroblastoma. Metastatic neoplasms to the adrenal glands are more common than the primary neoplasms. For instance, carcinoma of the breast and bronchogenic carcinoma produce the most frequent metastases to the adrenals. Metastatic tumors to the adrenal glands may, in rare instances, produce the clinical manifestations of Addison's disease.

References

Alpert, L.I., et al.: *Arch Pathol, 91:55*, 1971.
Bill, A.H.: *Surgery, 66:45*, 1969.
Black, B.M.: *Surg Clin North Am, 51:955*, 1971.
Brown, J.J., et al.: *Br Med J, 2:391*, 1972.
Catt, K.J.: *Lancet, 1:827*, 1970.
Chopra, I.J., et al.: *J Clin Endocrinol Metab, 31:382*, 1970.
Davies, A.G.: *Br Med J, 2:206*, 1972.
Dawson, M.A.: *Am J Med, 52:406*, 1972.
Decicco, F.A., et al.: *Arch Pathol, 94:65*, 1972.
DeGroot, L.J.: *Med Clin North Am, 54:117*, 1970.
DeLuca, H.F.: *Nutr Rev, 29:179*, 1971.
Doniach, I.: *J R Coll Physicians Lond, 6:299*, 1972.
Emerson, C.H. and Utiger, R.D.: *N Engl J Med, 287:328*, 1972.
Englund, N.E.: *J Clin Endocrinol Metab, 35:90*, 1972.
Hall, R.: *Br Med J, 1:743*, 1970.
Hartog, M.: *Br Med J, 1:679*, 1972.
Hoffenberg, R.: *Practitioner, 208:360*, 1972.
Kilman, J.W. and Klassen, K.P.: *Am J Surg, 121:170*, 1971.
McConahey, W.M.: *Med Clin North Am, 56:885*, 1972.
McKenzie, J.M.: *Metabolism, 21:883*, 1972.
Maddox, W.A., et al.: *Am Surg, 37:653*, 1971.
Melick, R.A.: *Br Med J, 1:204*, 1972.
Nabarro, J.D.N.: *Br Med J, 1:492*, 1972.
Omae, T., et al.: *Endocrinol Jap, 17:57*, 1971.
Psarras, A., et al.: *Br J Surg, 59:545*, 1972.
Raker, J.W.: *Adv Surg, 5:129*, 1971.
Reiss, 7. and Canterbury, J.M.: *Am J Med, 50:679*, 1971.
Robertson, P.W.: *Br Med J, 1:220*, 1972.
Russell, R.P., et al.: *Medicine, 51:211*, 1972.
Strahan, R.W., et al.: *Laryngoscope, 81:1388*, 1971.
Takita, H. and Mongaya, R.B.: *NY J Med, 70:2667*, 1970.
Van de Velde, R.L. and Friedman, N.B.: *Am J Pathol, 59:347*, 1970.
Wald, M.K.: *Pediatrics (Suppl. 2), 47:254*, 1971.
Wasserman, R.H. and Taylor, A.N.: *Ann Rev Biochem, 41:179*, 1972.

CHAPTER 25

FEMALE GENITAL TRACT

ANOMALIES AND HORMONAL INTERRELATIONSHIP

Anomalies of the Female Genital Tract

AGENESIS MAY OCCUR in the ovary; however, it is generally a unilateral agenesis. True hermaphroditism is due to the absence of gonadal tissue, i.e. ovarian or testicular tissue. Hermaphroditism is related to the genes that determine sex or to a defect of the endocrine system. Ovarian agenesis results in a female with male nuclei in all of the cells. The supernumerary ovary may be present in the mesovary or broad ligament. The rare ovotestis is located in the inguinal hernia. The ovotestis contains two kinds of cells, i.e. testicular cells and ovarian cells. Hypoplasia and hyperplasia may occur in the female genital structures.

Turner's syndrome consists of ovarian agenesis, dwarfism, retarded skeletal growth, open epiphyseal lines, osteoporosis, ocular anomalies, prominent skin folds in the neck, low estrogen, high gonadotrophin, and low 17-ketosteroids.

Pseudohermaphrodism is an endocrine defect due to the persistence of the wolffian apparatus. The uretha opens far anterior, and no vaginal opening exists. Cysts of the mesonephron and the hydatid cyst of the fallopian tube may develop following persistence of the wolffian apparatus. The latter represent thin-walled, clear, small cysts, which do not produce symptoms. Mesonephric remnants located in the wall of the cervix may give rise to an adenocarcinoma of the cervix. Gartner's duct cyst is a thin-walled cyst located in the vaginal wall. The latter arises from remnants of the wolffian duct. When the müllerian ducts fail to develop, there is an absence of the fallopian tubes, vagina, and cornua of the uterus. Failure of the müllerian ducts to fuse leads to notching of the fundus of the uterus and formation of a septum down the middle of the uterus, extending into and including the vagina, uterine cavities, and two crevices.

Agenesis may occur unilaterally or bilaterally in the fallopian tubes. Other anomalies of the fallopian tubes are atresia, accessory ostium or ampulla of the tubes, and hypoplasia of the fallopian tubes generally associated with a generalized hypoplasia of all female genital organs. Walthard's cell rests are located in the wall of the fallopian tube and form nodules on the outer surface of the tube. Walthard's cell rests are remnants of the wolffian duct that appear as large, transitional-like cells arranged in cell nests.

Menstrual Cycle and Hormonal Interrelationships

The anterior pituitary follicle stimulating hormone (FSH) causes maturation of the ovarian follicles. The granulosa cells of the ovarian follicle produce estrogen, which is responsible for growth and hyperemia of the endometrium and myometrium, and for the development of the secondary sex characteristics of the female. Estrogenic substances cause a depression of the anterior pituitary functions. Only one ovarian follicle will rupture, while all of the other follicles die. When one ovarian follicle ruptures, the endometrium ceases to proliferate and become secretory in nature. The mucosecretion is altered, and the basal temperature curve reaches an inverse peak and rises.

The corpus luteum is formed under the influence of the luteinizing hormone (LH), and the granulosa cells form large, luteinizing cells filled with fat. Estrogen is secreted along with progesterone. The progesterone causes inhibition of muscle contraction in the endometrium; ovulation is inhibited and the breast undergoes lobular development. Twenty-four to forty-eight hours prior to menstruation, the corpus luteum undergoes regression, constriction of arteries takes place, and ischemic necrosis and sloughing result.

The corpus luteum is rather large, i.e. 4 to 5 centimeters in diameter. When the corpus luteum undergoes degeneration, there is organization, hyalinization, and formation of the corpus albicans (white body). The endometrium has a dense stroma, small cells, and sparse glands. Frequent mitotic activity occurs in the columnar epithelial cells lining the glandular elements. The stroma becomes edematous, and proliferation ensues. The numerous glandular elements are composed of pseudostratified epithelial cells. No secretion is present during this phase. Mitosis occurs and produces crowding of cells. As ovulation approaches, the glandular elements outgrow the stromal tissue; however, there is still no secretion at this phase.

The secretory phase of ovulation is accompanied by the formation of vacuoles in the glandular elements, increased tortuosity, and papillary infolding of the epithelium. Secretion occurs into the lumen of the glands. The late secretory endometrium supports the development of the decidual cells. Hemorrhage occurs in the premenstrual endometrium, and the arteriole are shut off. The decidual changes result in formation of large decidual cells, and during menstruation all cells are shed.

In the anovulatory cycle, when the follicle does not rupture, estrogen continues to be secreted, and the endometrium remains in a state of proliferation. The ovarian follicle subsequently deteriorates and hemorrhage ceases. Hemorrhage is irregular and follows a cyclic pattern. No corpus luteum is formed, and the endometrium is not prepared for sloughing during the anovulatory cycle.

At puberty and at the menopause, there is hyperplasia of the endometrium due to excessive estrogen with absence of progesterone. The latter is due to the persistence of the ovarian follicles or failure of the ovarian follicle to rupture. Gross hemorrhage occurs, and the endometrium becomes a thickened and soft tissue with a pale, nodular surface. Numerous glands are present in a dense, stromal tissue. Cystic dilation may occur in the endometrial glands, termed a *Swiss-cheese endometrium*.

Following the menopause, the endometrium becomes atrophic and contains a thin, dense, cellular stroma. Glands are minimal, and the surface of the endometrium consists of low, columnar, epithelial cells.

Vaginal smears made during the follicle phase of the menstrual cycle reveal that the exfoliated cells contain a high level of estrogen and thus stain pink. The cells present in the secretions are loose, flat cells. Prior to ovulation, all exfoliated cells stain pink.

Progesterone causes agglutinated cells, changes in cytoplasm, and wrinkling of cells. Following the menopause, atrophic vaginal smears occur, which reveal squamous cells from the intermediate layer of the epithelium. Postmenopausal smears reveal cells that stain blue due to the absence of estrogen.

The corpus luteum normally supplies the progesterone required by cells; however, during pregnancy, the placenta takes over the function of producing progesterone. Parturition occurs because of decreased progesterone or increased production of estrogen. During parturition, the placenta stops the production of progesterone.

The earliest ovum is produced at seven and one-half days. This ovum remains three days in transit in the fallopian tube following fertilization. The ovum may implant on the ovary (trophoblast), in the fallopian tube forming an ectopic pregnancy, or in the peritoneal cavity. The trophoblastic cells are invasive cells, which are capable of destroying the endometrium, stroma, and epithelium. The decidual cells surround the trophoblasts, providing them with needed glycogen. The secretory endometrium contains large, glandular elements; the glands are readily destroyed by the invasive trophoblasts. The chorionic villi are trophoblastic buds covered by two layers of cells, i.e. inner Langhans' cells and outer syncytial cells. When the placenta ages, the villa become smaller and contain numerous Langhans' cells. The Langhans' cells disappear at term, and the syncytial cells appear as giant cells. Degeneration ensues when fibrin is deposited between the villi, resulting in ischemic necrosis of villi.

During the ectopic pregnancy, the ovum fails to reach the uterus prior to development. The ectopic pregnancy consists of an implanted ovum with invasion of the tissue by the trophoblastic cells. Good decidual formation is absent in the fallopian tubes. The trophoblasts invade the muscular wall and rupture as the mass grows. Rupture of the embryonic sac ensues, and the embryo is liberated into the lumen, accompanied by hemorrhage into the peritoneum (hematoperitoneum).

During a tubal abortion, the fallopian tube ruptures and the embryo and membrane are extruded into the peritoneal cavity, accompanied by hemorrhage. In a tubal abortion, the trophoblasts are vital and become secondarily implanted on the surface of the ovary. Nutrition to the embryo is poor in the latter situation, and death results, followed by absorption. The products of conception survive, whereas the embryo dies at a later date, followed by maceration, resorption, mumification, and deposition of calcium in the necrotic tissue. Lithopedion is a term indicating a dead fetus that has undergone calcification within the fallopian tube or peritoneal cavity. An abdominal or tubal pregnancy may, on occasion, survive to term. Approximately 600 instances have been reported of embryos surviving to term in the peritoneal cavity.

When an embryo is situated outside the uterine cavity, enlargement of the uterus takes place for a period of three months, and the uterus becomes softer than normal. Well-formed decidua located within the endometrium slough out when the embryo dies. When an abdominal pregnancy occurs, the placenta should be left intact because it will degenerate and undergo resorption if the fetus is removed.

Abnormalities occur in placental membranes. Deposition of fibrin occurs rather diffusely in the placental villi and decidua with time. Foci of calcification develop during late pregnancy and the villi become surrounded by fibrin, leading to necrosis and calcification. Fibrin plaques fill the villi, placentosis develops, and the exchange of electrolytes is reduced. The deposition of fibrin is responsible for false infarcts or bloodless areas of the placenta. The affected area is initially solid and red, but subsequently it turns into a pale, firm, and bloodless area of the placenta. A true placental infarct results from an interruption of the blood supply from the maternal side. The true placental infarct is characterized by a collapsed structure crowded with villi and by an absence of blood between the villi.

Nutrition to the endometrium determines the shape of the implanted trophoblast. Nutrition is also a vital factor in determining whether any deformities develop in the placenta. The placenta defusa is the lining of the endometrial cavity. An annular placenta is one that encircles the uterine cavity as a band. Double, triple, and accessory placenta may be formed. Extra lobes may develop on the placenta, which connect with other parts of the placenta by means of blood vessels crossing the uterine cavity and traversing the cervical os. When extra lobes of the placenta develop at the cervical os, they are termed *vasa preva* at delivery. Placental implants occur low in the uterus in $\frac{1}{2}$ percent of instances.

Trauma is capable of injuring the placenta, and hemorrhage may accompany trauma prior to separation. When the placenta covers the cervical os, a dangerous situation develops. The extra lobes of the placenta are left behind, producing hemorrhage at delivery. When the uterus contracts, hemorrhage is delayed for several weeks but subsequently occurs at a later date. The placenta separates along with fibrin. If the placenta becomes anchored, it cannot separate since a cleavage plane is absent. The anchored placenta is termed the *placenta accreta*.

A ruptured placenta containing a hematoma undergoes separation, and uterine hemorrhage occurs prior to delivery. A ruptured uterus is accompanied by an extensive ingrowth of uterine tissue into the wall with fibrosis. Uterine apoplexy develops when the muscle fibers of the uterus do not contract and relax.

Tumors of the placenta are the chorioangioma and the hemangioma. The latter neoplasms are responsible for hemorrhage in the placenta. Neoplasms generally develop on the fetal surface or deep within the placenta.

Infections of the placenta generally are due to an ascending infection through the internal canal following an early rupture of the membrane. Suppurative inflammation of the placenta may result from a postnatal sepsis. Microorganisms may reach the placenta through a maternal bacteremia. Viruses cross the placental membrane and are capable of infecting the fetus. Tubercle bacilli spread and infect the placenta. *Treponema pallidum* cross the placental membrane, producing congenital syphilis. Syphilitic infection of the placenta results in the production of large, pale, thick, and firm villi enlarged by perivascular fibrous tissue around thick-walled blood vessels.

Degeneration of the placenta accompanies erythroblastosis fetalis. In the edematous infant, the placenta becomes edematous and contains thick, shiny villi, which are enlarged because of the presence of edema fluid. The Langhans' cells persist, there are few syncytial vessels, and there are nucleated erythroblasts in the fetal blood vessels.

DISEASES AND NEOPLASMS OF THE OVARY

Histology of the Ovary

The stroma of the ovary is composed of theca cells. Theca cells are similar to fibroblasts; however, they are visible histologically only if stained by a fat stain. Theca cells are extremely rich in lipids. The surface of the ovary is covered by germinal epithelial cells, i.e. low cuboidal epithelial cells. The pluripotential cells of the ovaries are the granulosa cells and lutein cells. The pluripotential ovarian cells are capable of developing along any pattern.

Inflammation of the Ovary

Inflammation of the ovary accompanies advanced inflammation or rupture of the fallopian tube. Since the fallopian tube is in contact with the ovary, inflammation may produce a tuboovarian abscess, which is capable of destroying the entire ovary. When the inflammation involves only the outer surface of the ovary, it is generally secondary to an abdominal or ruptured appendicitis or ruptured diverticulitis. Oophoritis, i.e. inflammation of the ovary, is associated with mumps. Inflammatory diseases occur in the ovaries in conjunction with inflammation of the fallopian tube. Tuberculosis, bacterial infections, actinomycosis, and parasitic infections (echinococcosis) may develop in the ovaries. Endometriosis of the ovaries results in production of hemorrhagic, cystic lesions.

Ovarian Pregnancies.

Ovarian pregnancies may develop to full term. However, secondary calcification may take place in the ovarian pregnancy, i.e. lithopedion.

Ovarian Cysts (Nonproliferative Cysts, Retention Cysts)

Ovarian cysts are non-neoplastic retention cysts, which may be classified into the following groups: follicular cyst, luteal cyst, theca-lutein cyst, endometrial cyst (chocolate cyst), and the Stein-Leventhal syndrome. Cysts of the ovary are classified as non-proliferative (non-neoplastic) and proliferative (neoplastic) ovarian cysts.

The follicular cyst of the ovary is a retention cyst lined by granulosa cells and containing a clear fluid in the lumen of the cyst. The follicular cyst is accompanied by hyperplasia of the endometrium if this retention cyst persists. Sterility is also due to the follicular cyst and accompanies the endometrial hyperplasia. Follicular ovarian cysts develop from the graafian follicles. If the graafian follicle fails to rupture it becomes atretic, scarred, or cystic. Small, follicular cysts measuring 2 centimeters in diameter develop from the graafian follicle and are free of symptoms. The follicle cysts are thin-walled cysts located on the surface of the ovary. It has a smooth surface lining the lumen. Remnants of the granulosa layer form two to three layers of granulosa cells, which line the lumen of the follicular cyst.

When the corpus luteum undergoes a cystic change, it becomes enlarged up to 10 centimeters in diameter and forms the luteal cyst (corpus-lutein cyst). The lumen of this cyst is initially filled with hemorrhage; however, it subsequently contains a clear fluid, sanginous fluid, or yellow cystic fluid. Grossly, the luteal cyst has a yellow wall, which identifies its origin from the corpus lutein. Histopathologically, luteinized corpus granulosa cells line the cyst wall. Endometrosis may develop in the wall of the luteal cyst.

The theca-lutein cyst is a retention cyst of the ovary. This cyst forms due to a luteinizing change in the small cells of the theca lutein. The theca-lutein cells become enlarged, and fluid accumulates in the tissue and is surrounded by a cystic wall. The theca-lutein cyst is associated with the hydatidiform mole and the chorioepithelioma. The theca-lutein cyst of the ovary is accompanied by a high pregnancy test. The theca cells are stimulated to luteinize with the production of bilateral lutein cysts of the ovary.

The endometrial or chocolate cyst is located on the surface and hilus of the ovary. The endometrial epithelial lining may have endometrial stroma adjacent to the epithelium. The epithelial lining of the chocolate cyst may be lost, and the lumen of the cyst becomes filled with blood clots; therefore, the term *chocolate cyst* is used. The endometrial stroma lines the lumen and contains blood pigment laden macrophages. The chocolate cyst is prominent during the reproductive period.

The Stein-Leventhal syndrome is a syndrome or symptom complex associated with sterility. This syndrome results from a thickened tunica albiginica, which interferes with the rupturing of follicles. This syndrome produces bilateral changes; the ovaries are enlarged, with follicular cysts located under the surface of the thica albiginia.

True Neoplasms of the Ovary

True neoplasms of the ovary include the following: cystic ovarian tumors, benign solid ovarian tumors, malignant solid ovarian tumors, and tumors with endocrine function.

Cystic Ovarian Tumors

The serous cystadenoma of the ovary consists of a wall lined by a layer of cuboidal epithelium and a lumen containing clear fluid. The cystadenoma is a multilocular lesion with papillary projections extending from the wall into the lumen. This cyst occurs in females from forty to forty-five years of age. Two-thirds of the cystadenomas of the ovary develop bilaterally. Forty-five percent of the cystadenomas of the ovary undergo malignant transformation to the serous cystadenocarcinoma.

The serous cystadenoma begins as a simple cyst with a smooth and thin wall containing a clear fluid. Nodular thickenings develop in the inner aspect of the wall and are responsible for the term *cystadenoma*. The lining epithelium proliferates as the cyst grows in size. Large nodules of neoplastic tissue extend into the lumen of the cyst. The lumen contains a cloudy fluid filled with exfoliated epithelial cells. The papillary projections extending into the lumen contain a core of loose connective tissue. Malignant epithelial lining cells invade the wall of the cyst and appear on the serosal surface of the wall. The malignant cystadenocarcinoma spreads along the peritoneal surfaces where it acts as an irritant, producing exudation from the peritoneum. The exudation is accompanied by ascites, and the malignant cells grow on the peritoneal surface as well as within the fluid media in the form of tufts of neoplastic cells. Chronic inflammatory cells are present on the mesothelial membrane.

Another cystic ovarian tumor is the pseudomucinous cystadenoma of the ovary. This ovarian tumor is similar in appearance to the serous cystadenoma and may grow to a very large size. The pseudomucinous cystadenoma is a unilateral multilocular cyst, which occurs in the ovary of females from fifty to sixty years of age or as a postmenopausal cyst. This cyst is lined by tall, columnar, mucin-producing epithelium. The epithelial lining of this cyst has a teratomatous nature. The cystadenoma may rupture at surgery, and epithelial cells become implanted on the peritoneum. The implanted neoplastic cells proliferate and form the pseudomyxomatous peritoneii. The latter indicates an abdomen filled with mucinous material. The pseudomyxomatous peritoneii has a malignant clinical behavior pattern.

The pseudomucinous cystadenoma contains a thick, mucinous fluid and may undergo malignant transformation into a cystadenocarcinoma.

Dermoid cysts or cystic teratomas of the ovary are benign unilateral or bilateral cystic ovarian tumors, which occur during the reproductive stage when the fetus is in the wrong place. Grossly, the dermoid cyst has a thin, cystic wall containing bone tissue, cartilage, muscle, teeth, hair follicles, and sebaceous glands in the wall or projecting into the lumen. The lumen is generally filled with sebaceous material and hair. The epithelial tissue of the dermoid cyst of the ovary are derived from both the ectoderm and the mesoderm. The dermoid cyst may grow up to 20 centimeters in diameter.

The ovarian teratoid tumors may be classified as dermoid cysts and teratomas of the ovary.

The solid teratomas are composed of collections of the following tissues: skin, respiratory epithelium, sebaceous glands, intestinal epithelium, lung tissue, brain tissue, bone, and cartilage. When thyroid tissue predominates in the teratoid cysts of the ovary, the lesion is termed the *stuma ovarii*.

The solid teratoma of the ovary is a potentially or frankly malignant neoplasm. A single tissue component may undergo malignant transformation and metastasize to distant sites. The other tissues present in the solid teratoma are left behind as benign components of the teratoma. However, several tissue components of the teratoma may undergo malignant transformation and metastasize to distant sites.

The malignant teratoma of the ovary consists of components from all three germinal layers. This teratoma contains an enteric-like mucosa, nervous tissue, thyroid, cartilage, bone, and teeth located in stromal tissue. The teratoma develops during the reproductive age and has a malignant clinical behavior pattern.

Another cystic ovarian tumor is termed the *paralutein cyst*. The paralutein cyst is associated with pregnancy, the hydatidiform mole, and the chorioepithelioma. The paralutein cyst develops bilaterally as a multilocular cyst. It arises from atrophic immature follicles. The paralutein cyst has a poor lining surface, which is surrounded by luteinized theca cells. The paralutein cyst is stimulated to grow by gonadotrophins.

Benign Solid Ovarian Tumors

Connective tissue neoplasms of the ovary include the fibroma and adenofibroma. The adenofibroma develops on the surface of the ovary in the form of a papillary growth. Meig's syndrome is due to a benign ovarian tumor, i.e. the leiomyoma accompanied by ascites and accumulation of fluid in the pleural cavity. The fluid that accumulates during Meig's syndrome is a protein-free exudate. The neoplasm in Meig's syndrome originates as a germinal neoplasm arising from totipotential germinal epithelium.

The benign fibroma of the ovary is a solid tumor, which develops after the menopause. The fibroma is pedunculated and may undergo torsion and infarction.

The Brenner tumor of the ovary is a benign, nonfunctioning neoplasm arising from embryonal Walthard's cell rests remaining from the invagination of the primitive coelomic epithelium. This rare neoplasm occurs in older age groups, is unilateral in distribution, and approximately one-third are cystic in some portion of the tumor. The Brenner tumor has a dense consistency, is solid, firm and smooth, homogeneous, and a gray white color on cut section.

Histopathologically, the Brenner tumor is composed of dense, fibrous stroma and islets of epithelioid cells with central cyst formation. The lumen of the cysts contain colloidal material. The cells lining the lumen contain mucous and glycogen.

Meig's syndrome of the ovary is caused by a fibroma or other solid tumor present in the ovary and is accompanied by hydrothorax and, sometimes, ascites. Other solid ovarian neoplasms, i.e. the theca cell tumor, the granulosa cell tumor, and the Brenner tumor of the ovary, may also be accompanied by hydrothorax and ascites. The hydrothorax and ascites consist of a transudate.

Malignant Solid Ovarian Tumors

The adenocarcinoma of the ovary is commonly a cystic type of lesion. This carcinoma is either solid or cystic in nature. A serous or pseudomucinous adenocarcinoma may be made up of undifferentiated tall columnar cells. The undifferentiated adenocarcinoma is difficult to classify or identify.

The sarcoma is a rare ovarian neoplasm compared to the carcinoma. It may arise by malignant transformation from an ovarian fibroma or proliferate directly from the stromal tissue of the ovary. Histologically, it is generally a spindle cell sarcoma.

The dysgerminoma is not a hormone-producing neoplasm; however, this neoplasm is capable of provoking hormonal disturbances. The dysgerminoma causes hermaphrodism. The neoplasm is similar to the seminoma of the testicles. The dysgerminoma is composed of caviarlike cells that appear similar to epithelial cells, which have a pale cytoplasm and small lmphocytes. Diffuse luteinization of the ovary may cause masculinization. The theca cells of the ovary become lutein cells.

The dysgerminoma occurs in young females in their teens as well as from twenty to thirty years of age. The histopathology of the dysgerminoma is identical to the seminoma; however, its clinical behavior pattern is not as aggressive as the seminoma. The dysgerminoma grows to a large size and has an irregular, lobulated surface, which is solid and pink in color. Necrosis, degeneration, and hemorrhage produce a fleshy neoplasm.

Metastases to the Ovary

Metastatic neoplasms occur to the ovaries from distant, primary, malignant neoplasms. Malignant primary neoplasms of the breast and gastrointestinal tract may metastasize to the ovaries. Krunkenberg's tumor is a metastatic neoplasm from the stomach to the ovaries. This adenocarcinoma is composed of signet ring cells and proliferating fibrous stroma. Krunkenberg's tumor is similar in morphology to the anaplastic neoplasm of the ovary. However, the presence of mucous and signet ring cells identifies the neoplasm as arising primarily in the stomach or gastrointestinal tract with metastases to the right and left ovaries.

Neoplasms with Endocrine Functions

Functional ovarian neoplasms produce hormonal substances, i.e. estrogenic substances in the granulosa cell tumor and the thecoma. The granulosa cell tumor is more common than the thecoma and represents 3 percent of ovarian neoplasms. This tumor achieves a tremendous size and has a bilateral distribution. The granulosa cell tumor is homogeneous when small and firm and tan in color. Cystic degeneration occurs as the neoplasm becomes enlarged, and hemorrhage is responsible for a softening and mottled appearance. Microscopically, the neoplastic cells have the appearance of granulosa cells, i.e. they are small, dark cells with little cytoplasm and packed in solid sheets, forming follicular and glandular structures. Approximately one-third of the granulosa cell tumors of the ovary are malignant in their clinical behavior pattern. The neoplasms metastasize primarily to the viscera and less frequently to the serous cavities. The granulosa cells are unilateral neoplasms that undergo luteinization, forming large pale cells that produce a hemogeneous appearance and yellow color.

The hormone-producing neoplasms cause femininization, which results from the estrogen produced by the estrogen-producing cells of the ovary. The granulosa cell tumor develops either in small girls undergoing premature development or in older age groups, i.e. at the two extremes of life. The granulosa cell tumor may be classified into the microfollicular and macrofollicular neoplasms. The macrofollicular pattern appears similar to glands lined by granulosa cells. When this macrofollicular pattern contains Exner bodies, the neoplasm has a malignant clinical behavior pattern. However, the microfollicular pattern is more prone to develop into a highly malignant clinical behavior pattern than the macrofollicular granulosa cell tumor.

The thecoma is a less common functional ovarian neoplasm compared to the granulosa cell tumor. The thecoma arises from cells of the theca interna and develops into pale, spindle-shaped, small round cells. The thecoma is unilateral in distribution and grows to only 15 centimeters in diameter. Hyperestrinism is present with endometrial hyperplasia and extensive colic pain in the abdomen. Symptoms of hyperestrinism include excessive hemorrhage due to the hyperplasia. The hemorrhage occurs during the postmenopausal period. Persistence of proliferative activity causes precocious puberty. The thecoma is associated with the endometrial carcinoma in approximately 5 percent of instances of this neoplasm.

The thecoma occurs in older age groups who are still in the reproductive age. Microscopically, it is not possible to differentiate the theca cell tumor from the fibroma without utilizing special lipid stains. The thecoma is readily stained red with Sudan III.

When the granulosa cells and the theca cells are present in the mixed tumor of the ovary, both cells are responsible for feminization. Hormone-producing neoplasms also cause masculinization. The benign masculinizing neoplasms include the benign testicular adenoma of Pick, and the benign luteoma or adrenal rest tumor (masculinovoblastoma).

The testicular adenoma of Pick is a rare masculinizing neoplasm, which has a morphology similar to the seminiferous tubules of the testes. This adenoma develops in the region of the rete ovari. The luteoma (adrenal test tumor) is composed of luteinizing cells resembling the corpus luteum. This lipid neoplasm contains large, pale cells with vacuolated cytoplasm and small nuclei.

The malignant masculinizing neoplasm is termed the *arrhenoblastoma*. Ths neoplasm resembles the seminiferous tubules and is a malignant, hormone-producing tumor responsible for masculinization as a main symptom. The arrhenoblastoma is a firm, homogeneous, and yellow tumor. Microscopically, tubular and glandular structures are present. This neoplasm has a unilateral distribution and is less malignant in its clinical behavior pattern than the granulosa cell tumor.

The adrenal corticoid tumor also produces masculinization as a symptom. The neoplastic cells appear similar to adrenal cortical cells with brown granules. This neoplasm is not malignant in its behavior pattern. Masculinization generally occurs in prepubertal years but may occur at any time.

DISEASES OF THE FALLOPIAN TUBES

Introduction

There are three divisions to the fallopian tube, i.e. the intramural division located in the uterus, the isthmic division, and the ampulla. The fallopian tube is lined by tall columnar ciliated epithelium arranged into folds. The outer surface of the fallopian tube is partially covered by peritoneum. The lining of the fallopian tube differs from the lining present in the cervix, uterus, and ovary.

Inflammation of the Fallopian Tube

Gonorrhea is the most common cause of inflammation, i.e. salpingitis. The inflammation is superficial and accompanied by a purulent exudate in the fallopian tube. Hydrosalpinx is the presence of a watery exudate in the dilated fallopian tube. During salpingitis, a large number of eosinophiles become mobilized in the wall of the fallopian tube.

Salpingitis may involve the intramural portion of the fallopian tube, which is located in the uterus. The latter situation is termed *salpingitis ischmica nodosa*. The complications of salpingitis are sterile adhesions, pyosalpinx, and hematosalpinx. Hematosalpinx is the presence of blood filling a dilated fallopian tube. Hematosalpinx may be responsible for the tubal pregnancy or ectopic pregnancy in the fallopian tube. The fallopian tube may rupture during a tubal pregnancy, which is accompanied by a decidual-like cell reaction. Trophoblasts invade the fallopian tube and cause a rupture of the thin wall. The ectopic pregnancy is a cause of inflammation of the fallopian tube. Endometrosis is also responsible for causing inflammation in the fallopian tubes.

Tuberculosis of the fallopian tube is second in incidence only to pulmonary tuberculosis. The percent of instances of pulmonary tuberculosis is accompanied by involvement of the genital tract by way of the blood stream. Caseation necrosis occurs in the wall of the fallopian tube followed by numerous adhesions since the tuberculous lesions involve the wall of the fallopian tube. The tubercular fallopian tube is composed of a caseous, fibrous mass with obliteration of the lumen. During puerperal sepsis, the outer surface of the fallopian tube is initially involved by the infection; however, the mucosal surface is subsequently infected followed by spread of the infection through the entire wall of the tube. Inflammation of the fallopian tube, therefore, results from the following causes: gonorrhea, tuberculosis, endometriosis, ectopic pregnancy, and malignant neoplasms in the fallopian tube.

Carcinoma of the Fallopian Tube

Carcinoma of the fallopian tube is rare. It is extremely difficult to determine whether the carcinoma arises from the epithelial lining of the fallopian tube or from the endometriosis present. The carcinoma of the fallopian tube occurs in females between fifty and sixty years of age. It generally has a unilateral distribution; however, approximately one-third of the carcinomas occur bilaterally. Microscopically, this neoplasm is a papillary adenocarcinoma or solid undifferentiated carcinoma, which spreads by way of the lymphatics to the regional lymph nodes and by the blood stream to the liver and lungs.

Parovarian Cyst

The parovarian cyst is located between the fallopian tube and the ovary (mesovary). This cyst arises from the wolffian duct remnants. The cyst has a thin wall and a lumen filled with clear fluid. The cyst is approximately one centimeter in diameter. The morgagnian cyst is due to cystic dilation of the blind outer extremity of the wolffian duct.

Tumor of Round or Broad Ligament

The tumor of the broad ligament is a leiomyoma. The leiomyoma is a common neoplasm in the broad ligament and in the genital tract. The adenomyoma is composed of smooth muscle and glandular structures and is located in the broad ligament and fallopian tubes.

DISEASES AND NEOPLASMS OF THE UTERUS

Introduction

The endometrial lining of the uterus consists of endometrial straight tubular glands located in a stromal tissue. The proliferating endometrium is under the influence of estrogen during the first half of pregnancy. The estrogenic stage consists of proliferating endometrium, which is lined by tall columnar cells with basal nuclei. The stromal tissue is dense and is composed of round or spindle-shaped cells. During the second half of pregnancy, the endometrium is under the influence of progesterone. During this period, the endometrial glands become tortuous and dilated, and there is an increase in the number of glandular elements. The columnar lining cells contain a centrally located nucleus, and subnuclear vacuoles are present. There is a secretion from the surface of the secretory endometrium, which consists of a loose stroma and large cells.

The endometrium is a tissue under the influence of hormones. The endometrium becomes atrophic and contains a thin dense stroma with a few glands, following the menopause. When an imbalance of hormones exists, the endometrium becomes altered. For instance, too much estrogen or a lack of progesterone produces a hyperplastic endometrium.

Hyperplasia of the Uterus

Hyperplasia of the uterus results from estrogen stimulation and a failure to ovulate. A failure to ovulate also is responsible for polyp formation in the uterus. When the hyperplasia of the uterus regresses, the polyp continues to persist. The polyp may subsequently become the site of the development of an adenocarcinoma of the endometrium.

There are two types of endometrial hyperplasia, i.e. polypoid hyperplasia and cystic hyperplasia. Polypoid endometrial hyperplasia contains no secretory glands; however, there is an increase in glandular elements, and the stroma is dense. Cystic endometrial hyperplasia consists of dilated glands filled with inspissated secretion. Cystic hyperplasia develops near the menopause and has been termed *Swiss-cheese hyperplasia*. Large cysts may develop in the endometrium during the postmenopausal period in individuals who previously had endometrial hyperplasia. Hyperplasia of the endometrium and cyst formation in the endometrium never take place simultaneously. However, proliferation of the endometrium and hyperplasia may take place simultaneously. In some instances, hyperplasia of the endometrium appears rather severe in nature with proliferating adenomatous or polypoid masses present. However, these are not malignant neoplasms. It may be necessary to consider undertaking a hysterectomy when it is impossible to determine whether an atypical adenomatous hyperplasia is benign or malignant in nature. Squamous metaplasia may occur in the endometrial glands and must be differentiated from the squamous cell carcinoma. Hyperplasia of the endometrium contains only glandular elements and no stroma. Signs of malignancy include hyperchromatism and no stroma.

Inflammation of the Endometrium

Inflammation of the endometrium, i.e. acute endometritis, is caused by puerperal sepsis following invasion by *Streptococcus hemolyticus,* and septicemia. If chronic endometritis persists postabortion, retention of tissue and tuberculosis should be ruled out as the etiologic factors. Streptococci spread throughout the uterus by way of the blood stream to the fallopian tubes, endometrium, and cervix. However, endometrial and vaginal inflammation are relatively rare. The tissue appears to have some degree of resistance to infection.

Obstruction, trauma, and endometrial infection may occur in the postmenopausal patient. Endometritis may be due to acute or chronic inflammation of the endometrium. If complete obstruction occurs at the cervical os, suppuration and pyometria develop. Tuberculosis may be the etiologic factor in endometritis and salpingitis.

Squamous Metaplasia of the Endometrium

Squamous metaplasia may develop in the endometrium of elderly females without any significance. The presence of anaplastic squamous epithelial cells in the endometrium indicates an endometrial carcinoma and a malignant clinical behavior pattern. When squamous metaplasia develops to a noticeable extent, one must consider the development of an adenocarcinoma. The senile uterus consists of a periglandular stroma and a shrunken mucosa. Large cysts may develop in the senile uterus due to the estrogenic hormone following the menopause.

Benign Neoplasms of the Uterus

Myometrial benign neoplasms most commonly are smooth muscle tumors, i.e. the leiomyoma, fibromyoma, or fibroid tumor of the myometrium. Twenty percent of females over thirty years of age have fibroid tumors (leiomyoma). The leiomyoma is more common in the Negro than in the Caucasian. The fibroid tumor may be single or multiple and grows to 1,000 grams. The fibroid tumor is located beneath the endometrium and is or may be a subendometrial or submucosal neoplasm. The fibroid tumor may also be located in the wall of the uterus, i.e. as an intramural neoplasm and beneath the serosa as a subserosal neoplasm. The intramural and subserosal leiomyoma of the myometrium do not produce any clinical signs or symptoms. However, the submucosal leiomyoma is accompanied by signs and symptoms. The subendometrial location of a fibroid tumor produces symptoms consisting of hemorrhage from the overlying endometrium, and hyperplastic polyps simply due to mechanical pressure exerted by the neoplasm. The hemorrhage is the most common clinical symptom for the submucosal leiomyoma.

The fibroid tumor is a circumscribed nonencapsulated benign neoplasm composed of whorls of smooth muscle. The smooth muscle may undergo degeneration, hyalinization, form cysts, and undergo cystic degeneration and necrosis. The subserosal leiomyoma may become twisted and undergo infarction. Hemorrhagic infarcts in the leiomyoma appear as red, degenerating, and softened areas. The degenerating fibroid tumor is common during pregnancy. Ectopic endometrial leiomyomas may occur within the uterine wall. The ectopic leiomyoma is composed of both glandular elements and stroma, i.e. it is an endometriosis. The ectopic neoplasm located in the uterine wall may be composed of glands alone and is, therefore, an adenomyosis. If it is composed of stroma alone, it is termed *stroma endometrium*. Myometritis is associated with endometritis, and both accompany puerperal sepsis.

Leiomyomata are related to estrogen stimulation. Leiomyomata of the uterus are produced in guinea pigs by means of estrogen administration. The leiomyoma of the uterus grows to a large size when the individual is treated with estrogen therapy. The leiomyoma of the uterus may undergo malignant transformation and degenerate into a sarcoma in 1 percent of instances following the menopause. Sarcomatous degeneration of the leiomyoma results in a soft, fleshy mass from the original hard, solid tumor. The leiomyoma is, therefore, considered to be the estrogenic neoplasm of the ovary. The leiomyoma is also associated with endometrial hyperplasia. Benign polyps develop in the uterus and are composed of uterine glands and stroma.

Malignant Neoplasms of the Uterus

Malignant endometrial carcinomas are less common than carcinoma of the cervix. The endometrial carcinoma develops during the postmenopausal period in females who have never had any children. The endometrial carcinoma is a localized rather than an invasive carcinoma. The adenoma malignum is a neoplasm confined to the endometrium without any invasion of the myometrium. The adenocarcinoma of the endometrium is not a confined or localized neoplasm. The latter neoplasm metastasizes rapidly and significantly faster than the carcinoma of the cervix. The endometrial adenocarcinoma metastasizes to the lymph nodes, liver, and lungs. Ninety-six percent of all endometrial neoplasms are adenocarcinomas. The cure rate for carcinoma of the endometrium is 70 percent. The cure rate for carcinoma of the cervix is only 40 percent.

Uterine carcinoma produces a variant as a result of metaplasia termed the *adenoacanthoma*. The adenoacanthoma is an adenocarcinoma of the uterus combined with a squamous cell carcinoma due to metaplasia. The adenoacanthoma has the clinical behavior pattern of the malignant carcinoma.

Malignant transformation may occur in the benign uterine polyp. This transformation is in distinct contrast to the behavior pattern of the benign cervical polyp, which fails to undergo malignant transformation. Polyps of the endometrium may undergo malignant transformation by forming a polypoid growth, which spreads along the surface of the endometrial cavity. Therefore, the entire endometrium may be converted to adenocarcinoma. Invasion of the myometrium by the adenocarcinoma occurs only as a late occurrence. Histopathologically, the well-differentiated adenocarcinoma is composed of irregular glandular structures, which crowd out the endometrial stroma. In advanced adenocarcinoma, the endometrial carcinoma acquires its own fibrous tissue stroma, which is not endometrial stromal tissue. The glandular elements of the adenocarcinoma are lined by either columnar epithelium or tall ciliated epithelium.

The endometrial sarcoma is a malignant connective tissue neoplasm, which develops in older females. The sarcoma arises from endometrial stroma and has a rather poor prognosis. The endometrial sarcoma metastasizes by way of the blood stream and lymphatics. Four percent of malignant uterine neoplasms are endometrial sarcomas. Sarcomas may occur in the uterus in combination with an adenocarcinoma. The latter neoplasm is termed the *carcinosarcoma* of the uterus. Sarcomas arise in 50 percent of instances of leiomyomas of the uterus. The leimyosarcoma does not arise from the benign leiomyoma. It arises directly from nonneoplastic smooth muscle of the uterus. The leimyosarcoma consists of elongated spindle cells showing anaplasia and abundant mitosis.

Endometriosis of the Body of the Uterus

Endometriosis is the presence of endometrial tissue in areas other than the lining of the uterus. When endometrial tissue is located deep within the myometrium, the condition is termed *adenomyosis of the uterine wall*. Islands of endometrial tissue located within the myometrium produce hypertrophy of muscle and nodular areas that are due to either cysts or hemorrhage. Endometriosis are not circumscribed but consist of either areas grouped together or scattered and poorly defined areas.

During endometrosis of the uterus, there is no submucosa present in the endometrium. The surface epithelial cells simply rest directly on muscle tissue. The stromal and glandular tissue extends into the muscle tissue for only a short distance. Microscopically, endometriosis consists of endometrial stroma plus a few glandular structures, dilated with blood. Islets of endometrial tissue may undergo cystic changes along with the endometrium.

Endometriosis may be the cause of hematosalpinx if the endometrial glands are present in the fallopian tube. The following represent the main theories for the formation of endometriosis: Samson theory, Mayer theory, and Novak theory. The Samson theory states that endometriosis is caused by a dislocated endometrium, which is the result of pressure upon the endometrium. The Mayer theory states that the endometriosis arises from multipotential cells. The Novak theory states that the endometriosis arises from cells that represent embryonic rests.

Adenomyosis of the Uterine Wall and Other Sites

The etiology of adenomyosis is obscure. Endometrial tissue (ectopic) may be located in the opening of the fallopian tubes, ovary, and on the peritoneum in the abdominal cavity. Stromal adenomyosis consists of only stromal cells ectopically located without any glandular elements. Ectopic endometrial tissue generally consists of glandular tissue plus stroma. Cyclic changes, pain, hemorrhage, inflammation, and adhesions occur during adenomyosis. Following the menopause, the symptoms of adenomyosis subside and scarring results.

Neoplasms of the Corpus Uteri Associated with Pregnancy

Neoplasms of the uterus associated with pregnancy include the placental polyp, benign hydatidiform mole, and the choriocarcinoma. The placental polyp is, in reality, a pseudo-neoplasm, which is associated with pregnancy. When a portion of the placenta is retained, it is termed the *placental polyp*.

The benign hydatidiform mole is associated with pregnancy and develops following an abortion. The hydatidiform mole is a rare neoplasm and has an incidence of 1 in 24,000 ovarian pregnancies. At five weeks *in utero*, the fetal vascular supply develops. The villi blood vessels of the placenta are also formed at this time. If the embryo dies, no blood vessels are formed in the villi. The connective tissue of the villi persist and live. However, the placental villi live without blood vessels since nutrition is absorbed through the villi, which become edematous. Large vesicular masses develop, which are joined by stalks having the appearance of grapelike clusters. Cysts form in the stalks of grapelike clusters and measure 3 centimeters in diameter. The stroma of the villi become cystic. The hydatidiform moles can be cured by scrapping the uterine lining. However, the mole may undergo malignant transformation into the choriocarcinoma in 5 to 15 percent of instances. If the trophoblastic cells are active, the hydatidiform mole usually remains a benign neoplasm. The patient may expel or pass grapelike structures in the form of clusters of small cysts or edematous chorionic villi. The hydatidiform mole consists of edematous connective tissue lined by trophoblastic cells.

The hydatidiform mole is initiated at the placental site with growth of the neoplasm taking place through the wall of the uterus. Grossly, the mole appears as a hemorhagic, cystic mass. Microscopically, villi are absent, and the neoplasm consists of trophoblastic cells, undifferentiated Langhan's and syncytial cells, which destroy the adjacent tissue.

The choriocarcinoma is a highly malignant and rare neoplasm associated with pregnancy. The choriocarcinoma may develop as a malignant neoplasm from the onset, or it may arise by malignant transformation from the benign hydatidiform mole. Metastases take place to the lungs by means of hematogenous spread from the persisting villi. The metastases may not occur for months to years following the pregnancy. The choriocarcinoma grows by expansion and may grow into the vagina. Metastases develop following the spread of the choriocarcinoma into the vagina.

DISEASES OF THE CERVIX UTERI

Introduction

The ectocervix is composed of a nonkeratinizing stratified squamous epithelium. The endocervix is composed of tall columnar epithelial cells. In the child, the cervical lining is composed of a thin layer of epithelial cells. However, in the adult the cervical lining is composed of a thick layer of epithelial cells, and in senescence the cervical lining becomes atrophic. Alterations take place in the epithelium of the cervix as a result of estrogen. Estrogen is responsible for cell maturation and keratinization of the cervical epithelium. Progesterone influences the cervical epithelium by producing more cellular proliferation and less keratinization compared to estrogen.

The menstrual stage can readily be detected by examining exfoliated cells present in a cervical smear. During the estrogen stage, the smear consists of large, flat, epithelial cells with eosinophilic keratin and small pyknotic nuclei. During the progesterone stage, the cervical smear reveals smaller cells with large nuclei. The lower layer of cervical epithelial cells becomes crowded and stains basophilic rather than eosinophilic. During senescence, no hormones are pesent; therefore, only small parabasal cells containing large, basophilic nuclei are present.

Pregnancy and the Cervix

Alterations take place in the cervical tissues during pregnancy. The cervix develops more stroma than normal, more vascularity, and larger glands in the endocervix during pregnancy. The glands of the endocervix become hypertrophic and contain more mucin. The cells of the superficial endocervical and ectocervical layers form decidualike cells, which appear swollen and undergo hyperplastic and proliferative alterations. The latter hyperplasia and proliferation are frequently difficult to differentiate from the histology of malignancy because of the increase in the thickness of the basal cell layer and other atypical cellular changes due to pregnancy.

Cervicitis

Acute cervicitis accompanies gonorrhea. Chronic cervicitis is a common lesion with an obscure etiology. The latter may be present following birth, trauma or trichomoniasis, and is due to hormonal changes and alterations in the pH of the cervical secretions. Chronic cervicitis appears clinically as a red lesion with cervical erosion generally present at the mucocutaneous junction, and endocervical and ectocervical junctions. No ulcerations are present in the cervix. The stroma immediately beneath the red lesion is infiltrated with numerous chronic inflammatory cells, and the endocervical glands are occluded and dilated, forming cystic cervicitis or the Nabothian cyst. When the endocervicitis is of long standing, the endocervical and glandular epithelial cells may undergo squamous metaplasia. The squamous metaplasia consists of columnar epithelial cells located on top of squamous cells. The squamous metaplasia does not represent a malignant lesion and should be differentiated from early malignancy. Cervicitis is capable of spreading throughout the genital tract.

Cervicitis and endocervicitis are more common in childbearing women. The inflammatory exudate that develops during cervicitis is quite variable in composition. A low grade, nonpathogenic microorganism may be responsible for provoking inflammation. Excessive mucous is secreted by the glands, and a vaginal discharge is present. The excessive mucous and injured epithelial cells result in a chronic destruction of the epithelium, producing cervical erosions. The destruction of the squamous epithelium normally present in the vagina leads to its replacement by columnar epithelium originating from the endocervix. During the regenerative process, squamous epithelium proliferates and undermines the columnar epithelium. The columnar epithelium is exfoliated and replaced by squamous epithelium.

Chronic cystic cervicitis is associated with erosions and alterations in the endocervical epithelium and glands. Chronic cervicitis consists of proliferation of glandular elements, dilatation, and cyst formation.

Epidermidalization

Epidermidalization or squamous metaplasia occurs in the cervical glands. Benign squamous cells develop within the cervical glands. Squamous epithelium grows into the endocervical region, or the reserve cells located below the columnar cells may develop into squamous metaplasia, producing epidermidalization of the endocervix. Carcinoma of the endocervix may develop in the sites of epidermidalization of the endocervix.

Tuberculous Cervicitis

Cervicitis may be caused by tuberculosis of the fallopian tube. The cervicitis develops secondary to pulmonary tuberculosis. Condyloma acuminatum may involve the cervix by the development of an infectious and autoinoculable papillary growth caused by a filterable virus.

Benign Adenomatous Tumor of the Vagina

The benign adenomatous tumor of the vagina is termed the *meonephric tubular adenoma*. This adenoma develops from embryonal remnants of the wolffian duct. Wolffian duct remnants located within the vagina may also develop into Gartner's cyst.

Cervical Polyps

Endocervical polyps are benign, highly vascular lesions located on the endocervix. The stroma is lined by tall columnar cells and some glands. Endocervical polyps may form in regions of the endocervix and consist of edematous tissue, inflammation, and proliferation of connective tissue, which is covered by squamous or columnar epithelium. The endocervical polyp is accompanied by hemorrhage and a long-standing chronic endocervicitis and endocervical stenosis. Endocervical stenosis is also a complication of radium therapy.

Some investigators report that the endocervical polyp never undergoes malignant transformation. However, a few instances have been reported in which malignant transformation has occurred within the endocervical polyp. The endocervical polyp, however, is not to be considered as a premalignant or premalignant lesion of the cervix.

Carcinoma of the Cervix

Carcinoma of the cervix is the second most common malignant neoplasm of the female. Carcinoma of the breast is the most common neoplasm. Carcinoma of the cervix is responsible for 20 percent of the deaths in women. Carcinoma of the cervix is three times as common as carcinoma of the endometrium. Carcinoma of the cervix develops in women who have had children. Women who are married to uncircumsized males, early in life, have a high incidence of carcinoma of the cervix. Carcinoma of the cervix is high in Negroes, moderate to average in Caucasians, and low in Jewish women. Carcinoma of the cervix develops before the menopause, i.e. around forty years of age.

The lymphatics of the cervix become involved early during carcinoma of the cervix. The carcinoma involves the pelvic tissues, i.e. the frozen pelvis develops in which the uterus and adnexea are adherent to the pelvic walls, producing immovable structures.

The earliest detectable malignancy of the cervix is the carcinoma *in situ*. Carcinoma *in situ* is confined to the epithelium of the cervix with a good, limiting, and intact basement membrane. Carcinoma *in situ* arises at the mucocutaneous junction. Carcinoma *in situ* and invasive carcinoma of the cervix may have no symptoms. It may be impossible to palpate the carcinoma; therefore, no clinical clue is present to the diagnosis of carcinoma.

When the carcinoma is detected and diagnosed in its *in situ* stage, it has a 100 percent cure rate. When carcinoma *in situ* is left untreated, it will invade the surrounding tissues within five to seven years. When spread of the carcinoma of the cervix occurs to parametrial tissues, the cure rate is only 6 to 7 percent. Ninety-six percent of malignant neoplasms of the cervix are epidermoid carcinomas. The prognosis of epidermoid carcinoma is good following early and adequate therapy, i.e. removal of the cervix. Carcinoma *in situ* is composed of hyperchromatic epithelial cells and hyperplasia of the basal cell layer so that the epithelium is composed primarily of basal cells. Mitotic figures are evident at the surface of the epithelium, and there is anaplasia and loss of polarity.

Brody classified the squamous cell carcinoma of the cervix into grades 1, 2, 3, and 4. Grade 1 squamous cell carcinoma consists of 0 to 25 percent undifferentiated cells. Grade 2 squamous cell carcinoma consists of 25 to 50 percent undifferentiated cells. Grade 3 squamous cell carcinoma consists of 50 to 75 percent undifferentiated cells. Grade 4 squamous cell carcinoma consists of 75 to 100 percent undifferentiated cells. Carcinoma *in situ* of the cervix is classified as grade 0. It may be difficult to differentiate between benign squamous cell metaplasia and carcinoma *in situ*, as well as between atypical hyperplasia of pregnancy and the squamous cell carcinoma.

In addition to the latter histopathologic classification, the squamous cell carcinoma of the cervix has a clinical classification, i.e. stage 1, 2, 3, and 4. In stage 1, the lesion is limited to the cervix. In stage 2, the neoplasm extends outside the cervix; however, it fails to invade the pelvic wall. In stage 3, the neoplasm invades the pelvic wall and the vagina. In stage 4, the frozen pelvis has developed with the formation of a hard, nonmovable mass and all pelvic structures are infiltrated with the neoplasm. Carcinoma of the cervix grows by infiltration of the rectal, iliac, and periaortic lymph nodes, and the liver. Death is caused through renal failure and toxemia. Carcinoma of the cervix also undergoes invasion and obstruction around the ureter with development of pyelonephritis. When toxemia is present, necrosis develops in the central portions of the carcinoma, producing and releasing toxic material into the bloodstream.

Adenocarcinoma of Cervical Glands

Adenocarcinoma of the cervix may arise from the cervical glands. One out of ten carcinomas of the cervix are adenocarcinomas; therefore, this malignant neoplasm is not common.

Exfoliative Cytology in the Diagnosis of Carcinoma of the Cervix

Exfoliative cytology is important in the early diagnosis of carcinoma of the cervix. Papanicolaou smears should be a standard part of every annual physical examination for females. The Papanicolaou smear and stain reveals keratinization of epithelial cells. The immature cervical epithelium has no keratinization. The malignant cervical epithelial cell has no keratinization. However, the malignant cervical epithelial cell has an altered ratio of nucleus to cytoplasm. The malignant cell contains an enlarged nucleus and decreased amount of cytoplasm. The nucleus is hyperchromatic and contains chromatin clumps and numerous nucleoli, and there is a tendency for the malignant cells to stick together in the cervical smear.

The diagnosis of carcinoma of the cervix can be made initially by means of exfoliative cytology. However, the cytology diagnosis should be followed immediately by a surgical biopsy from the involved cervix. A wedge-shaped piece of tissue should be removed from the lesion, including stromal tissue. The treatment of early squamous cell carcinoma of the cervix, carcinoma *in situ,* or stage 1 carcinoma of the cervix consists of total hysterectomy including the removal of lymph nodes followed by irradiation. During advanced carcinoma of the cervix, radium may be inserted into the cervix as one aspect of therapy.

DISEASES AND NEOPLASMS OF THE VULVA AND VAGINA

Venereal Lesions of the Vulva and Vagina

Gonorrhea causes an infection of the urethra, Bartholin's glands, and Skene's glands. However, gonorrheal infection does not involve the vagina in adults. In children, gonorrheal infection does involve the vagina. The cervix and uterine tubes are infected during gonorrhea, but the endometrium is unaltered. The acute inflammation due to gonorrhea consists of suppuration and edema in the vulva and vagina of children.

Gonorrhea is responsible for an inflammation that spreads superficially along the epithelium of the vagina, resulting in vaginitis, cervicitis, endometritis, and salpingitis. Gonorrhea in children is responsible primarily for causing vaginitis and cervicitis. The disease is always more severe in the mucosal tissue of children because it consists of only a few layers of epithelial cells. Therapy consists of the administration of estrogen in adults, in order to produce changes in the mucosa, plus antibiotics.

Bartholin's glands are the site of infection by the gonococci, as well as by other microorganisms. Bartholin's abscess, therefore, develops when there is a blockage of the duct to Bartholin's gland. The Bartholin cyst is a simple cystic lesion with the lumen filled with clear fluid. The Bartholin cyst develops when the purulent material is resorbed following the gonorrheal infection.

Syphilis may occur in the vulva and vagina. Primary syphilis produces the syphilitic chancre, and secondary syphilis is responsible for producing the flat condylomata lata, i.e. chronic inflammation and proliferation of epithelium in the form of gross, warty lesions of the vagina. Condylomata lata lesions produce drainage onto the vulva, cervix, and vagina. Tertiary syphilis is rare in the vulva and vagina. The tertiary lesion of syphilis is a superficial lesion with ulceration of the skin. The tertiary lesion of syphilis in the vulva and mucous membranes is termed the *syphiloma*.

Lymphopathia venereum is a venereal lymphogranuloma that involves the vulva and inguinal lymph nodes. The diagnosis of the vulval infection is accomplished by means of the Frei test, i.e. an intracutaneous diagnostic test for lymphopathia venereum based upon a reaction to an antigen. Injection of the antigen results in a red, indurated area in the skin within twenty-four to forty-eight hours. Symptoms of this venereal disease include development of papilla, ulcerations, lymphadenopathy, drainage of exudate, and elephantiasis. Perirectal tissue subsequently becomes involved as a complication of the venereal infection.

Granuloma inguinale is a granulomatous venereal disease of the female genitalia caused by *Donovania granulomatis (Calymmatobacterium granulomatis)*. Deep, purulent ulcerations develop in the female genitalia accompanied by scar formation following resolution and healing of the skin lesions. Granuloma inguinale produces ulcerations primarily in the inguinal region and perineum.

Chancroid produces a soft chancre and is a venereal disease of the female genitalia and inguinal lymph nodes caused by *Hemophilus ducreyi*. This venereal disease occurs in both males and females and is ten times more common in Caucasians than Negroes. Chancroid-produced, small ulcerations develop upon an inflamed and edematous base from a pustule formed from a papule. Nonspecific ulcerations may be caused by other microorganisms in females. In some instances, chancroid lesions in older females fail to reveal hemophilus organisms upon culturing the lesion.

Vaginal Tuberculosis

Vaginal tuberculosis or tuberculosis of the female genitalia develops secondary to pulmonary tuberculosis. Ten percent of instances of pulmonary tuberculosis show genital involvement following hematogenous spread. Tuberculosis also spreads to the uterus and cervix in addition to the vagina.

Chronic Vaginitis

Chronic vaginitis accompanied by a white discharge is due to infection by *Trichomonas vaginalis*. A hanging drop and cervical smear are useful examination methods for arriving at the diagnosis of chronic vaginitis. Chronic endocervicitis is caused by trichomoniasis. During trichomoniasis, the cervical smear reveals desquamation of the superficial cells, with clumps of leukocytes located on epithelial cells; *trichomona vaginalis* are present.

Condyloma acuminatum is a projecting, warty growth of the vulva, i.e. a viral disease (viral wart) of the vulva. Condyloma acuminatum may or may not be associated with gonorrhea. Other types of viral warts develop in the urethra of older women. These are generally the squamous cell papilloma and are not due to the virus causing condyloma acuminatum.

Monilia vaginitis is a nonspecific inflammation in the vagina of children and in adults during the postmenopausal period. The acute inflammatory reaction occurs in the vagina due to infection by *Candida albicans*.

Kraurosis Vulvae and Leukoplakia of the Vulva

The postmenopausal patient may be affected by senile vaginitis and kraurosis of the vulva. Kraurosis vulvae is atrophy of the squamous epithelium of the vulva, producing a thick, shrunken, and parchmentlike tissue in the vulva. During kraurosis vulvae, the surface of the epithelium is shiny, fragile red, and inflamed. There is a fibrosis of the subepithelial connective tissue accompanied by the development of surface cracks in the epithelium. The surface cracks may readily become infected. Itching (pruritis) is commonly present, and scratching leads to trauma and secondary infection.

Leukoplakia of the vulva is a thickening of the squamous epithelium, with hyperkeratosis and parakeratosis, and dyskeratosis. An inflammatory exudate underlies the leukoplakia of the vulva. Leukoplakia or squamous cell carcinoma may develop on top of kraurosis vulvae and leukoplakia vulvae, which should, therefore, be classified as a precancerous or procancerous lesion. Leukoplakia of the vulva has a high rate of malignant transformation. The rate of malignant transformation from leukoplakia of the vulva is greater than malignant transformation in leukoplakia of the skin and lips. Benign papillomas never develop in the vulva.

Bowen's Disease of the Vulva and Vagina

Bowen's disease (carcinoma *in situ*) is an intraepithelial malignancy of the vulva and vagina. Bowen's disease is limited to a single area whereas carcinoma *in situ* may be multicentric and involve several areas of the vulva and vagina. Early squamous cell carcinoma is also limited to a single area of the vulva or vagina. The prognosis of Bowen's disease is good. Diagnosis of

Bowen's disease is accomplished by observing the following histopathologic findings: nests of anaplastic cells, hypoplastic cells showing a loss of polarity, mitosis, variation in size and shape, and variation in staining characteristics.

Benign Neoplasms of the Vulva and Vagina

Benign neoplasms of the vulva and vagina include the fibroma, hemangioma, leiomyoma, hiradenoma (benign sweat gland tumor of vulva), and Gartner's cyst. Gartner's cyst is not a true neoplasm and arises from embryonic remnants of the wolffian duct.

Malignant Neoplasms of the Vulva and Vagina

Carcinoma of the vulva has a higher incidence than carcinoma of the vagina. Carcinoma may arise in the clitoris, producing a thickening and ulceration of the surface of the vulva. Metastases from carcinoma of the vulva or vagina spread to the inguinal lymph nodes. When the clitoris or upper vagina is involved by carcinoma, the metastatic lesions occur in the iliac lymph nodes.

The vagina and cervix of children may be involved by a mesodermal mixed tumor termed *sarcoma botyroides*. Sarcoma botyroides is a pedunculated, polypoid mass located in the vagina and cervix of children. This neoplasm is composed of fibroblasts, striated muscle, and cartilage. Metastasis occurs rather early and is generally widespread and fatal.

Squamous cell carcinoma of the vulva occurs in individuals between fifty and sixty years of age. It is a highly malignant carcinoma, which spreads by means of the bloodstream to the inguinal, iliac, and aortic lymph nodes. A spreading carcinoma of the vulva is responsible for destruction and infiltration of the skin by the neoplasm. An adenocarcinoma may rarely arise from Bartholin's glands.

Nevi and Malignant Melanoma of the Female Genitalia

Benign nevi may occur in the female genitalia. A pigmented skin lesion may represent a congenital nevus. The congenital nevus may not necessarily be present at birth but may develop as a pigmented lesion at a later date. The nevus cell comprising the benign nevus are derived from the nerve endings or neural cells and from the melanocytes. There are three types of benign nevi of the female genitalia: the intradermal nevus, the junctional nevus, and the compound nevus. The junctional nevus is a variety of nevi that may undergo malignant transformation and has definitive potentialities for malignant transformation. The compound nevus also has the potential for malignant transformation.

Pure, junctional nevi are characteristically located on the genitalia, rectum, lower extremities, hands, and face.

The malignant melanoma of the female genitalia is accompanied by very widespread metastases. The malignant melanoma causes the most widespread metastases of any malignant neoplasm. Metastatic lesions develop in the heart, brain, and any site throughout the body.

TOXEMIA OF PREGNANCY

Toxemia of pregnancy, i.e. the presence of an exotoxin, endotoxin, or noxious substance in the circulating blood during pregnancy, involves the premature aging and degeneration, clumping, excessive hyalinization, and calcification of the syncytial masses. Infarcts of the placenta are common during toxemia of pregnancy. Glomerular alterations include hyalinization and thickening of the basement membrane of the glomeruli. If toxemia of pregnancy persists along with hyalinization of the basement membrane of glomeruli, the result is the development of eclampsia. Eclampsia is the presence of coma and convulsions during or immediately after pregnancy. During eclampsia, there is degeneration of the convoluted tubules of the kidney, hemorrhage and necrosis of the liver, and necrosis of the renal cortex.

The syncytial cells are generally invasive in nature and capable of destroying the tissues of the endometrium and decidua. The syncytial cells invade the myometrium at the placental site. Syncytial cells are capable of producing a syncytial endometritis. This endometritis is not an inflammation or neoplastic alteration. Pleomorphic cells invade the muscle tissue but do not destroy areas of the myometrium. The pleomorphic cells gain access to the venous channels and produce emboli in the lungs composed of syncytial cells. The syncytial cells degenerate following delivery.

References

Aaro, L.A., Jacobson, L.J., and Soule, E.H.: *Obstet Gynecol, 21*:659, 1963.
Abell, M.R.: *Am J Obstet Gynecol, 86*:470, 1963.
Afonso, J.F., Martin, G.M., Nisco, F.S., and de Alvarez, R.R.: *Am J Obstet Gynecol, 84*:667, 1962.
Boutselis, J.G., Bair, J.R., Vorys, N., and Ullery, J.C.: *Am J Obstet Gynecol, 85*:994, 1963.
Breen, J.L. and Neubecker, R.D.: *Obstet Gynecol, 21*:669, 1963.
Burdick, C.O. and Warner, P.O.: *Obstet Gynecol, 23*:396, 1964.
Chamlian, D.L. and Taylor, H.B.: *Obstet Gynecol, 36*:659, 1970.
Corscaden, J.: *Gynecologic Cancer,* 3rd ed. Baltimore, Williams and Wilkins, 1962.
Diaz-Bazan, N.: *Obstet Gynecol, 23*:281, 1964.
Emge, L.A.: *Am J Obstet Gynecol, 83*:1541, 1962.
Ferguson, J.H. and Maclure, J.G.: *Am J Obstet Gynecol, 87*:326, 1963.
Foss, G.L.: *Br Med J, 2*:1907, 1960.
Gall, S.A., et al.: *JAMA, 207*:2243, 1969.
Gardner, H.L. and Fernet, P.: *Am J Obstet Gynecol, 88*:680, 1964.
Girouard, D.P., Barclay, D.L., and Collins, C.G.: *Obstet Gynecol, 23*:513, 1964.
Gore, H. and Hertig, A.T.: *Clin Obstet Gynecol, 5*:1448, 1962.
Grady, H.G. and Smith, H.C. (Eds.): *The Ovary.* Baltimore, Williams and Wilkins, 1963.
Graham, J.B., Sotto, L.S.J., and Paloucek, F.P.: *Carcinoma of the Cervix.* Philadelphia, Saunders, 1962.
Greene, R.R., Holzwarth, D., and Roddick, J.: *Am J Obstet Gynecol, 88*: 1001, 1964.
Greenwald, P., et al.: *N Engl J Med, 285*:390, 1971.
Herbst, A.L., et al.: *N Engl J Med, 284*:878, 1971.
Hertig, A.T. and Gore, H.: Tumors of the female sex organs, Parts I, II, and III. *Atlas of Tumor Pathology,* Washington, D.C., Armed Forces Institute of Pathology, 1960.
Hertig, A.T. and Gore, H.: *Am J Roentgenol, 87*:48, 1962.
Hughesdon, P.E.: *J Obstet Gynaecol Br Commow, 66*:566, 1959.
Hurlbutt, F.R. and Nelson, H.B.: *Obstet Gynecol, 21*:730, 1963.
Johnson, L.D., Easterday, C.L., Gore, H. and Hertig, A.T.: *Cancer, 17*:213, 1964.
Malhotra, S.L.: *Br J Cancer, 25*:62, 1971.
Malinak, L.R. and Miller, G.V.: *Am J Obstet Gynecol, 91*:251, 1965.
Marcus, C.C. and Marcus, S.L.: *Am J Obstet Gynecol, 81*:752, 1961.
Newman, H.F. and Northrup, J.D.: *Am J Obstet Gynecol, 84*:1816, 1962.
Novak, E.R. and Woodruff, J.D.: *Gynaeological and Obstetrical Pathology,* 5th ed. Philadelphia, Saunders, 1962.
O'Hern, T.M. and Neubecker, R.D.: *Obstet Gynecol, 19*:758, 1962.

O'Malley, B.W.: *N Engl J Med, 284*:370, 1971.
Plummer, G. and Masterson, J.G.: *Am J. Obstet Gynecol, 111*:81, 1971.
Richardson, G.S.: *N Engl J Med, 286*:645, 1972.
Ryan, G.M.: *Am J Obstet Gynecol, 84*:198, 1962.
Samuels, B., Bradburn, D.M., and Johnson, C.P.: *Am J Obstet Gynecol, 82*:393, 1961.
Scully, R.E.: *Hum Pathol, 1*:73, 1970.
Snaith, L.M. and Barns, T.: *Lancet, 1*:712, 1962.
Vellios, F., Stander, R.W., and Huber, C.P.: *Am J Clin Pathol, 39*:496, 1963.
Whelton, J. and Kottmeier, H.L.: *Acta Obstet Gynecol Scand, 41*:22, 1962.
Wilkins, L., Grumback, M.M., Van Wyk, J.J., and Shepard, T.H.: *Pediatrics, 16*:287, 1955.
Woodruff, J.D., Williams, T.J., and Goldberg, B.: *Am J Obstet Gynecol, 87*:679, 1963.
World Health Organization: Five years of research on human genetics. *WHO Chron, 24*:248, 1970.

CHAPTER 26

THE BREAST

INTRODUCTION

Embryology and Endocrinology of the Breast

THE MAMMARY gland is an accessory sex organ that is endocrine dependent, i.e. it is dependent on the pituitary. The mammary gland is a rudimentary gland in the male and a quiescent gland in the female. The mammary gland is a modified skin appendage and collection of glandular elements. The prepubertal and male breasts consist of connective tissue and collapsed straight ducts. The ducts undergo budding and proliferation when under the influence of estrogen. A special type of lobular connective tissue develops in the breast, which is stimulated by estrogen. The latter breast is composed largely of fat lobules surrounded by a connective tissue, which differs from the connective tissue of the normal breast. The specialized type of lobular connective tissue, stimulated by estrogen, is a loose connective tissue containing stellate fibroblasts. The fibroblastic cells proliferate along with the proliferation of ducts and development of hyperemia.

Embryologically, the breast is derived from modified skin appendages and modified sweat glands. Accessory breast tissue may develop in the axilla or along the milk line running from the axilla to the inguinal region. Multiple nipples develop along the milk line. The normal thick epidermis disappears along the milk line, and blood vessels pass close to surface epithelium. In the pectoral region, an area of increased vascularity is due to the accessory breast tissue.

The breast is composed of three types of epithelial cells, i.e. the ampulla, the ductal epithelium, and the lobular epithelium.

The ampulla contains Paget cells, which are derived from the epidermis. The ductal and lobular epithelial cells of the breast have the capacity to develop from ductal cells to lobular cells and vice versa. The ductal cells of the breast of the newborn proliferate, and budding takes place from the tubules. Estradiol produces ductal hyperplasia plus hyperplasia of the periductal connective tissue.

The normal ducts of the breast consist of one layer of cuboidal cells and a flattened layer of cells located beneath the cuboidal cells. A few myoepithelial cells are located beneath the cuboidal cells to help empty the ducts. Witch's milk may be present in the first born following a long and difficult labor. When labor is prolonged, the fetus remains in contact with hormones for a greater period of time, and the result is the presence of witch's milk three to four days after birth and lasting for one or two weeks. The witch's milk is due to prolactin derived from the mother before birth.

At three and one-half to four years of age, the male and female breasts are similar. However, senile involution occurs in the male breast up to puberty. During adolescence, the breasts are similar to the breast tissue present at birth. At puberty, a node develops beneath the nipple and remains until nineteen to twenty-one years of age. The puberty node is a normal structure, and males and females respond alike to the node. However, lobular development never appears in the male breast. Lobular development begins in the female following the first menstruation.

The breast is stimulated by estrogen. Estrogen is responsible for the production of periductal connective tissue and general growth of the breast. Prepartum secretion is present during the middle of pregnancy; however, lactation does not take place. Prepartum secretion is nonfunctional and should not be considered as lactation since lactation only occurs as a postpartum secretion. After nine months, the uterus has completed its function and the breast begins its function. The uterus and breast are not in step with each other since the breast function occurs postpartum and not prepartum. When the pituitary gland functions normally, estrogen alone is capable of stimulating lobular development in the breast. Estrogen sensitizes the breast to the action of the mammogenic hormone from the pituitary gland. Estrogen influences all of the mesenchymal tissues of the breast and aids in the formation of the basement membrane. The elements and hormones present in the bloodstream must diffuse through the blood vessel and basement membrane. Estrogen influences the matrix and connective tissue that surround and support the lobules of the breast. Estrogen, therefore, influences intralobular connective tissue. Estrogen also determines whether the pituitary hormone will stimulate the breast.

Breast tissue passes through the following cycles: the menstrual cycle, the pregnancy cycle, and the lactation cycle. Senile involution of the breast occurs during the postnatal period, menstruation, castration, and following pregnancy and lactation. The regressive phases of the breast are, therefore, endocrine dependent.

Progesterone sensitizes the breast to the action of the mammogenic hormone of the pituitary gland. Progesterone is responsible for proliferation of connective tissue cells and ducts of the breast. Under the influence of progesterone, the lobules of the breast become swollen and edematous, and there is an increase in the quantity of intracellular substances. Progesterone disappears during cystic disease of the breast.

The anterior pituitary hormone is responsible for glandular hyperplasia accompanied by a budding outgrowth from the ducts of the breast. Following pregnancy, the alveoli, stroma, and lobules are formed, and the glands of the breast never regress. As soon as the placental influence is removed, lactation begins in the breast. The latter is accompanied by an increased secretion of the alveoli of the breast. Lactation is, therefore, defined as a postpartum secretion of the breast. During the first four days of postpartum lactation there is engorgement, which may be quite painful; however, no milk is present or secreted. If the fetus is born dead, estrogen may be administered to inhibit lactation. Once lactation has begun, testosterone may be administered to inhibit pain. The nipple may disappear as a result of swelling (massive) from a complication, i.e. lymphedema. The breasts should be wrapped during the postpartum engorgement associated with lactation.

The endocrine gland secretions produced by the various glands have the potential to influence the growth and development of the mammary glands. The mammogenic hormone has not been isolated from the pituitary gland.

The pseudosecretion phase of the breast is accompanied by a prolifierative phase in the uterus. A storage phase occurs in the uterus during early senile changes. The thyroid, breast, and uterus are secretory organs and endocrine-dependent organs. The latter secretory organs undergo declines during various periods of life. The thyroid gland declines at an early age simply by withholding iodine, resulting in involution of the thyroid. The prostate and breast undergo involution in the presence of high estrogen levels in the blood. During senility, the cells of the breast disappear and the storage function persists as the secretory phase terminates. Fibrocystic disease of the breast is due to storage and diminished secretion. One percent of males and 6 percent of females develop nodules in the thyroid similar to fibrocystic disease of the breast. The breast is an endocrine-dependent organ that undergoes aging cycles.

The function of the ductal system of the breast is to deliver and store milk within the ducts similar to the storage of milk in the acini. Abnormalities of the ductal system of the breast increases with age at the expense of the lobular structures. The aging abnormalities represent a form of involutional cystic disease.

Congenital Anomalies of the Breast

There are only a few congenital anomalies of the breast, which include an absence of the breast, absence of the nipples, smaller or larger breasts compared to the normal, accessory breast tissue, accessory nipples, and accessory breast tissue without any nipples. It is rather common to find accessory breast tissue in the axilla without accessory nipples.

Inflammatory Lesions of the Breast

Mammary abscesses may bind the breast for a period of twenty-four hours. Within forty-eight hours following breast abscesses, the breast undergoes involution. During lactation, $\frac{1}{2}$ to 1 percent of females have abscesses of the breast, i.e. lactation mastitis. The latter may occur in primipara lactation mastitis, which occurs prior to the birth of a subsequent child. The primipara lactation mastitis generally takes place one to two months postpartum in the primipara. The breast abscess may be a residual inflammation and fail to heal. The residual abscess of the breast may be the seat of a carcinoma of the breast. The diagnosis is difficult when the carcinoma of the breast arises in the residual abscess.

Mastitis is generally a rare, inflammatory lesion of the breast during the early days of lactation. Mastitis follows the entry of microorganisms through the ducts of the breast. *Staphylococcus aureus* produces a diffuse phlegmonous inflammation in the breast accompanied by pain, fever, and localized abscess formation beneath the skin of the breast.

Plasma cell mastitis is an infiltration and accumulation of plasma cells periductally, and peritubularly particularly around the periphery of dilated ducts. Plasma cell mastitis produces an accumulation of giant cells and eosinophiles in addition to plasma cells in the tissues of the breast. Following the birth of numerous children, there may occur a dilatation of the ducts of the breast with maintenance of the storage of milk. However, secretion of milk stops as a result of inspissated material that develops in the dilated ducts beneath the nipple. The inspissated material is responsible for obese breasts and may readily become the seat of chronic infection.

Chronic cystic mastitis presents as a hard lump in the breast. Upon palpation, the stroma of the breast produces the hard mass rather than the glandular tissue or epithelium. Chronic cystic mastitis is a microscopic and clinical disease entity. A lump in the breast may represent a papilloma or fibroadenoma. However, a hard lump in the breast should lead one to consider chronic cystic mastitis. The breast is composed mainly of fat tissue and is considered a rather quiescent organ unless the individual is pregnant. Neonatorium mastitis is an inflammation due to infection of the breast of the newborn.

Nodules in the breast are associated with hyperestrogen. Stimulation of the breast tissue causes an increase in estrogen and decrease in progesterone. Increased estrogen is accompanied by epithelial irregularities. A lump in the breast may also be associated with a missed period. In order to obtain aid in the diagnosis of a lump in the breast a needle can be injected into the lump. This aids in the diagnosis of cystic disease of the breast. Cystic disease of the breast occurs during the menopause or following the birth of children during a sudden stoppage of the pregnancy. The cessation of pregnancy is accompanied by a sudden withdrawal of estrogen. Cystic disease of the breast disappears during pregnancy; however, this represents only a suppression of the disease and not complete resolution. A decrease in the quantity of estrogen in the blood causes formation of cystic disease of the breast. Cystic disease of the breast represents an involutional phenomenon due to the isolation of the breast tissue from its normal endocrine dependence. Fibrocystic disease or cystic involution may develop in any of the endocrine-dependent glands of the body.

Tuberculosis of the breast occurs secondarily to lymphatic extension from mediastinal tuberculosis. Tuberculosis of the breast is accompanied by sinus tracts. Carcinoma may develop in areas of chronic sinus tracts present during tuberculosis of the breast. Tuberculosis of the breast and lactation mastitis are rare; however, plasma cell mastitis has a greater frequency than tuberculosis of the breast.

Chancre or gumma of the nipple plus a positive Wassermann fail to preclude the possibility of a neoplasm of the breast. Antileutic treatment should be given in the chancre or gumma of the nipple; however, penicillin is not indicated because it produces shrinkage of breast tissue and may prevent the proper diagnosis and therapy for neoplastic diseases of the breast. Arsphenamines cause shrinkage of a gumma of the breast without altering a neoplasm. Penicillin therapy reduces secondary inflammation of the breast and also causes the breast neoplasm to shrink, making the diagnosis more difficult. Syphilitic lesions of the breast should not be biopsied without antileutic treatment for a minimum of forty-eight hours. The procedure should be followed for syphilitic lesions throughout the body in order to protect the physician, dentist, nurses, and technicians in the operating room. Biopsy of a suspected syphilitic lesion should be undertaken only during a noncontagious stage of syphilis.

Irradiation of other portions of the body for treatment of neoplasia may result in secondary ulcerations of the breast and/or radiation dermatitis of the skin overlying the breast. Ulcerations of the breast may represent a late reaction to irradiation, a spread of the primary breast neoplasm, or the irradiation may produce an entirely new neoplasm of the breast.

Infantile mammary hypertrophy may develop in the female. The mammary hypertrophy is due to the granulosa cell tumor, estrogen, malignant tumors of the ovary, lesions of the hypothalamus, and post infectious encephalitis. Mammary hypertrophy cannot be experimentally produced in animals.

Gynecomastia in Males

Gynecomastia in the male is caused by mumps, Klinefelter's syndrome, hepatic injury, chorioepithelioma, malignant neoplasms of the testes, the adrenal cortical tumor, industrial hazards, and methyl testosterone. Mumps reduces the male hormone, and Klinefelter's syndrome produces grade one atrophy in the testes; however, the sertoli cells persist and estrogen is secreted. Cirrhosis and protein deficiency of the liver results in gynecomastia, hepatitis, and jaundice. The lowered metabolism of steroid hormones results in an inability to remove accumulated estrogen. Chorioepithelioma located at any site in the body such as in the mediastinum produces mammary hypertrophy. Adrenal cortical neoplasms cause masculinization or gynecomastia or a variety of different effects. Industrial hazards consist of numerous commercial chemicals including the production of estrogen by chemists. Methyl testosterone when administered orally has an adverse effect on the liver, i.e. it produces an iatrogenic reversible liver injury. At puberty some enlargement of the male breast occurs. However, this is not a gynecomastia and should not be treated. There is no lobule formation in the male breast, which appears to be an argument against the theory that estrogen is responsible for the formation of the lobules of the breast. Gynecomastia of the breast is accompanied by epithelial hyperplasia, increase in periductal stroma, and an absence of lobules.

Cystic Disease of the Breast

Cystic disease of the breast or Schimmelbusch's disease is the result of an exaggerated estrogen level in the following: young unmarried women, married women with children, and women who have not nursed their children. Cystic disease of the breast produces a painful enlargement of the breast prior to the menstrual period. Excessive progesterone stimulation may be a factor in the production of this cystic disease. The disease becomes prominent at the menopause in multiparous women. Endometrial hyperplasia accompanies cystic disease of the breast that occurs at the menopause.

Cystic disease of the breast develops in females over fifty years of age. Cystic disease produces a breast composed of fat and dilated ducts. Adenosis produces bilateral nodules in the breast with the formation of the late involutional cyst.

The cut surface of a gross specimen of cystic disease of the breast reveals a diffuse, nodular, and shotty consistency to the breast tissue. The cystic breast consists of pale, homogeneous, smooth, and rubbery tissue with palpable nodules (cysts). Wormlike masses or casts extrude from the cut surfaces of the ducts of the breast. The casts present in the ducts of the breast consist of a thick, milky or dry, puttylike material.

Microscopically, cystic disease of the breast consists of an increase in intralobular, specialized connective tissue, cystic dilatation of ducts, fibrosis or hyalinization of connective tissue, and widely separated ducts or proliferating ducts within the connective tissue of the breast. The ductal epithelium is predominantly flat but may consist of tall cells. There is an apocrine transformation of the ductal epithelium of the breast. Proliferating ductal epithelium produces papillary buds extending into the lumen of the duct. Adenomatous formation of cells results from the proliferation of ductal epithelium to fill the lumen of the ducts. The dilated ductal system of the breast, therefore, is filled with solid epithelium. Pleomorphism develops in the ductal epithelium that fills the lumen. The diagnosis of cystic disease of the breast with active ductal hyperplastic epithelium or carcinoma *in situ* can be made upon histopathologic examination of breast tissue. Chronic inflammatory cells are present in the interstitial tissue; however, cystic disease of the breast is not an inflammatory condition. The ductal hyperplasia is quite variable in the various ducts of the breast; however, it does produce masses of glandular structures composed of pale, epithelial lining cells.

Cystic disease of the breast, Swiss cheese of the uterus, and the colloid adenoma of the thyroid are unrelated to neoplasia. The lobules of the breast disappear in the absence of endocrine and structural support. It takes much more structural support to keep the breasts functioning normally than it does to maintain the uterus. Cystic disease of the breast may commonly coexist with carcinoma of the breast.

Mastidia is the presence of pain in the breasts. The tenderness and pain that are present result from a localized disturbance.

Adenosis

Adenosis of the breast is due to a relative hyperestrogenism with a long-standing, chronic endocrine imbalance resulting in dense, nodular breasts. Adenosis of the breast occurs in 2 percent of females and has six times the incidence of mammary carcinoma. It is not possible to aspirate any material from adenosis of the breast because the nodularity is due to fibrosis of the breast. The bilateral nodularity is due to late involutinal cysts. Extensive fibrosis of glandular elements of the breast is termed *scirrhosing adenosis*. The rare scirrhous carcinoma develops from scirrhosing adenosis of the breast.

Benign Neoplasms of the Breast

Benign neoplasms of the breast are not related to the endocrine glands and the secretions that control the breasts. The papilloma and fibroadenoma are the common benign neoplasms of the breast. The breast papilloma is due to an abnormal, rapid, and persistent proliferation of epithelium from the lobular end or bifurcation of the lobular ducts. The prelobular epithelium gives rise to the papilloma of the breast. The intracystic papilloma is not influenced by estrogen, but it is accompanied by a bloody discharge. Carcinoma of the breast rarely is accompanied by a bloody discharge. The intracystic papilloma of the breast may undergo malignant transformation in approximately 6 to 7 percent of instances.

Fifty percent of intracystic papillomas of the breast produce a bloody discharge at the nipple. When the nipple remains intact, the breast lesion is not a malignant neoplasm. Approximately four percent of all carcinomas of the breast are accompanied by a bloody discharge, whereas fifty percent of intracystic papillomas are accompanied by either a bloody or sanguinous discharge. A milky or serous discharge from the nipple is unrelated to malignant neoplasia. Galactorrhea is the presence of a milky secretion arising from the breast one year after breast-feeding the child. A bloody discharge is significant only for the intraductal papilloma or intraductal carcinoma. The papilloma of the breast is fragile and bleeds readily.

The fibroadenoma of the breast is a benign neoplasm composed of a growth of tubules and branches with periductal tissue and ducts. The fibroadenoma differs from the papilloma since the former is under the influence of estrogen. The fibroadenoma develops in the female's breast in individuals from sixteen to twenty-six years of age. The fibroadenoma increases rapidly during early pregnancy and again at the menopause. The fibroadenoma undergoes involution, dilatation of the ductal system, and infarction. The fibroadenoma may undergo hyalinization and ossification. Cystic changes may occur in the ducts of the fibroadenoma, and this benign neoplasm may rarely undergo malignant transformation to a sarcoma. The benign giant myxoma of the breast may also undergo sarcomatous transformation at the menopause.

The fibroadenoma consists of a specialized proliferating connective tissue, is well circumscribed, and therefore, is easily surgically enucleated. The fibroadenoma is homogeneous, pale, contains small lobules and papillary projections, and is a well-defined neoplasm.

The periductal fibroadenoma of the breast involves numerous ductal elements. There is extensive connective tissue proliferation involving the smaller ductal branches. Grossly, the periductal fibroadenoma is firm, and the neoplasm may grow rapidly into a large lesion.

The cystadenoma of the breast originates in the larger ducts and produces masses of tissue within the affected ducts. The papilla projections that occur in the ducts of the breast are composed of tall columnar epithelial cells with pale cytoplasm covering the projections. The cystadenoma of the breast has a tendency to undergo malignant transformation. The lipoma and fibroma are common benign connective tissue neoplasms of the breast.

Malignant Neoplasms of the Breast

Carcinoma of the breast is the most common neoplasm of females. Approximately 110,000 new instances of carcinoma of the breast occur annually. Ten thousand women die annually from carcinoma of the breast. Twelve to fifteen percent of instances of breast carcinoma are too advanced at the time the definitive diagnosis is made to be treated properly and eradicated. Carcinoma of the breast is responsible for 25 percent of all cancer deaths in women.

Carcinoma of the breast is more common in women who have difficulty in nursing or in women with few children and no nursing. The more nursing difficulties, the greater the incidence of breast cancer. Radical mastectomy may produce a five-year cure rate from carcinoma of the breast. However, the breast carcinoma may return in seven to eight years following the mastectomy. Carcinoma of the breast metastasizes to bone in 50 percent of instances of this neoplasm. Axillary metastases also occurs in 50 percent of instances of breast carcinoma. Seven to thirteen percent of females with carcinoma in one breast also have carcinomatous involvement in the other breast.

Carcinoma of the breast may possibly be related to the following contributing factors: a carcinoma factor may be transmitted in the milk of the human breast; heredity; a milk factor; and estrogenic stimulation. Carcinoma of the breast is common in women who have never given birth and to multiparous women who did not nurse their children. Carcinoma of the breast occurs toward the menopause, and 44 percent of instances of this neoplasm develop in the upper outer quadrant of the breast. There has been a 40 percent increase in the incidence of carcinoma of the breast since 1960. Eighty to eighty-five percent of females with lesions of breast carcinoma report to a physician for diagnosis and treatment, i.e. one out of every three females with carcinoma of the breast seeks treatment for the lesion.

The principal sites for the development of carcinoma of the breast are the outer upper quadrant (44%) and the central zone of the breast because epithelial cells are more common in these locations. The remaining areas of the breast consist of fat tissue. Carcinoma of the breast develops in females around forty-five to fifty years of age primarily as a solitary mass in the breast. The breast is higher than normal and the nipple is retracted. Transillumination of a breast containing a carcinoma reveals a darkly cast shadow when viewed in a dark room. When hemorrhage is present in the breast, transillumination reveals a dark shadow. Transillumination of fibrocystic disease of the breast reveals no shadows.

Retraction of the nipple is present during carcinoma of the breast; however, it may also be due to a congenital malformation. Carcinoma of the breast results in atrophy of fat tissue and retraction of the skin covering the breast. Breast carcinoma is accompanied by a large fibrous tissue reaction with fibrosis of the breast.

Seventy-five percent of carcinomas of the breast are adenocarcinoma, and scirrhous or desmoplastic carcinomas. Infiltrating scirrhous carcinomas of the breast are grade 3 carcinomas. Carcinoma of the breast is complicated by lymphangitis. Inflammation of the lymphatics results from the highly malignant neoplastic cells.

Seventy-five percent of breast carcinomas cause contraction of the overlying skin and hard and enlarged axillary glands. Carcinoma of the breast is a rapidly progressive neoplasm. Breast carcinoma will generally measure 1 centimeter in diameter three months after initiation; however, after an eight-month period of growth, it reaches three and one-half centimeters. Twenty-five percent of carcinomas of the breast are composed of lobules, ducts, and adenoid tissue. The intraductal carcinoma of the breast bulges outward on the cut section. The gelatinous breast carcinomas are soft and also bulge outward on the cut surfaces. A better prognosis and better cure rate exist for breast carcinomas that grow inward.

Spread of Carcinoma of the Breast

Carcinoma of the breast spreads to the pleural cavity. Lymphatics penetrate through the chest wall and carry malignant cells to the pleural fluid. The pleura contains an exudative type of fluid that supports the growth of metastatic malignant cells from carcinoma of the breast. Bones are common sites for metastases from carcinoma of the breast. The red marrow bones and flat bones are principal sites of metastases. The viscera are also involved by metastatic breast carcinoma.

Paget's Disease of the Nipple

Paget's disease of the nipple or carcinoma of the nipple is not a highly malignant neoplasm. Clinically, Paget's disease of the nipple appears as a scaly or red granular nipple, which appears blood tinged. This carcinoma is preceded by eczema of the nipple. The eczema appears like burnt skin that has sloughed off. Ductal epithelial cells and preductal cells proliferate into the ducts of the breast and epidermis.

Microscopically, atypical squamous epithelial cells predominate in this carcinoma of the nipple. The nuclei of the latter squamous cells are large, and mitotic figures are present in the epithelial cells, which are termed Paget cells. Paget cells consist of clear cytoplasm with intracellular bridges, vacuoles in the cytoplasm, and large nuclei and nucleoli. Smears made from the nipple secretions reveal Paget cells and are an aid in the diagnosis of Paget's disease of the nipple. The carcinoma of the nipple contains Paget cells that are highly malignant in their clinical behavior pattern.

The lymphatics that drain the breast, skin, and body wall pass deep to the plexus located outside the chest wall. Therefore, the pectoral muscles must be removed in order to find the deep lymphatics located close to the chest wall. Metastases occur to the inguinal region and to the opposite breast; however, the axillary lymph nodes are also involved by the spread of Paget's disease of the nipple. The internal mammary lymphatics that are located inside the chest cavity may be involved by the spread of Paget's disease of the nipple.

References

Arthes, F.G.: *Cancer, 28*:1391, 1971.
Berg, J.W.: *Cancer, 28*:1453, 1971.
Bloom, H.J.G. (Ed.): *Symposium on the Prognosis of Malignant Tumors of the Breast,* New York, Hafner, 1962.
Bulbrook, R.D., Hayward, J.L., Spicer, C.C., and Thomas, B.S.: *Lancet, 2:* 1238, 1962.
Chopra, H.C., et al.: *Cancer, 28*:1406, 1971.
Cooper, W.G. and Ackerman, L.V.: *Surg Gynecol Obstet, 77*:279, 1943.
Copeland, M.M.: *Am Surg, 29*:304, 1963.
Cromar, C.D.L. and Dockerty, M.B.: *Mayo Clin Proc, 16*:775, 1941.
Cutler, M.: *Tumors of the Breast,* Philadelphia, Lippincott, 1962.
Cutler, S.J., et al.: *Cancer, 28*:1376, 1971.
Frantz, V.K., Pickren, J.W.:, Melcher, G.W., and Auchincloss, H.: *Cancer, 4*:762, 1951.
Geschickter, C.F.: *Diseases of the Breast,* 2nd ed. Philadelphia, Lippincott, 1945.
Grady, H.G.: *Schweiz, Z F Path Bakt, 18*:685, 1955.
Haagensen, C.D.: *Diseases of the Breast,* Philadelphia, Saunders, 1971.
Handley, R.S. and Thackray, A.C.: *Br Med J, 1*:61, 1954.
Hasson, J. and Pope, C.H.: *Surgery, 49*:313, 1962.
Hill, R.P. and Miller, F.N.: *Cancer, 7*:318, 1954.
Horn, R.C.: In Lewison, E.F.: *Breast Cancer and Its Diagnosis and Treatment,* Baltimore, Williams and Wilkins, 1955.
Huggins, C. and Taylor, G.W.: *Arch Surg, 70*:303, 1955.
Huseby, R.A. and Thomas, L.B.: *Cancer, 7*:54, 1954.
Karnauchow, P.N.: *Am J Pathol, 30*:1169, 1954.
Kraus, T. and Neubecker, R.D.: *Cancer, 15*:444, 1962.
Lewison, E.F.: *Breast Cancer and Its Diagnosis and Treatment,* Baltimore, Williams and Wilkins, 1955.
McClanahan, B.J. and Hogg, L.: *Cancer, 7*:586, 1954.
Mirra, A.P., et al.: *Cancer Res., 31*:77, 1971.
Newman, W.: *Ann Surg, 157*:591, 1963.
Ochsner, A.: *Postgrad Med, 33*:133, 1963.
Orr, J.W. and Parish, D.J.: *J Pathol, 84*:201, 1962.
Pollard, H.M.: *Cancer, 28*:1368, 1971.
Priori, E.S., et al.: *Cancer, 28*:1462, 1971.
Sandison, A.T.: An autopsy study of the adult human breast, *National Cancer Institute, Monograph No. 8,* U.S.P.H.S., 1961.
Schlom, J. and Spiegelman, S.: *Proc Natl Acad Sci USA, 68*:1613, 1971.
Seman, G., et al.: *Cancer, 28*:1431, 1971.
Strax, T.: *Cancer, 28*:1563, 1971.
Thiessen, E.U.: *Cancer, 28*:1537, 1971.
Treves, N.: *Cancer, 11*:1083, 1958.
Vessey, M.P., et al.: *Cancer, 28*:1395, 1971.
Wynder, E.L., Bross, I.J., and Hirayama, T.: *Cancer, 13*:559, 1960.
Zippin, C. and Petrakis, N.L.: *Cancer, 28*:1381, 1971.

CHAPTER 27

MALE GENITAL SYSTEM

VENEREAL DISEASES OF THE MALE GENITALIA

Gonorrhea

INFECTION of the male genitalia may be due to *Neisseria gonococcus*. The incubation period for gonorrhea is three to six days, approximately four days. The infection spreads in a superficial manner along the mucosa of the male genitalia. Gonorrhea is accompanied by a regional lymphadenopathy, and the infection is responsible for the production of urethritis, periurethritis, prostatitis, seminal vesiculitis, colliculitis, and nontesticular epididymitis. Gonorrhea infection not only involves the male genitalia but spreads to the joints, producing a gonorrheal arthritis (suppurative arthritis). Gonorrheal infection produces a bacteremia that may be responsible for subacute or acute bacterial endocarditis and death. Gonorrhea may spread to the inguinal skin and rarely to the groin, producing a purulent or pyogenic inflammatory reaction. *Neisseria gonococci* react in the tissues similarly to the staphylococci or other cocci. Gonorrheal infection is responsible for a bulbovaginalitis and conjunctivitis in the newborn.

Syphilis

Syphilis of the male external genitalia is accompanied by the chancre in the primary stage of this venereal disease. Syphilis has an incubation period of twenty-one days, with the syphilitic infection spreading by way of the blood stream. Syphilis produces inguinal lymphadenopathy late in the course of this venereal disease. Syphilis of the male genitalia occurs primarily in young individuals between twenty-two and thirty-two years of age.

Lymphopathia Venereum

Lymphopathia venereum is another venereal disease that affects the male genitalia and is rather prominent in Negroes and sailors in the United States. South America lymphopathia venereum produces a small eschar lesion on the male genitalia, which has the gross appearance of a flea bite. The latter variety of lymphopathia venereum is classified as a reticuloendothelial disease that produces a bulbolymphadenopathy. This venereal disease produces rectal strictures; however, the strictures are more common is females than males. Lymphopathia venereum may involve all tissues in the body and is capable of producing encephalitis. The incubation period for the disease is three weeks. The Frei test is utilized for a definitive diagnosis of lymphopathia venereum of the male genitalia. Tubercles or a granulomatous reaction occurs in infected genital tissues and in the inguinal glands with central suppuration.

Chancroid

The chancroid infection produces a soft chancre in the male genitalia due to infection by *Hemophilus ducreyi*. The chancroid has an incubation period of four to five days. This venereal disease produces skin lesions on the male genitalia, which begin as pustules that rapidly expand and eventually ulcerate, producing a soft chancre without indurated edges. Regional lymphadenopathy accompanies the chancroid of the male genitalia. Any lesion located on the penis should be considered as a potential syphilitic chancre or chancroid lesion, and serology should be undertaken immediately.

Granuloma Inguinale

The venereal disease granuloma inguinale is responsible for the production of minor ulcerations on the penis; however, the disease primarily affects the soft tissues of the genitalia. The etiology of granuloma inguinale is *Donovania granulomatis*, which produces deep, purulent ulcerations of the skin of the external genitalia. This venereal disease is a granulomatous disease with a Donovan body inclusion located within macrophages. The

Donovan body represents a viral, parasitic, or bacilli inclusion body in the macrophage. A definitive diagnosis is made following examination of smears obtained from ulcerations of the groin. The Donovan inclusion bodies are readily apparent in the macrophages of the granulomatous inflammation.

DISEASES OF THE URETHRA

Anomalies of the Urethra

Anomalies of the urethra accompany other anomalies of the genital tract. There may be failure of closure of the urethra. Hypospadias is a developmental anomaly in which the urethra opens on the ventral surface of the penis or on the perineum. Epispadius is a congenital defect in which the urethra opens on the dorsum of the penis.

Urethritis

Urethritis is a common disease and a complication of gonorrhea leading to strictures in the urethra. The endotoxins produced by *Neisseria gonococcus* are responsible for the damage that occurs, rather than the microorganisms. The gonococci invade the glands, causing urethritis, fibrosis, and stricture with obstruction of the urethra.

Diverticulitis of the Urethra

Diverticulitis is either a congenital defect of the urethra or is the result of inflammation and stricture of the urethra. Calculi may be located in the urethra since they pass from the upper urinary tract into the urethra. Neoplasms and cysts may develop in the periurethral glands and generally include polyps, adenomas, papillomas, and only rarely the carcinoma.

DISEASES AND NEOPLASMS OF THE SCROTUM

The scrotum may have secondary anomalies, such as maldevelopment of the scrotum, failure of fusion producing clefts and openings, and inflammation of the scrotum secondary to trauma.

Superficial fungal infection of the scrotum is due to *Tinia cruris*. This ringworm infection produces a reticulosis of the skin and ulceration of the scrotum. Reticulosis is an increase in the number of histiocytes and other reticuloendothelial elements.

Filariasis is a parasitic infection of human tissues caused by *Wuchereria bancrofti*. This filarial parasite is a 10-inch worm (microfilaria) present in the bloodstream of the infected individual. *Wuchereria bancrofti* causes obstruction of the lymphatics, and when the microfilaria decays, elephantiasis develops. Edema develops in the scrotum and legs during elephantiasis. The skin and subcutaneous tissues of the scrotum undergo a marked thickening and swelling. The scrotum eventually becomes indurated and folded. The scrotum may weigh 15 kilograms or more during elephantiasis.

The scrotum may be affected by the following cystic alterations: hydrocele, spermatocele, varicocele, and hematocele depending upon the contents of the scrotum. The hydrocele is an inflammatory reaction with the accumulation of fluid between the layers of the tunica vaginalis. The hydrocele may accompany a hernia, follow surgery and trauma, and result as a complication of gonorrhea or other venereal disease. The hydrocele transilluminates as a clear cyst. The contents of the hydrocele include the following substances: globulin, fibrin, and albumen in 200 to 400 cc of a watery fluid.

The spermatocele of the testes is a cystic lesion with a clear or turbid fluid containing spermatozoa occupying the lumen of the cyst. Some of the spermatozoa are degenerating or dead. The spermatocele is a cyst lined with an epididymis cell layer. The cyst may grow to 1 to 3 centimeters in diameter. Twenty percent of males over sixty years of age develop the spermatocele.

The hematocele is a hydrocele containing blood in the lumen rather than a clear fluid. The fluid is a serosanguinous exudate. The hematocele develops following surgery, trauma, and malignant disease of the testes. The varicocele of the testes results following a varicosity of the pampiniform plexus (pampinocele). Twenty percent of older males have the varicocele, which fails to produce any clinical symptoms, and therapy is unnecessary.

Neoplasms of the scrotum are rare. However, hydrocarbons, paraffins, oil, and grease stimulate the development of a squamous cell carcinoma of the scrotum and penis.

DISEASES AND NEOPLASMS OF THE TESTES

Anomalies of the Testes

Anomalies develop in the testes, epididymis, and spermatic cord. The main testicular anomalies are malposition of the testes and failure of the testes to descend completely from the abdomen (cryptorchidism). Undescended testes may become the site for the development of neoplasms and, therefore, should be corrected or removed surgically. Cryptorchidism results in an absence of fertility (sterility) or in malignancy. Malignancy develops in testicular tissue and is twenty times greater in incidence than the development of sterility. At the present our knowledge is obscure concerning what role the endocrine system plays in controlling the descent of the testes. During cryptorchidism, the affected male is less masculine, i.e. masculinization is delayed. Perhaps the hormones that control the descent of the testes are deficient or absent during cryptorchidism.

Testicular Atrophy

Atrophic testes are caused by the failure of the testes to descend from the abdomen. When the testes fail to descend (ectopic testes), they may be displaced to the pelvis or to a location outside the inguinal canal. Late descent of the testes may take place at thirteen to seventeen years of age.

The undescended testes are classified into atrophic grades 1, 2, and 3. Grade 1 atrophy indicates that the sertoli cell syndrome is present. In the latter syndrome the interstitial leyden cells, the sertoli cells, and the basement membrane all persist. The sertoli cell syndrome results from high fevers and drug reactions. Cryptorchidism may be accompanied by grade 3 atrophy, and mumps may be accompanied by grade 1 or grade 3 atrophy of the testes. A grade 3 testicular atrophy is seen in undescended testes after an infarction of the testes or following mumps. In a grade 3 testicular atrophy all testicular tissue is absent, and fibrosis and hyalinization result. All sertoli cells are absent in the grade 3 atrophy. The testes undergo atrophy with age, debilitation, avitaminosis, hypothyroidism, hypothalamic and pituitary disorders. Atrophy of the testes may be produced by administration of the stilbestrol (diethylstilbestrol) hormone.

Inflammation of the Testes

Inflammation in the testes is due to an interference with the blood supply. Orchitis, i.e. inflammation of the testes is either acute or chronic and occurs secondarily to inflammation in other sites of the genitourinary tract. Tuberculosis affects the testes following hematogenous spread from pulmonary and organ tuberculosis. Tuberculosis produces epididymitis following lymphatic spread. Tuberculosis may begin in the epididymis and secondarily involve the testes. Gonorrhea produces epididymitis by direct extension from tuberculosis in the genitourinary tract. However, syphilis and mumps produce an orchitis.

Syphilis affects the testes after an initial period of two to three months. The epididymis is involved secondarily since syphilis begins in the testes. Syphilis of the testes is diagnosed only following a dark field examination and treponema immobilization test. Fifty percent of individuals with a chancre have a positive serology. The diagnosis of primary syphilis is made by removing the crust from a chancre and squeezing the exudate from the chancre into a hanging drop preparation for dark field examination. During secondary syphilis, 98 percent of infected individuals have a positive serology. Individuals with tertiary syphilis have a negative serology. The only definitive diagnostic test for tertiary syphilis is the treponema immobilization test. The levidati silver impregnation stain for spirochetes is not a satisfactory test for syphilis. The treponema pallidum are very difficult to stain, except when using the Giemsa stain. Gumma may develop in the testes during tertiary syphilis with the production of a large, irregular area of gummatous necrosis in the testes.

Torsion, Infarction, and Volvulus of the Testes

The testes may revolve freely in the scrotal sack. The revolving testes are prone to torsion and infarction. If an operation is not performed very early during torsion, the 360 degree revolution of the testes will block the blood supply and cause an infarction of the testes. Traumatic torsion of the testes leads to gangrene. Torsion of the testes is accompanied by the following symptoms: pain, acute onset of the inflammation and swelling, tenderness, and dark and congested testes. An accurate and detailed history is important in arriving at the diagnosis of torsion of the testes. Torsion of the testes is uncommon. Volvulus of the testes is a twisting of the testes, causing obstruction of the blood supply. Pain results following the twisting of the testes.

Irradiation of the Testes

Heavy irradiation of the testes results in grade 3 atrophy in which all testicular tissue is absent. Light irradiation of the testes is followed by the regeneration of testicular cells. Irradiation may produce a grade 4 atrophy indicating that all interstitial cells are absent. Grade 8 atrophy indicates that the offspring is a monster.

The testes are radiosensitive tissues; however, regeneration may take place if the irradiation is not excessive and irreversible in nature. The testes have the capacity to undergo regeneration, including the eventual restoration of the sex cells. Ovarian tissue, however, is incapable of regeneration following irradiation. It takes a greater amount of irradiation to destroy the ovaries than the testes. However, the testes have the capacity for regeneration.

Age Changes in the Testes

The testes maintain their fertility up to eighty or more years of age. Atrophy of the testes takes place in older males; however, it is not known what specific changes are the result of aging. The functional state of the testes requires future investigation because many questions remain unanswered. Castration should be investigated with fresh tissue, since the latter is the only method of obtaining reliable information.

Klinefelter's Syndrome

In Klinefelter's syndrome the testes are small and softened. Sertoli cells are present; however, there is a hyalinization of the basement membrane and tubules with marked hyperplasia of Leydig's cells. Patients with this syndrome have gynecomastia, and secondary atrophy of the testes due to an alteration in the pituitary gland. The gynecomastia results following a high estrogen titer, which suppresses the gonadotrophic hormone of the pituitary. The gonadotrophic hormone also produces the secondary atrophy of the testes. Klinefelter's syndrome occurs in young boys due to excessive estrogen that inhibits the pituitary gland and, therefore, is the cause of the gynecomastia present in this syndrome.

The testes pass through two stages prior to testicular atrophy. The serotoli cells persist during the first stage where intermediate atrophy takes place along with the development of gynecomastia. During the second stage, complete testicular atrophy ensues with fibrosis of the testes. The alterations in the testes during atrophy may have some correlation to carcinoma of the prostate.

Benign Neoplasms of the Testes

Benign neoplasms are rare in the testes. The fibroma and angioma may, however, originate in the epididymis.

Malignant Neoplasms of the Testes

Malignant neoplasms may arise in testicular tissue and occur secondarily in the epididymis. The most important neoplasms of the testes are the seminoma, teratoma, and embryonal carcinoma of infancy. The seminoma is a testicular neoplasm similar to the dysgerminoma of the ovary. The cut surface of the seminoma is whitish in color and has a potato like appearance because the sex cells stand apart like caviar. The seminoma arises from the cells of the seminiferous tubules. The seminoma is a soft, fleshy neoplasm, which may attain a relatively large size. The highest five-year survival rate for the seminoma occurs following a unilateral orchectomy and irradiation of the peritoneal lymph nodes. The seminoma is a rare neoplasm among the civilian population. In the Armed Forces the incidence of malignant testicular neoplasms is one in 10,000 military men between the ages of eighteen and thirty years. The seminoma accounts for 50 percent of all testicular neoplasms.

The seminoma spreads by way of the genitourinary tract and metastasizes by way of the retroperitoneal lymph nodes to the lungs. The seminoma metastasizes rather late, whereas the chorioepithelioma and malignant teratoma metastasize early. The seminoma is sensitive to radiation therapy. However, the chorioepithelioma and malignant teratoma are not very sensitive to radiation therapy.

The teratoma of the testes is less common than the seminoma and occurs in younger males. The teratoma of the testes is composed of cartilage, intestinal epithelium, and brain. The epithelial tissues in the teratoma frequently become cystic. The teratoma has the second best survival rate of all of the testicular neoplasms. The teratoma may contain five mixed germinal layers (three germ layers, trophoblasts, and secondary cells) or any one type of tissue may predominate. An example of the one cell type is the chondroma of the testes or brain tissue located within the testes. When numerous tiny cysts develop in the testicular teratoma, the neoplasm assumes the appearance of a fibrocystic disease of the testes. A portion or the entire testis may be replaced by the teratoma during adult life. However, enlargement of the testes does not occur until adult life regardless of the fact that the teratoma of the testes is congenital in origin. The teratoma of the testes is a firm neoplasm, larger than the seminoma, and it may contain cystic areas.

The malignant teratoma resembles the tissues of the female genital tract, i.e. the chorioepithelioma of the female. However, the malignant teratoma of the testes is a rather small neoplasm, which contains mixed germinal tissues. The malignant group of neoplasms of the testes develop in a young age group, i.e. in males between twenty and forty years of age. The malignant testicular neoplasms, therefore, develop during the most active reproductive period of the male. Hormones may, therefore, have some importance in the development of testicular malignant neoplasms. The malignant teratoma metastasizes primarily to the lung, producing a soft, spongy mass containing hemorrhage.

The embryonal carcinoma of infancy is a highly malignant neoplasm of the testes. Chorionic tissue is the tissue of origin of the testes. All types of tissues are present in the testes because it arises from three germ layers. The fertilized ovum produces five germ layers, i.e. three germ layers plus the trophoblasts and secondary cells, which are reserved for future generations. The trophoblastic tissue gives rise to the chorionic tissue from which the testes develop.

The embryonal carcinoma is a teratocarcinoma of the testes.

It is composed of a cellular white, neoplastic mass that replaces the testicular body of infants, resulting in displacement of the epididymis and rete testes (a network of canals at the termination of the straight tubules). The embryonal carcinoma consists of solid areas of trabecular carcinoma and many small cysts.

Neoplasms of the testes may produce hormones. A pregnancy test is a useful method of determining the metabolism and variations in gonadotrophic hormones. The seminoma has the least amount of gonadotrophic hormone; whereas, the chorioepithelioma has the greatest amount of gonadotrophin.

Spermatogenesis

Malnutrition is accompanied by atrophy of the testes and a decrease in spermatogenesis, inflammation, fatigue, and anxiety. Normal production of semen amounts to 0.6 or 0.5 to 1 cc per twenty-four-hour period. Spermatozoa are opalescent grey white in color and motile for twenty-four hours. A decrease in the motility of spermatozoa is an important factor in sterile males. The number of sperm varies but is approximately 150,000 sperm per cubic centimeter of semen. The morphology of the sperm may also vary. Abnormal forms of spermatozoa occur, i.e. spermatozoa may contain a split head and split tail.

DISEASES AND NEOPLASMS OF THE PENIS

Anomalies of the Penis

Anomalies of the penis accompany the other anomalies of the male genitalia. Phimosis is the presence of a tight foreskin, which becomes inflamed and painful, causing constriction of the glans penis. Chronic phimosis represents an underlying or predisposing factor for the production of carcinoma of the penis.

Inflammation of the Penis

Inflammatory lesions of venereal etiology, such as syphilis, involve the frenum of the glans penis. Herpes simplex infection is a viral disease that involves the glans penis. Granuloma inguinale of the groin is a venereal disease that spreads to the penis.

Benign Neoplasms of the Penis

Benign neoplasms are rare in the penis but may include the fibroma, lipoma, verruca (squamous), angiomata, and condylomas.

Malignant Neoplasms of the Penis

The main malignant epithelial neoplasm of the penis is the squamous cell carcinoma. The carcinoma of the penis is generally preceded by inflammation of phimosis. However, carcinoma of the penis is absent when circumcision has been undertaken. Carcinoma of the penis may appear clinically as a verrucous lesion or ulcerative lesion, which may grow to a large size. Sarcomas of the penis are extremely rare.

Carcinoma of the penis generally develops in males after fifty years of age. Carcinoma of the penis metastasizes to the inguinal lymph nodes. When carcinoma develops in an uncircumsized individual, it is associated with the smegma, i.e. the secretion of the sebaceous glands. Shale oil or paraffin industry workers may develop carcinoma of the scrotum following contact with the oil and paraffin. However, carcinoma of the penis does not develop in such workers.

Carcinoma *in situ* or grade 1 squamous cell carcinoma of the penis corona may develop in noncircumsized individuals. Bowen's disease also occurs in the penis and may remain as a localized lesion for ten to fifteen years. Bowen's disease is an intraepithelial carcinoma of the penis, which may be treated with radium and may apparently heal completely. However, in five years following the radium therapy, ulceration and fibrosis may occur and are due to the irradiation. Carcinoma *in situ* of the penis may remain localized for as long as fifteen years. However, amputation of the penis may be necessary if the carcinoma expands and infiltrates into the depths of the penis.

DISEASES AND NEOPLASMS OF THE PROSTATE GLAND

Introduction

The prostate gland surrounds the urethra and is capable of obstructing the flow of urine, i.e. production of anuria. The obstruction and anuria may have a sudden onset in older males affected with prostatism (hypertrophy or chronic disease of the prostate gland). When the urinary flow ceases, a thickening occurs in the muscularis of the urinary bladder, accompanied by dilatation of the ureter, urinary retention, and uremia. The latter findings develop in a progressive fashion over a twenty-year period, terminating in anuria. Fibrosis subsequently develops around the urethra and in the submucosa, replacing the normal mucous glands in the area.

Hypertrophy of the Prostate

Diffuse hypertrophy of the prostate involves the lateral lobes of the prostate gland. Median bar obstruction and fibromuscular hypertrophy accompany the involutional changes in the prostate gland. Seventy-five percent of males over eighty years of age have a diffuse prostatic hypertrophy. The involutional changes begin in the prostate (and ovary) at forty years of age. All of the endocrine-dependent organs undergo aging at approximately the same time, except the testes. The testes appear to avoid the aging process at forty years of age when compared to the prostate and ovary. However, the testes undergo aging along with the vital organs rather than with the endocrine-dependent organs. If the testes are surgically removed, involution of the prostate takes place rather than prostatic hypertrophy.

Prostatic hypertrophy and prostatic carcinoma are associated with an arrest of the gonadocytes' potential to become spermatocytes. In individuals over forty years of age and in the presence of arrested gonadocytes, hypertrophy or carcinoma may develop in the prostate gland. The prostatic duct persists during aging of the prostate gland; however, the acini are converted into ducts. It is the dilatation of the latter newly formed ducts that is responsible for obstruction of urinary flow. With age there is an involution of secretory elements of the prostate gland along with fibromuscular changes in the stroma. An increase in fibromuscular hypertrophy accompanies the epithelial involution or atrophy of the prostate gland.

Ectasia, i.e. dilation of ducts and not hyperplasia, follows cystic involution of the prostate gland. Fibromuscular proliferation of the stroma of the prostate gland results in the obstruction to urinary flow. Therefore, two alterations take place in the prostate gland during aging, i.e. cystic involution and a fibromuscular reaction. The two alterations are subsequently followed by a diffuse prostatic hypertrophy and a fibroblastic change and epithelial hyperplasia. The epithelial hyperplastic reaction is considered as a precancerous lesion of the prostate gland.

Fibromuscular nodules may develop around the urethra in males between forty-five and fifty-five years of age, producing prostatic obstruction, i.e. the phenomenon termed *prostatism*. Prostatism is accompanied by retention of urine or difficulty in evacuation of the bladder and indicates urinary flow disease. The prostate gland contains dilated glandular structures, and fibrocystic and fibromuscular changes following the administration of gonadotrophic hormone. Prostatic hypertrophy is accompanied by epithelial alterations, i.e. increased secretion of glandular elements and infolding of epithelial cells; however, no proliferation of epithelial tissue is evident. During prostatism, a nodule develops in the floor of the bladder, causing a constriction at the neck of the bladder, hydronephrosis, pyelonephritis, and uremia.

Hyperplasia and chronic inflammation occur in older males and may result from an estrogen-androgen imbalance. Fifty percent of males eventually develop nodular hyperplasia of the prostate gland and 10 to 15 percent of males develop carcinoma of the prostate.

Benign Neoplasms of the Prostate Gland

Benign neoplasms of the prostate gland are uncommon. However, they may rarely include the adenoma of the acinar tissue and the leiomyoma of fibromuscular tissue.

Malignant Neoplasms of the Prostate Gland

The majority of neoplasms of the prostate gland are malignant in their clinical behavior pattern. The etiology of malignant prostatic neoplasms is obscure. Carcinoma of the prostate gland has all of the same urinary findings described for prostatic enlargement.

Carcinoma of the prostate gland accounts for five percent of all carcinomas in males. Carcinoma develops in the posterior lobe or prostate bar of the prostate gland. Grossly, it is rather firm, cartilagenous, or woody to palpation. The cut surface reveals a nodular growth pattern. The glandular tissue does not bulge from the cut surface of the neoplasm in a prostatic carcinoma. In contrast, the glandular tissue in prostatic hyperplasia bulges from the cut surface of the neoplasm. Yellow streaks of tissue and hard nodules are visible grossly, and the prostatic carcinoma may be described either as a scirrhous (hard) or medullary (soft) carcinoma from its gross appearance.

Microscopically, carcinoma of the prostate gland has a variable structure; however, it primarily consists of a mixture of glands and acini. Some carcinomas are highly cellular, whereas other carcinomas are predominantly fibrous tissue with few cellular elements. The mature prostatic neoplastic cells have scarce mitotic figures. The clinical behavior pattern of the prostatic carcinoma is not one of a highly malignant and aggressive nature. During carcinoma of the prostate, the normal nodularity of the gland disappears. The histopathology of the individual malignant cell may fail to resemble the atypical neoplastic cell. Therefore, the histopathologic diagnosis of prostatic carcinoma may be extremely difficult to make from a frozen section alone. Fixed tissue sections must be examined before a final diagnosis can be made.

The prostatic carcinoma frequently invades early, therefore, the initial diagnosis is made after metastases have taken place. Metastases occur along the urogenital route to the spine and pelvic bones. Fifty percent of instances diagnosed as carcinoma of the prostate gland show involvement of the pelvic bone. If the initial lesion discovered in a male is an osteolytic lesion, carcinoma of the prostate gland should be considered in the differential diagnosis. Proliferation of bone tissue subsequently occurs during prostatic carcinoma, producing with time a sclerosis of the involved bone. Prostatic carcinoma is responsible for a thickened and sclerotic pelvic bone. Paget's disease of bone may also produce a sclerotic pelvic bone. However, the latter may be differentiated because only alkaline phosphatase is increased in the blood during Paget's disease; both alkaline and acid phosphatases are increased in the blood during carcinoma of the prostate, which has metastasized to bone tissue. Prostatic carcinoma metastasizes by way of the perineural lymphatics and vertebral veins, which supply the seminal vesicles.

The base of the urinary bladder is invaded by carcinoma of the prostate in one-third of the instances of this neoplasm. Urinary obstruction may be the result of a primary neoplasm of the bladder or secondary invasion from a prostatic carcinoma.

Alkaline phosphatase is altered in the bloodstream during a variety of diseases that are associated with osteoblastic activity. However, prostatic carcinoma with metastatic bone lesions is the only disease that is accompanied by an increase in the acid phosphatase in the blood stream. The cells lining the prostatic acini produce the acid phosphatase. Acid phosphatase is also increased in the urine during prostatic carcinoma with bone metastases. The increase in acid phosphatase in the blood occurs prior to any bone metastases that may be diagnosed radiographically. It is impossible to diagnose prostatic carcinoma simply from the presence of increased alkaline phosphatase (alone) in the bloodstream.

One in nine males over seventy years of age may have occult carcinoma of the prostate gland. Yellow nodules develop in the prostate gland during occult carcinoma. The nodules measure 1 to 2 mm in diameter and are located only in the posterior portion of the prostate gland. The occult carcinoma of the prostate gland as well as the occult carcinoma of the thyroid gland are generally found only at autopsy.

Diagnosis of the prostatic carcinoma can be made following a rectal examination and punch biopsy of the neoplasm. When a hospitalized patient with a carcinoma of the prostate develops a severe backache, it is generally due to metastasis of the carcinoma to the spine. Diagnosis can be made by means of the blood (clinical chemistry) tests and radiographic examinations in older male patients whose chief complaint is a backache. The differential diagnosis of the older male patient is generally a metastatic carcinoma from the primary carcinoma of the prostate.

Metaplasia of the suburethral glands may be due to a transurethral resection. The resulting metaplasia has the appearance of a pseudomalignant lesion.

Treatment of carcinoma of the prostate includes castration and peroneal prostatectomy. Estrogen is of value in therapy because it produces a smaller neoplasm and alters the rate at which metastases occur. Orchidectomy is of value in therapy because it also alters the rate of metastases. Stilbesterol administered four times daily inhibits prostatic carcinoma for a period of time.

Other prostatic malignancies are rare. The sarcoma of the prostate is a rare, fatal, and highly malignant neoplasm. The prostatic sarcoma develops in a much younger age group when compared to the carcinoma of the prostate gland.

References

Bates, P.L., Wilets, A.J., and Cokely, H.J.: *J Urol, 71*:114, 1954.
Berry, N.E. and Reese, L.: *J Urol, 69*:286, 1953.
Campbell, J.C.: *Br J Urol, 27*:106, 1955.
Capers, T.H.: *Am J Clin Pathol, 34*:139, 1960.
Clark, B.G. and Bamford, S.B.: *JAMA, 172*:1750, 1960.
Commission on Clinical Oncology of the Union Internationale Contre Cancrum: TNM Classification of Malignant Tumors. Geneva, *International Union Against Cancer,* 1968.
Dean, A.L.: *J Urol, 75*:505, 1956.
Elkin, M. and Mueller, H.P.: *Cancer, 7*:1246, 1954.
Farman, F. and McDonald, D.F.: *Geriatrics, 16*:63, 1961.
Flocks, R.H.: *J Urol, 101*:741, 1969.
Franks, L.M.: *J Pathol, 68*:603, 1954.
Franks, L.M.: *Cancer, 13*:490, 1960.
Gersh, I.: *J Urol, 66*:450, 1951.
Gopel, H.: *Chirurg, 31*:59, 1960.
Graham, J.B. and O'Conor, V.J.: *J Urol, 72*:946, 1954.
Greene, L.F. and Simon, H.B.: *JAMA, 158*:1494, 1955.
Hagerty, R.F. and Taber, E.: *Am Surg, 34*:244, 1958.
Putschar, W.G.J. and Manion, W.C.: *Am J Pathol, 32*:15, 1956.
Scorer, C.B.: *Br J Surg, 49*:357, 1962.
Semple, J.E.: *Br Med J, 1*:1640, 1963.
Staubitz, W.J., Lent, M.H., and Oberkircher, W.J.: *Cancer, 8*:371, 1955.
Thomas, G.J. and Bischoff, A.J.: *J Urol, 72*:411, 1954.
Vernet, S.G.: *Urol Nephrol (Paris), 63*:391, 1962.
Jewett, H.J., et al.: *JAMA, 203*:115, 1968.

Kane, J.T.: *NY J Med, 57*:3989, 1957.
Marmell, M., and Ultman, R., and Weintraub, S.: *J Urol, 70*:776, 1953.
Mellinger, G.T.: *Surg Clin North Am, 35*:1413, 1965.
Rubin, P.: *JAMA, 210*:320, 1072, 1969.
Strahan, R.W.: *J Urol, 89*:875, 1963.
Ward, J.A., Krantz, S., Mendeloff, J., and Haltiwanger, J.A.: *J Clin Endocrinol Metab, 20*:1622, 1960.
Wentzell, R.A.: *Urol, 73*:845, 1955.
Wilson, M.C., Horton, G.R., and Horton, B.F.: *J Urol, 71*:721, 1954.

CHAPTER 28

THE SKIN

Introduction

THE SKIN is composed of layers of dense collagen and elastic tissue covered by keratinized stratified squamous epithelium. Rete ridges extend from the surface epithelium into the subjacent connective tissue, resulting in a very irregular junction separating the epidermis from the dermis. A zone of fatty tissue attaches the skin to the underlying tissue. The skin has a variable thickness depending on location. The thickness of the dermis varies from one area to another. The morphology (gross and microscopic) of the skin is, therefore, related to its function. The thickness of the skin is also related to its function. The epidermis of the skin has various degrees of hornification (keratinization) depending upon the function of the area of the skin. The skin of the palms and soles has a thick layer of keratin due to the degree of mechanical friction encountered by these surfaces. The rate of epithelial cell renewal varies according to specific areas of the skin because it is dependent upon function. The dermis is subjected to different forces during function; therefore, this tissue is different in arrangement and morphology. The subcutaneous tissue consists of connective tissue or muscle depending upon the functional demands. For instance, the subcutaneous scrotal tissue consists of smooth muscle. Whenever functional demands are present, the dermis consists of dense connective tissue beneath the stratified squamous epithelium of the skin. In specialized situations throughout the body, the mucous membranes of the urinary tract, bladder, ureter, and pelvis are supported by a dense, tough zone of connective tissue and elastic fibers that are loosely bound to the muscular layer. The skin may be stretched because elastic fibers are present, although some areas of the skin appear to be immobilized. The strongest opposition to friction or mechanical demands is present in the keratinized epithelium of the skin. In the latter epidermis, the junction between epithelium and the connective tissue is irregular due to the long rete ridges and high connective tissue papillae. A thick epithelium, which undergoes maturation to produce keratin, has a high biochemical cellular activity and a good blood supply.

Sebaceous glands and hair follicles are present in the skin as a normal component. Vitamin A is essential for maintenance of the skin. The requirement for vitamin A increases with the age of the skin. Vitamin A is essential for the maintenance of the skin because it plays a role in mitotic activity (cell division) of epithelial cells. Deficiency of vitamin A results in hyperkeratosis (hyperkeratinization) and epithelial hyperplasia of the epidermis. Vitamin A deficiency is responsible for atrophy of sebaceous glands and hair follicles as well as atrophic changes in the stratified squamous epithelium. The regenerative cycle in the skin is dependent upon proliferation of epithelial cells in the basal cell layer (stratum germinativum), followed by maturation of epithelial cells. The latter mechanism results in fully differentiated, adult functioning epithelial cells. The adult functioning stage is followed by desquamation or shedding of epithelial cells. The rate of shedding is equivalent to the rate of cell division (mitosis) of the basal cells; therefore, the epithelium of the skin maintains a constant thickness.

DISEASES OF THE SKIN

Scleroderma

Scleroderma is a rare disease accompanied by thick and stiff skin. The disease occurs in two forms, i.e. localized and systemic scleroderma. In the local form, the skin is generally tight and stretched about the joints of the fingers. The circumscribed form may develop into diffuse scleroderma. The skin becomes fixed, atrophic, and indurated. Diffuse scleroderma progresses slowly, but it is a fatal disease. Diffuse scleroderma involves the mucous membranes (mouth, esophagus), serous membranes, and fascia. Scleroderma is associated with atrophy and pigmentation in the skin. Diffuse scleroderma may be associated with calcinosis and myosclerosis. The mouth is frequently involved, and the tongue becomes atrophic, stiff, and boardlike so that the patient has difficulty in eating. Speech defects become prominent due to the immobility of the tongue. The changes restrict the movements of the tongue to such a drastic degree that the extrinsic and intrinsic forces that maintain the alignment of teeth are no longer balanced. The soft palate, esophagus, and larynx become atrophic, firm, and stiff. Dysphagia accompanied by choking frequently develops in the scleroderma patient. The patient develops limitation of the lip musculature with an inability to close or open the mouth. The muscles of mastication become atrophic, and there may be unilateral or bilateral atrophy of the maxilla and mandible.

Cheilitis Venenata

Cheilitis venenata represents all of the various allergic reactions that may occur in the lips. This form of allergy (hypersensitivity) is due to lipstick (fatty acids, oils, or perfume), cigars and cigarettes, moustache waxes, and various foods. Clinically, the symptoms that develop begin with itching, and formation of vesicles develops within twenty-four hours. The lips become red and inflamed. The epithelium may exfoliate if the hypersensitivity is severe.

Glossitis Venenata

Glossitis venenata is a hypersensitivity reaction of the tongue due to sensitization to a mouthwash, lozenges (penicillin and other drugs), cough drops, lipstick, etc. A painful, red, swollen, and inflamed tongue occurs in glossitis venenata.

Angioneurotic Edema

This edema is characterized by a rapidly swollen lip, cheek, tongue, and soft palate. The angioneurotic edematous reaction is believed to be an allergic manifestation that produces a hypersensitivity of the neurovascular apparatus. There is dilatation of capillaries, increased capillary permeability, and diffusion of large quantities of fluid into the affected tissues.

Pityriasis Rosea

Pityriasis rosea is an acute disease of the skin of obscure etiology. The disease is self-limiting and lasts for approximately six weeks. It is characterized by patches of scaling and begins with the herald spot or patch on the trunk. The patches on the skin have a pale red color, and the primary lesion (herald spot or patch) is often the most conspicuous because of its size and more brilliant color. Adherent scales cover the pale red patches. The scales are silver to grey in color.

Psoriasis

Psoriasis is a chronic inflammatory disease of the skin characterized by red brown papules or plaques covered by silvery white scales. The following areas of the body are commonly affected: extensor surface of elbows and knees, scalp, region of the sacrum, upper chest, face, abdomen, and genitalia. As a rule, the lesions of psoriasis are symmetrical. The lesions begin as papules and plaques, which are dry, sharply delineated, slightly elevated, and covered by silvery white scales arranged in layers. The early lesions are pinpoint, flat, and sharply defined. When the scales are forcibly removed or removed following trauma, multiple bleeding points may develop. The etiology of psoriasis is obscure. There appears to be an inherited predisposition for psoriasis. The disease has also been attributed to neurogenic factors and metabolic disturbances.

Lichen Planus

Lichen planus is a subacute or chronic inflammatory disease of the skin characterized by small, multiple, purple papules. The disease has a long history persisting for months to years. The initial lesions consist of pinpoint, flat, and sharply defined angular patches. The papule is covered by a thin, horny film. The papules may be discrete focal lesions in the skin; however, when numerous, the papules coalesce and lose their identity. Lichen planus involves the flexor surfaces of the wrists, forearms, and legs above the ankles. The lesions are symmetrical and generally limited to these sites. Lesions may also be generalized or cover large areas of the back; however, the disease rarely involves the face, scalp, palms, or soles. Lichen planus occurs in several forms, i.e. hypertrophic, atrophic, annular, and bullous. The etiology of lichen planus is obscure. A history of neurogenic disorders can be obtained from numerous patients with this skin disease. Mental strain, grief, and anxiety precede the development of the skin lesions. Instances of carcinoma of the skin have been reported as developing in lichen planus. However, it is not possible to ascertain that lichen planus is a precancerous condition of the skin. Lichen planus should not be considered a premalignant skin disorder.

Darier's Disease (Keratosis Follicularis)

Darier's disease is a chronic disease of the skin characterized by an extensive eruption, which originates in the form of papules. The papules become covered by a crust and coalesce, forming foci of papillomatous masses. The initial lesion represents a keratosis of the orifices of follicles. The lesions of keratosis follicularis occur on the face, neck, scalp, and extremities. The disease progresses and may involve rather large areas of the body. The etiology of Darier's disease is obscure. The disease, however, begins in childhood, and heredity may be an important factor.

Keratosis follicularis is a dermatologic disease that is accompanied by lesions in the oral cavity and, less frequently, on the larynx, pharynx, and vulvae. Histopathologic findings reveal a benign dyskeratosis characterized by corps ronds and grains located in lacunae or intraepithelial vesicles directly above the basal cell layer of the epidermis.

Reiter's Syndrome

Reiter's syndrome is characterized by conjunctivitis, arthritis, and urethritis. The arthritis is nongonorrheal in origin. Hemorrhagic eruptions, papules, vesicles, and pseudomembranous lesions are present in the skin and mucous membranes of the body. The etiology of Reiter's syndrome is obscure. The arthritis affects the weight-bearing joints of the lower extremities. The syndrome is nonfatal.

Chronic Discoid Lupus Erythematosus

Discoid lupus erythematosus is a localized, chronic collagen disease of the skin. It is common in young females. Chronic discoid lupus may spread to form disseminated lupus erythematosus. The primary lesion consists of several elevated red macules covered by a greasy scale. The initial lesion grows peripherally to a larger, well-delineated, round or oval lesion. The discoid variety spreads over the bridge of the nose and both cheeks to form a lesion with the shape of the spread wings of a butterfly. The central areas of the butterfly lesion may become scarred while the periphery of the butterfly continues to progress. Lesions of chronic discoid lupus erythematosus occur on areas of the skin exposed to sunlight. The etiology of chronic discoid lupus is obscure. The disease may be preceded by acne, erysipelas, prolonged exposure to sunlight, trauma, and variola. Chronic discoid lupus is accompanied by lesions on the oral mucosa in 25 to 50 percent of patients affected with the disease.

Pemphigus

Pemphigus is an acute and chronic dermatologic disease characterized by development of bullae. There are five varieties of pemphigus. Pemphigus acutus occurs in individuals with a history of injury, infected wound, or prior vaccination. The skin bullae are accompanied by chills, temperature, malaise, and albuminuria. The skin eruption consists of bullae of varying sizes, which may cover rather large areas of the body. The bullae contain clear fluid.

Pemphigus vulgaris is the most common form of pemphigus in the United States. The vulgaris type produces severe bullous lesions accompanied by itching and burning. Bullae are located on the lips, face, neck, axilla, groin, trunk, and extremities. The bullae may occur in a localized area or become widespread. Bullae are soft and contain clear fluid. The bullae rupture and release either clear fluid with an offensive odor, or seropurulent and hemorrhagic exudates. This disease is characterized by exacerbations and remissions. Crusts form following the rupture of the bullae. The disease runs a rapid and fatal course without treatment. ACTH and cortisone therapy prevent a fatal termination.

Pemphigus foliaceus is a rare variety of pemphigus, which is characterized by flaccid bullae on normal-appearing skin. The bullae rupture early, leaving a raw, denuded surface. Contents of the bullae may be purulent or hemorrhagic. Crusts develop after rupture of the bullae. Crusts are readily removed from the skin following the slightest force. The form of pemphigus may last for a few months to years.

Pemphigus vegetans is accompanied by malaise, fever, and impairment of health followed by bullae on the skin. The skin lesions develop about the vulva, anogenital region, and umbilicus of females. The bullae closely approximate each other and are covered by a mucuslike secretion. The scalp, axilla, hands, and feet may also be affected by lesions of pemphigus vegetans. The bullae become ulcerated, vegetative masses, thus changing from the bullae to the papillary or warty lesion. Granulations proliferate from the ruptured bullae, discharging a fetid purulent exudate. The lesions show periods of partial remission and exacerbations. Many instances of pemphigus vegetans terminate fatally.

Pemphigus erythematosus is a benign chronic pemphigus characterized by bullae on the extremities, trunk, and face. The bullae rupture and crust formations produce a crusted dermatitis. The disease undergoes exacerbations and remissions. Patches may be present on the face, new bullae on the trunk with old crusted lesions on the extremities. The etiology of pemphigus erythematosus is unknown.

Benign mucous membrane pemphigoid is accompanied by cutaneous lesions in 50 percent of instances. This mucous membrane disease has a chronic benign clinical behavior pattern. The conjunctiva may be involved (pemphigus of conjunctiva) during benign mucous membrane pemphigoid, with blindness resulting. Bullae develop in a subepithelial location, and there is an absence of acantholysis of epithelial cells. A severe inflammatory infiltrate is present in the connective tissue. Severe scarring may occur in mucous membranes of the mouth. The bullae collapse, and a characteristic white, thickened epithelium with partial ulceration rests upon an erythematous base. Scarring then develops and is more common than in other forms of pemphigus or in other diseases producing bullae. In addition to the oral cavity, the throat, nose, vagina, and anus may be similarly affected with bullae and erosions during benign mucous membrane pemphigoid.

Erythema multiforme is an acute, recurrent, inflammatory disease of the skin characterized by papules and, occasionally, by bullae. The disease occurs on the hands, forearms, face, and neck and is part of a self-limiting, generalized disease that lasts for approximately four weeks. The mild form of erythema multiforme produces superficial lesions of the skin, which have a high recurrence rate. One form of erythema multiforme results from infectious diseases of known etiology. Another form of this disease is a cutaneous manifestation of visceral diseases or follows the ingestion of drugs or injection of serum. The severe bullous type of erythema multiforme may terminate fatally. Erythema multiforme is associated with fever and sore throat. The clinical manifestations include edematous macule, flat papule, and flat nodules. Bullae are only occasionally produced. There is a multiplicity of lesions in erythema multiforme. The lesions of erythema multiforme are generally symmetrically distributed over the dorsal surface of the hands and feet, extremities, face, and neck. The skin eruptions begin as small macules, which enlarge and develop into papules or nodules. The lesions are well delineated and blue to purplish red in color. Erythema multiforme has a variable duration lasting from a few days to weeks.

Ectodermosis erosiva pluriorificialis, Stevens-Johnson syndrome, and Behcet's disease have a marked similarity. No definitive etiologic factors have been demonstrated for any of the three diseases, which probably represent variants of erythema multiforme exudativum.

Ectodermosis erosiva pluriorificialis is a variant of erythema multiforme. The disease is characterized by fever, chills, headache, skin eruptions on the extremities, stomatitis, conjunctivitis, and occasional involvement of the nasal, vaginal, urethral, and anal mucosa. Ocular involvement accompanies dermal symptoms.

The ocular manifestations may be extremely severe and cause partial to total blindness. The ocular lesions consist of a bilateral vesicular conjunctivitis. The eruption on the skin consists of macules, papules, vesicles, and purpura. Some investigators believe that ectodermosis erosiva pluriorificialis is a specific disease entity rather than a variant of erythema multiforme exudativum. The conjunctivitis and keratitis are not as severe as in Stevens-Johnson syndrome.

Stevens-Johnson syndrome is a form of erythema multiforme with ocular, skin, and oral involvement. This syndrome has characteristics of acute pemphigus and of the bullous form of erythema multiforme. The mortality rate is approximately 20 percent. The disease runs an acute course, and the ocular involvement leads to complications that may result in blindness. The acute phase consists of macular and papular skin eruptions, conjunctivitis, and stomatitis. The histopathologic features of Stevens-Johnson syndrome are similar to those of pemphigus acutus and erythema multiforme. Bullae are present, but acantholysis is absent. The acute systemic symptoms of this syndrome are headache, malaise, nausea, pharyngitis, arthralgia, prostration, and high fever. Cutaneous vesicular lesions are present and may contain hemorrhagic fluid. The skin involvement is a generalized maculopapular eruption. The ocular involvement includes conjunctivitis, ulceration of the cornea, and photophobia. Complications may lead to loss of vision or severe corneal scarring. Genital lesions include a nonspecific urethritis, balanitis, and ulcers of the vagina. No joint lesions have been reported in Stevens-Johnson syndrome.

Behcet's disease is characterized by ocular, genital, skin, and oral lesions. Ulcerative lesions occur on the genitalia, and retinitis and iridocyclitis represent the ocular lesions. Behcet's disease resembles ectodermosis erosiva pluriorificialis but has been considered a separate disease. It may also be considered a form of erythema multiforme. This syndrome is accompanied by ulcerations of the genitalia and the following ocular lesions; conjunctivitis, iritis, and keratitis. The genital lesions are herpetic ulcers of the penis and scrotum. The cutaneous lesions are similar to the eruptions present in erythema multiforme exudativum. Arthritis and joint pains develop in many patients with Behcet's disease.

The mucocutaneous-ocular syndromes represent interesting and well-recognized clinical manifestations in which the outstanding feature is the simultaneous involvement of the skin, oral cavity, and other mucocutaneous regions.

Erythema nodosum is an acute inflammatory disease of the skin, characterized by numerous, painful, subcutaneous nodules. The subcutaneous nodules are pale red or pink, vary in size, and are often located on the anterior aspects of the lower portion of the legs. Subcutaneous nodules may be located on the upper extremities, abdomen, and face. The nodules are painful, soft, and may present a blue appearance similar to a contusion. Erythema nodosum is more common in females and occurs during the spring and autumn seasons. Erythema nodosum occurs following specific infections and the ingestion of sulphonamides, bromides, and iodides. It is considered as a separate and distinct disease entity rather than a form of erythema multiforme. Erythema nodosum is related to erythema multiforme. The disease is probably due to a bacterial allergy or is based upon a nonspecific allergic basis. Systemic symptoms of erythema nodosum include fever, malaise, muscle and joint pain, and polyarthritis.

Epidermolysis bullosa is a rare, hereditary disease of the skin, characterized by bullae that result from slight trauma. In the simple form of epidermolysis bullosa, the cutaneous bullae develop following trauma. The bullae may be located on any area of the skin that has been the site of trauma. The simple form produces skin lesions in early life, and they may be resolved with the onset of puberty. A second form of the disease is termed *dystrophic epidermolysis bullosa*. The dystrophic variety produces lesions on the elbows, hands, knees, and feet. The dystrophic bullae may contain a hemorrhagic fluid. The affected area undergoes scarring with pigmentation. Crusts cover the ruptured bullae. The nails are affected by dystrophic changes. The simple form of epidermolysis bullosa is inherited as a Mendelian dominant characteristic, whereas the dystrophic form is due either to dominant or recessive characteristics.

Senile keratosis may occur on the lips and is related to smoking. This disease has been termed *smoker's burn*. The lesions are elevated and either well delineated or lacking a sharp outline. When the lesion on the lip becomes indurated (hard) clinically with the invasion of the underlying tissue, the lesion is generally undergoing malignant transformation.

Bowen's disease is a precancerous, epithelial skin lesion that indicates an intraepithelial squamous cell carcinoma to some individuals and a premalignant dyskeratotic lesion to other individuals. The lesion is a firm papule covered by a keratinized layer or crust. The lesion may persist for years; however, approximately one-fifth of these lesions undergo transformation into invasive squamous cell carcinoma with development of metastases. The lesions of Bowen's disease occur on the extremities, abdomen, and buttocks.

Queyrat's erythroplasia is a rare, precancerous, cutaneous lesion. The lesions occur on the glans penis, prepuce, and vulva. The cutaneous lesions are well delineated, red velvety areas on the skin. The etiology of Queyrat's erythroplasia is unknown. Squamous cell carcinoma frequently develops in cutaneous lesions of Queyrat's erythroplasia. The precancerous lesions of Queyrat's erythroplasia appear to be an early stage of leukoplakia having histopathological features of a squamous cell carcinoma *in situ.*

NEVI AND MELANOMA OF THE SKIN

Nevi are of epithelial origin and may be considered as pigment cell neoplasms that are either present at birth or develop later in life. Heredity appears to be an important factor in the development of the various forms of nevi. The nevus is benign and arises from melanoblasts. Two clinical types of nevi exist, i.e. the flat junctional nevus with or without hair, and the pigmented or nonpigmented hairy nevus. Nevi are yellow, brown, or bluish black in color. They range in size from a pinhead to very large areas. Nevi may be flat, raised, or pedunculated. They may be smooth or covered by greasy scales. Soft, raised nevi are located in the face, trunk, thighs, and buttocks. They may be nonpigmented or contain very minimal pigmentation. *Junctional nevi* is a term used to indicate that nevus cells are located in nests or groups within the connective tissue papillae of the upper cutis and in the rete ridges. Therefore, nevus cells are always present in the upper cutis and epidermis of the junctional nevus. Junctional nevi are commonly located on the soles, palms of the hands, between fingers and toes, and genitalia; however, they may be located anywhere on the skin. The junctional nevus may be the forerunner of the malignant melanoma and is, therefore, a potentially premalignant lesion. However, a sharp delineation between the junctional nevus, intradermal nevus, and compound nevus is not possible in all instances of nevi. The junctional nevus is a flat, hairless, smooth lesion with a light brown or dark brown color. Rarely, instances of the malignant melanoma develop from the junctional nevus.

The intradermal nevus is the most common type of nevus or pigmented mole in which no nevus cells are attached to the epidermis; however, nevus cells are located in the dermis. The pigmented nevus cells reach the dermis by dropping off from the epidermis. Intradermal nevi are frequent in Caucasians, less frequent in Negroes. The lesions are flat or slightly raised brown nodules. Hairs may or may not be present in the center of the nevus. The intradermal nevus is present at birth or it may appear shortly thereafter. Intradermal nevi are more prominent at puberty. Intradermal nevi are generally small; however, they may attain an enormous size. The intradermal nevus is a mature quiescent nevus that remains quiescent for the remainder of adult life. The intradermal nevus of the face is a raised, globular, brown, and hairy lesion. Malignant melanoma does not occur in the nevus containing hair.

The compound nevus consists of a combination of elements from the junctional nevus and from the intradermal nevus. It represents 98 percent of the nevi present during childhood. The compound nevus is not common in adults. The junctional element of the compound nevus is responsible for classifying this nevus as a potentially premalignant adult lesion.

The blue nevus is a rare, sharply delineated, and indurated (hard) papule. It has a dark blue or bluish black color, is slightly elevated, and is either oval or round. The blue nevus occurs predominantly in females and is generally a single lesion. The blue nevus is commonly located on the face, dorsum of the hands, forearms, and dorsum of the feet. The blue nevus may occur as a linear lesion as well as a circumscribed nodule. The blue nevus begins in childhood and persists throughout adult life. The blue nevus is a lesion that resembles the globular appearance of the malignant melanoma and is, therefore, the most common lesion to be mistaken for melanoma. The blue nevus is not a true Mongolian spot. The Mongolian spot is a congenital pigmented spot on the lower sacrococcygeal region, buttocks, and any other site on the body. The Mongolian spot lacks the sharp border present in the blue nevus. A malignant blue nevus is exceedingly rare.

Juvenile melanoma is a benign neoplasm of the skin that is histologically similar to the malignant melanoma; however, it fails to metastasize. When melanomas occur in children, they do not have a malignant clinical behavior pattern or result in death prior to puberty. The term *juvenile melanoma* indicates both benign and malignant lesions of children. Following puberty, the melanoma of the skin behaves like the adult malignant melanoma, therefore, indicating some endocrine or hormonal basis for the clinical behavior pattern. The juvenile melanoma appears as a red or brownish red, raised, soft lesion. It may occur on the cheeks of children.

Malignant melanoma (melanocarcinoma) is a highly malignant neoplasm that causes death due to its ability to metastasize rather readily in its development. Melanoma is the most malignant cutaneous neoplasm due to its rapidly fatal course. The malignant melanoma arises from the melanoblasts in the skin, choroid, and, rarely, from the conjunctiva. The malignant melanoma rarely develops prior to puberty. The average age for the development of malignant melanoma is fifty years. The incidence of melanoma is similar in males and females. It is four times more common in Caucasians than Negroes. Fair-skinned and blond individuals have the highest incidence of melanoma. The Negro is believed to have a relative immunity to neoplasms of the skin. Malignant melanomas account for 20 percent of skin cancers (carcinomas) developing on the exposed body surfaces such as the face, extremities, and feet. A history of trauma or the use of electrocoagulation in the treatment of nevi has been considered an important etiological factor. Fifty percent of malignant melanomas develop in preexisting nevi. The malignant melanoma develops from the junctional and compound nevus. The junctional portion of the compound nevus gives rise to the malignant melanoma. The intradermal portion of the compound nevus is not the important derivative or precursor to the development of the malignant melanoma.

Clinically, the malignant melanoma begins as a small, black, blue, or light brown nodule in the skin. The lesion may be flat, raised, papillary, or ulcerated. When metastases develop, pigmented lines may be visible following the distribution of the lymphatics. Metastases may occur in the adjacent and regional lymph nodes; however, the first metastases may be located in the parenchymal organs. The more rapidly metastasizing malignant melanomas may be nonpigmented. Occasionally, primary multiple melanomas may develop in an individual. The pigmented lesions may be crusted, hairy, and inflamed. Many malignant melanomas develop from the apparently normal skin of the palms, soles, genitalia or any exposed surface of the skin. It is possible for malignant transformation to occur from nevi, lentigines, and malignant lentigo.

The neoplastic cells of the malignant melanoma may appear histologically like the cells in an undifferentiated squamous cell carcinoma or fibrosarcoma. Although the melanoblasts are commonly loaded with melanin pigment, there is great variation from cell to cell and from neoplasm to neoplasm. Hematogenous spread results in metastatic lesions in the skin, intestines, liver, heart, and brain. The prognosis of malignant melanoma is very grave with a 10 to 12 percent five-year survival rate.

Amelanotic melanoma is a variant of the malignant melanoma. The amelanotic lesion has all of the clinical and histopathologic features of the malignant melanoma with the exception of the melanin pigment in the melanoblasts. The presence of melanin pigment is not an important clinical feature or histopathologic criterion for the diagnosis of malignant melanoma. In the amelanotic melanoma, apparently, the melanoblasts are incapable of producing pigmented material from dopa, perhaps due to a deficiency of the oxidizing ferment that it normally contains.

References

Allen, A.C. and Spitz, S.: *Cancer, 6*:1, 1953.

Blank, H. and Rake, G.: *Viral and Ricksettsial Diseases of the Skin, Eye and Mucous Membranes of Man.* Boston, Little, 1955.

Demis, D.J., et al.: *Clinical Dermatology,* 4 vols. Hagerstown, Har-Row, 1972.

Eisen, A.Z., et al.: *J Invest Dermatol, 25*:145, 1955.

Helwig, E.B. and Mostofi, F.K.: *The Skin,* Baltimore, Williams & Wilkins, 1971.

Jeghers, H. and Mescon, H.: Pigmentation of the Skin. In MacBride, C.M. (Ed.): *Signs and Symptoms: Applied Pathologic Physiology and Clinical Interpretations,* 4th ed. Philadelphia, Lippincott, 1964.

Kligman, A.M.: *Arch Dermatol, 18*:231, 245, 1955.

Lever, W.F.: *Histopathology of the Skin.* 4th ed. Philadelphia, Lippincott, 1967.

McCreight, W.C. and Montgomery, H.: *Arch Dermatol, 61*:1, 1950.

Mohs, F.E.: *JAMA, 138*:564, 1948.

Montagna, W.: *The Structure and Function of Skin,* 2nd ed. New York, Acad Pr, 1962.

Montagna, W. and Ellis, R.A.: *The Biology of Hair Growth.* New York, Acad Pr, 1958.

O'Brien, J.P.: *J Invest Dermatol, 15*:95, 1950.

Pillsbury, D.M., et al.: *Dermatology.* Philadelphia, Saunders, 1956.

Rothman, S.: *Physiology and Biochemistry of Skin.* Chicago, U of Chicago Pr, 1954.

Shaffer, B.: *JAMA, 161*:1222, 1956.

Strauss, J.S. and Kligman, A.M.: *Arch Dermatol, 82*:779, 1960.

CHAPTER 29

THE MUSCULOSKELETAL SYSTEM

INFECTIONS OF BONE

ACUTE OSTEOMYELITIS. Osteomyelitis of bone and bones is produced by various pyogenic microorganisms. The most common organisms provoking osteomyelitis are *Staphylococcus aureus,* beta-hemolytic streptococcus and pneumococcus. The microorganisms reach bone tissue by the following means: through a fracture, spreading from adjacent tissues, or by way of the bloodstream from a distant inflammation. The microorganisms may be cultured from the blood of infected subjects. When the site of inflammation is localized to the periosteum, the infection is termed *periostitis.* When the site of inflammation is present in bone tissue, the term *osteitis* is used. During osteomyelitis, the periosteum, bone marrow, and bone tissue are all involved. Acute osteomyelitis occurs in childhood and is rare in adults. Suppuration develops in the medullary cavity of the long bones and spreads widely, accompanied by bone pain, fever, and leukocytosis. Radiographic examination of the infected bones during the early stage of osteomyelitis fails to reveal any significant alterations in bone tissue. The suppuration may burrow through a thin cortex in the metaphysis (shaft of long bone) to reach the periosteum. The periosteum is not attached very strongly to the shaft of the infected long bone. The infection spreads to form a subperiosteal abscess, which encompasses a large area of the shaft in pus.

The epiphysial plate (cartilage) is a barrier to the spread of osteomyelitis from the metaphysis (extremity of shaft) to the epiphysis (extremity). Areas of bone tissue adjacent to the pus and colonies of microorganisms become necrotic, and the dead bone is separated from the living bone to form a sequestrum. In severe instances, the entire diaphysis (shaft) may become necrotic and become separated from the epiphysis in the form of a large sequestrum. The portion of a sequestrum covered by pus remains unaltered; however, resorption of bone may take place if granulation tissue is present adjacent to an area of the sequestrum. When the acute osteomyelitis passes into the subacute phase, new bone is deposited beneath the periosteum to shield the dead bone. The newly deposited bone is termed an *involucrum*. The involucrum contains perforations termed *cloaca* through which the pus drains. The presence of a sequestrum is responsible for the continuation of the infection and retardation of the healing process. The sequestrum, which is surrounded by pus, cannot undergo dissolution. A chronic osteomyelitis may develop in some instances and cause draining sinus tracts for many years. Complications of acute osteomyelitis include septicemia, pyemia, septic arthritis, altered growth, chronic osteitis, chronic bone abscess (Brodie's abscess), and rarely, amyloidosis. Brodie's abscess is a circumscribed, local, chronic osteomyelitis.

TUBERCULOSIS OF BONE. The human type of tubercle bacillus is the primary cause of tuberculosis of bone tissue. The disease involves the vertebrae and ends of the long bones. The bony trabeculae are destroyed in the affected bone, and tuberculous granulation or caseous tissue replaces the lost bone tissue of the diaphysis or epiphysis. The infection of bone tissue is generally the result of the spread of the tubercle bacilli by way of the blood stream from a pulmonary lesion, lymph node, or other primary site.

POTT'S DISEASE (TUBERCULOSIS OF THE VERTEBRAE). Tuberculosis of the vertebrae occurs in children and young adults as a destructive process. Several vertebrae are involved and destroy the intervertebral discs. The destroyed vertebrae collapse. The infection may spread to the periosteum, and caseation necrosis forms a caseous pus by infiltration with polymorphonuclear leukocytes. Paravertebral abscesses develop at the front and sides of the vertebrae. Compression of the spinal cord with formation of the cold abscess may result, and the pus burroughs along the psoas sheath to terminate on the thigh. Involvement of the cervical vertebrae is accompanied by formation of a retropharyngeal abscess.

SYPHILIS OF BONE TISSUE. Congenital or acquired syphilis produces an osteitis or periostitis. Syphilis produces a proliferative process with irregular production of bone tissue and syphilitic lesions, which originate in the periosteum. Secondary syphilis may be accompanied by periostitis with painful swellings over the long bones and the skull followed by some subperiosteal bone formation. Tertiary syphilis is accompanied by gummatous periostitis.

Congenital syphilis produces osteochondritis in the long bones. Bone formation is altered, and the epiphysis is easily separated from the long bone. Periostitis may occur in congenital syphilis, and subperiosteal new bone is produced on the shaft of the long bones.

DISORDERS OF BONES DUE TO VITAMIN DEFICIENCY AND EXCESS

VITAMIN C DEFICIENCY. Vitamin C deficiency (rare) produces scurvy with alterations in bone tissue resulting from a generalized defect in fibrous proteins, i.e. the bone matrix and collagen. Scurvy, therefore, results in abnormal growth of bones and impaired healing of bone tissue following trauma. Bone alterations occur early in the disease and are due to an absence of bone matrix plus the failure of calcified cartilage to undergo resorption. Calcification is not disturbed during scurvy.

Subperiosteal hemorrhages may develop at the ends of the long bones, and subperiosteal new bone formation is commonly laid down at these sites.

VITAMIN D DEFICIENCY. Deficiency of vitamin D results in increased formation of osteoid tissue, i.e. the uncalcified matrix of bone. Rickets in children is accompanied by increased osteoid tissue in addition to defective mineralization of epiphyseal cartilage. Bone matrix produced after the onset of vitamin D deficiency remains uncalcified, and trabeculae of bone are composed of a central core of calcified bone surrounded by osteoid tissue. In both osteomalacia of adults and rickets of children, an excessive quantity of bone matrix is produced, which fails to calcify.

Rickets is a systemic disease of infancy characterized by formation of osteoid (not calcified) bone, which results in softening of bones. Disturbances develop in the ossification of both endochondral and membranous bones. Swelling occurs in bones at the epiphyseal lines and at the costochondral junction of the ribs. A row of swellings at the costochondral junctions is termed *rachitic rosary*. The long bones become bent, bowlegged, knock-kneed and shorter than normal. Curvature of the spine and flattened pelvis are due to rickets.

The clinical features that accompany rickets appear to result from failure to fix the calcium and phosphorus that are vital for the osteoblasts to deposit bone apatite. The osteoblasts, however, undergo normal proliferation, and osteoid tissue is normally produced.

Osteomalacia, if mild, results in occasional bone pain. There is failure or delayed healing of fractures. The callus of the heal-softening of bones and radiographically decreased density of bone tissue. Severe osteomalacia is accompanied by weakening and softening of bones and radiographically decreased density of bone tissue. The most prominent alterations occur in bones with the greatest rate of bone remodeling, i.e. in cancellous bone. Microscopically, the bones with osteomalacia show osteoid tissue encompassing mineralized bone trabeculae.

HYPEPRVITAMINOSIS D. Excessive administration of vitamin D causes increased blood calcium and an increase of calcium and phosphorus in the urine. Widespread metastatic calcification and renal calculi may develop. Where calcium is not consumed in the diet, the increased blood calcium is the result of diminishing calcium in the bone tissue and the addition of calcium to the blood.

SKELETAL LESIONS IN ENDOCRINE DISORDERS

PRIMARY HYPERPARATHYROIDISM. Excessive parathyroid hormone acts directly on bone tissue. Primary hyperparathyroidism causes increased resorption of bone tissue. Osteoclasts and Howship's lacunae are abundant on the surface of bone trabeculae. Osteoblasts are also prominent; therefore, resorption and apposition of bone are both active processes during hyperparathyroidism. The bone marrow is subsequently replaced by fibrous connective tissue, and the disease is termed *osteitis fibrosa*. New formation of bone trabeculae occurs in loose, fibrous vascular tissue. A large number of giant cells are present in the connective tissue, forming the brown tumor or giant cell tumor of hyperparathyroidism. When the parathyroid tumor is excised from the neck, the serum calcium drops, osteoclastic activity becomes normal, and the bone tissue becomes normal.

SECONDARY HYPERPARATHYROIDISM. Chronic renal failure, associated with a decrease in serum calcium, may produce alterations in bone tissue. The bone changes are identical to those seen in primary hyperparathyroidism.

ACROMEGALY. Enlarged mandible and enlarged hands and feet are due to acromegaly. During acromegaly, there is subperiosteal proliferation and endochondral ossification in specific bones (ribs, vertebrae, and digits) of the skeleton. The overgrowth of bone tissue is readily discernible in the skull, face and mandible, and extremities. Acromegaly is due to an adenoma of the pituitary gland, which develops after completion of bone growth.

CUSHING'S SYNDROME. This syndrome is accompanied by osteoporosis. The vertebrae contain decreased or an absence of the cortical plate, and the individual bone trabeculae are small and thin. This syndrome is primarily an adrenal cortical disturbance; however, identical skeletal alterations result following excessive dosages of cortisone therapy. Prolonged cortisone therapy produces alterations in the basophils of the pituitary gland.

CRETINISM. Cretinism produces retardation of endochrondal growth due to hypoplasia or lack of development of the thyroid gland. The epiphyses of the long bones are deformed and may be delayed in their closure. Ossification is also delayed in cretinism.

HYPERTHYROIDISM. A hyperplastic and overactive thyroid is associated with a mild osteoporosis of the skeleton. Bone resorption occurs at a greater rate than bone apposition. The bony alterations in hyperthyroidism are dependent upon the grade of the severity of the disease since nodular goiters produce less severe manifestations than diffuse thyroid, and hypertrophy and hyperplasia of the thyroid gland.

BONE DISORDERS OF OBSCURE ETIOLOGY

OSTEOPOROSIS. Osteoporosis is a decrease in the quantity of calcified bone tissue in a given amount of skeletal tissue. The matrix of skeletal tissue appear to be normally mineralized. This disorder may be due to either decreased bone apposition or increased bone resorption, or a combination of these conditions. The etiology is obscure. However, there is an increase in the incidence of fractures, deformities, and altered bone and bones. The following forms of osteoporosis may develop: localized, generalized, disuse atrophy and immobilization osteoporosis, and senile osteoporosis. Hormonal alterations such as insufficient or absence of estrogen appear to produce osteoporosis. However, the etiology of osteoporosis is obscure. Histopathologically, the bones show thin trabeculae and a decrease in cortical bone. The following diseases are associated with generalized osteoporosis: Cushing's syndrome, acromegaly, and thyrotoxicosis.

PAGET'S DISEASE OF BONE. Paget's disease of bone is a chronic osteodystrophy of bone tissue of unknown etiology, which occurs after forty or fifty years of age. Males are affected more than females. The alkaline phosphatase level of the blood is increased, otherwise the blood biochemistry is normal. This unusual bone disease is characterized by increased osteoblastic activity simultaneous with osteoclastic resorption of bone. The overgrowth of new bone tissue consists of a poorly calcified bone containing rather irregular spicules of bone. An individual bone may be affected in a small percentage of instances; however, the vertebrae, cranium, sternum, femur, tibia, sacrum, pelvis, and jaws are commonly involved. The condition is not considered a diffuse disease of bone tissue, rather it is a multifocal bone disease. Advanced instances of Paget's disease are accompanied by tenderness and bone pain, bowing of the lower extremities, and an increase in skull size and an increase in jaw size. Osteogenic sarcoma may develop in 3 percent of advanced or terminal instances of this bone disease.

The bones of the skeleton become thickened but are soft, porous, and therefore, light in weight. The skull shows a severe thickening of the calvarium, which is a progressive change. Microscopically, simultaneous apposition and irregular resorption of bone are present. The marrow becomes fibrotic, and the vascularity of the bone marrow is increased. Early microscopic findings of Paget's disease reveal activity of both the osteoclasts and osteoblasts. Initially, the bone resorption is marked and the bone lighter than normal. The bone is subject to bowing and/or fracture. As the disease progresses, the bone trabeculae are commonly thickened with the development of the mosaic pattern. The pathognomonic and diagnostic mosaic pattern consists of numerous, irregular, cement lines, which result following repeated resorption and apposition of bone. In the advanced stages, the bone becomes heavier but weaker than normal. The weakened bone makes it susceptible to fracture. Osteoarthritis may follow bone deformities, resulting in abnormal stresses on the major joints.

FIBROUS DYSPLASIA. Monostotic and polyostotic fibrous dysplasia are benign, fibro-osseous lesions of bone of obscure etiology. On rare occasions, the polyostotic form of fibrous dysplasia of bone is associated with pigmentation of the skin, precocious sexual maturation in girls, and precocious skeletal development. The latter symptom complex is termed *Albright's syndrome*. Monostotic fibrous dysplasia generally occurs in a rib, mandible, maxilla, skull, femur, and tibia. Polyostotic fibrous dysplasia frequently occurs in the femur and tibia, although many bones may be affected.

The lesions of fibrous dysplasia are accompanied by a thin cortex. The bone marrow and trabeculae are replaced by a white, firm, fibro-osseous tissue with a gritty consistency. Focal cystic degeneration and areas of cartilage may be present in lesions of fibrous dysplasia. Radiographically, the area of fibrous dysplasia has a ground-glass appearance with fine mottling due to the presence of woven bone. Fibrous dysplasia of the skull and jaws generally tends to contain more dense bone tissue than lesions in other sites. Therefore, upon radiographic examination, they appear more mottled and may contain areas of sclerosis.

Microscopically, the marrow and spongiosa are replaced by loose fibrous connective tissue with spindle-shaped cells. In the latter, stroma are small, curved, and irregular trabeculae of poorly calcified, nonlamellar, woven bone tissue. The bone trabeculae are irregularly scattered throughout the fibrous stroma. Osteoblasts are not present along the borders of individual bone trabeculae. The newly deposited trabeculae fail to undergo maturation to mature, lamellar bone tissue. Pain and bone deformity begin during childhood and adolescent years with the fibrous dysplasia following a slowly progressive course.

DEVELOPMENTAL ABNORMALITIES OF BONE TISSUE

OSTEOPETROSIS. Marble bone disease or Albers-Schönberg disease (osteopetrosis) is a hereditary, Mendelian recessive disorder of bone tissue characterized by a great increase in the thickness and excessive density of all bones. The bone marrow is obliterated, and a severe osteosclerotic anemia develops. In spite of the increased thickness and excessive density of the bones, fractures and brittle, chalky bones are present. The base of the skull, femur, tibia, pelvis, and vertebrae are the most commonly affected bones. Complications include deafness and impaired vision following involvement of the skull.

OSTEOGENESIS IMPERFECTA. Osteogenesis imperfecta is a familial and hereditary condition that develops during intrauterine life. A mesenchymal hypoplasia with marked alterations in the bones is present at birth. The mesenchymal hypoplasia produces fragile bone with repeated spontaneous fractures. As a result of numerous irregular fractures, the bones are shortened and have an altered morphology. In osteogenesis imperfecta, fractures and callus formation may occur before birth. The cranium is softened, and there is deficient ossification of cranial bones. The bones have a thin cortex and decreased quantity of cancellous tissues. Bone trabeculae are sparse and thin. Healing (callus) occurs following the numerous fractures; however, the bone is poorly ossified. The proliferation of cartilage cells (chondrocytes) in the epiphyseal plate is unaltered, and ossification of cartilage matrix in the zone of ossification proceeds in a normal fashion. However, there is a decreased quantity of bone formed. Deafness due to otosclerosis may develop in adults with osteogenesis imperfecta.

ACHONDROPLASIA. The developmental abnormality of bone is a frequent form of dwarfism, resulting from the failure of endochondral ossification. Dwarfism is present at birth, and the characteristic features include the following: head appears large, extremely short but thick bones in all extremities, nose is sunken, and skin of the extremities is folded. The bones of the head and trunk develop to a normal size. The soft tissues undergo excessive growth. The short thick bone in the extremities results from deficient endochondral growth and ossification.

PRIMARY NEOPLASMS OF BONE TISSUE

Primary neoplasms of bone tissue are of mesenchymal origin. The neoplasms arise from fibrous tissue (fibroma and fibrosarcoma), cartilage (enchondroma and chondrosarcoma), bone (osteoma, osteoid osteoma, benign osteoblastoma, osteosarcoma, and parosteal osteosarcoma), unknown origin (giant cell tumor—benign and malignant), vascular tissue (hemangioma, glomus tumor, and hemangio-endothelioma), fat cells (lipoma and liposarcoma) marrow elements (solitary plasmacytoma and myelomatosis), marrow stroma (reticulum cell sarcoma) and neural tissue (schwannoma, neurofibromatosis, ganglioneuroma, and neurofibrosarcoma).

Certain benign neoplasms of bone may progress to malignancy. This group includes the osteocartilaginous exostosis, enchondroma, giant cell tumor, solitary plasmacytoma, and neurofibromatosis.

The osteoma occurs as a bony prominence on bones of the skull and jaws and may protrude into the orbit, paranasal sinuses, and oral cavity. The osteoma is benign and consists of connective tissue and spongy bone trabeculae or of very dense, compact bone.

The osteogenic sarcoma is a malignant neoplasm of bone arising from the undifferentiated, bone-forming mesenchyme. This sarcoma is the most common primary malignant neoplasm of bone tissue. It occurs more often in males than females from ten to twenty-five years of age. The most common site is in the metaphysis of long bones, around the knee, and upper end of the femur and humerus. The neoplasm produces severe pain and swelling, but the patient is in good health provided no metastases have taken place. Spread of the osteogenic sarcoma occurs by way of the bloodstream to the lungs, viscera, and other bones. The prognosis is poor with a five year survival rate of from 5 to 20 percent.

Osteocartilaginous exostosis is a very common benign neoplasm or bony mass. It is comprised of an inner core of cancellous bone covered by cartilage and perichondrium. The exostosis may be single or multiple and arise predominantly from the metaphyses of the femur, humerus, and tibia.

The enchondroma is a benign, cartilagenous neoplasm arising within the medullary cavity of small bones of the hands and feet. The cartilagenous growth may be single or multiple and appears radiolucent. Symptoms include pain unassociated with fracture, enlargement of long bones, swelling, and pathological fracture in the phalangeal lesions.

Chondrosarcoma is a malignant neoplasm of bone that either begins as a primary growth or starts as a benign, cartilagenous neoplasm that undergoes malignant transformation. This neoplasm occurs within and on the surface of bones. It occurs in males twices as often as in females from forty to seventy years of age. The neoplasm arises in the ribs, pelvis, and the proximal femur. Chondrosarcoma has been difficult to diagnosis, and biopsies should be taken from the proliferating edge and not from the calcified or degenerated cartilage. The chondrosarcoma has a chronic or prolonged course with metastases developing by way of the blood stream to the lungs. The neoplasm spreads along veins in a retrograde fashion. Prognosis is poor to guarded because of misdiagnosis by pathologists.

The fibrosarcoma is a rare, malignant tumor of bone. It occurs both within and on the surface of bones in adults. It affects the metaphysis of long bones around the knee joint. The endosteal fibrosarcoma occurs within the medullary cavity of bones and has a poor prognosis. The peripheral fibrosarcoma on the surface of bones has a prognosis that is directly related to the degree of cell differentiation. Highly collageneous, peripheral fibrosarcomas metastasize late and have a good prognosis. Undifferentiated, pleomorphic, peripheral fibrosarcomas metastasize early and have a poor prognosis.

Giant cell tumors of bone produce an osteolytic lesion in the end of a long bone of individuals from twenty to forty years of age. Fifty percent of the giant cell tumors develop around the knee, i.e. in the lower end of the femur or upper end of the tibia. Approximately 50 percent of the giant cell tumors are treated successfully by local excision. However, one-third recur and 15 to 20 percent are malignant either initially or following recurrence and metastasize to the lungs. Some giant cell tumors that appear microscopically benign have been known to metastasize later.

METASTASES TO BONE TISSUE. Metastatic neoplasms of bone tissue are more frequent than primary bone neoplasms. The most frequent sites of metastases to bone tissue are the vertebral column, pelvis, humerus, femur, skull, and ribs. The following neoplasms metastasize to bone tissue most often: carcinomas of the breast, prostate, lung, ovary, thyroid, testis and kidney, hypernephromas and melanomas. Secondary neoplasms to bone are often multiple, generally destructive (osteolytic), and accompanied by pathologic fractures. It is possible for carcinoma cells to infiltrate the bone marrow and stimulate the osteoblasts to produce an osteosclerotic (bone-producing) metastatic neoplasm. Osteosclerotic secondary neoplasms are associated with carcinomas of the prostate and breast. Osteosclerotic metastatic neoplasms may result in osteosclerotic anemia when a large portion of the bone marrow is replaced by new bone formation.

INFLAMMATION OF JOINTS

Acute arthritis may result from infection of gonococci, pneumococci, or typhoid bacilli. However, with adequate antibiotic treatment, only a transient, nonsuppurative arthritis develops, which results in minimal joint damage. Acute staphylococcal and streptococcal arthritis are examples of suppurative arthritis and are common in the hip and knee of children and young adults. Gonococcal arthritis follows untreated gonorrhea since gonococci are carried from the urethra by the blood stream to other parts such as tendons, joints, and other fibrous tissues.

Tuberculous arthritis is decreasing in modern times. Children and young adults are commonly affected, and the hip and knee joints are the primary sites of involvement. Joint infection takes place by way of the bloodstream from primary or reinfection tuberculosis in the lungs or lymph nodes or other sites throughout the body. Early antibiotic treatment causes the arthritis to remain localized to the synovium, and function is readily restored. Where tuberculosis is treated early it is unusual to see massive joint destruction, discharging sinuses, and spontaneous ankylosis.

Syphilitic arthritis occurs on the secondary stage of syphilis and is accompanied by transient pain and stiffness of the joints. Fluid may accumulate bilaterally in the knee joint. In tertiary syphilis, gumma of the joint capsule may develop.

JOINT INFLAMMATION OF OBSCURE ETIOLOGY

Rheumatic fever is characterized by a fever, pancarditis, and arthritis unrelated to rheumatoid arthritis. The large joints of the body are affected by infiltration of leukocytes and an exudate into the joint, and subsequently, chronic inflammatory cells are present in the synovium.

Rheumatoid arthritis is a generalized disease of the body that generally occurs in individuals between twenty-five and forty but may occur at younger and older ages. Any and all synovial joints may be affected by this disease of unknown etiology. The joints of the hands and feet are generally involved in a bilateral distribution. The synovium undergoes marked hypertrophy with proliferation of synovial cells and dense infiltration of lymphocytes and plasma cells. A layer of granulation tissue termed a *pannus* grows over and alters the joint cartilage. Muscles become atrophic, and tendons may become involved by granulation tissue similar to the pannus over the cartilage. Subcutaneous nodules develop generally over the elbow in 20 percent of instances, which consist of a zone of fibrinoid necrosis surrounded by fibroblasts in a palisade arrangement.

Osteoarthritis is a degenerative joint disease and the commonest form of joint disease in adults over forty years of age. Many instances of osteoarthritis in adults are free of symptoms or are accompanied by minor symptoms. Osteoarthritis is found chiefly in the elderly and primarily affects the large, weight-bearing joints. The articular cartilage is altered, and it looses its smooth surface. The latter is followed by fibrillation of the matrix of the joint cartilage and thinning or loss of cartilage over small areas. At the margins of the joint, osteophytic masses develop, which are formed by proliferating cartilage cells. The latter produce the lipping of the joint so common to osteoarthritis.

Arthritis may be associated with gout, a disorder of purine metabolism. This type of arthritis is a chronic, degenerative joint disease, which initially occurs in individuals over forty years of age. Males are affected more often than females. The great toe joints, knee, elbow and finger, and other toe joints are generally involved. Urate deposits (sodium biurate) occur in the articular cartilage of the involved joints. Degeneration of articular cartilage ensues, and osteoarthritis type of changes cause the disability in gouty arthritis.

Synovial tumors may develop and include the benign, giant-cell tumor of the tendon sheath (villonodular synovitis) and the synovial sarcoma. The rare, synovial sarcoma is highly malignant and occurs outside a joint in young adults. Metastases are common to the lungs, lymph nodes, and parenchymal organs. Prognosis is bad and the mortality rate is high.

VOLUNTARY MUSCLE. Traumatic myositis ossificans is a benign lesion of voluntary muscle resulting from a single or multiple injury. There is proliferation of fibrous connective tissue within the affected muscle, and metaplastic bone tissue is laid down in this fibroblastic proliferation. Bone may form directly in the connective tissue, or cartilage may be laid down and later undergo ossification. Bacterial myositis of voluntary muscle results following gas gangrene, suppuration, Zenker's degeneration, and viral and parasitic myositis.

References

Al-Sarraf, M.: *Arch Pathol, 91:*550, 1971.
Dahlin, D.C., et al.: *Cancer, 25:*1061, 1970.
Dent, C.E.: *Proc R Soc Med, 63:*401, 1970.
Goldenberg, R.R., et al.: *J Bone Joint Surg, 52A:*619, 1970.
Goldstein, G.: *Ann Rev Med, 22:*119, 1971.
Harris, W.H. and Heaney, R.P.: *N Engl J Med, 280:*193, 1969.
Huvos, A.G., et al.: *J Bone Joint Surg, 54:*1047, 1972.
Lichenstein, L.: *Bone Tumors,* 4th ed. St. Louis, Mosby, 1972.
McGrath, P.J.: *J Bone Joint Surg (Brit), 54:*216, 1972.
O'Brien, W.M.: *Clin Exp Immunol Suppl, 2:*785, 1967.
Pollak, V.E., et al.: *Arch Intern Med, 103:*200, 1959.
Rawson, A.J., et al.: *Ann Intern Med, 62:*281, 1965.
Roberts, W.C., et al.: *Arch Intern Med, 122:*141, 1968.

Sandow, A.: *Pharmacol Rev, 17*:265, 1965.
Skorneck, A.B. and Ginsburg, L.B.: *N Engl J Med, 258*:1079, 1958.
Skosey, J.L.: *Med Clin North Am, 54*:141, 1970.
Sobel, H.J., et al.: *Am J Pathol, 65*:59, 1971.
Thomas, L.: *Fed Proc, 32*:143, 1973.
Thomas, T.V.: *Ann Thorac Surg, 13*:499, 1972.
Tursi, A., et al.: *Clin Exp Immunol, 6*:767, 1970.
Ziff, M.: *Fed Proc, 32*:131, 1973.

CHAPTER 30

THE NERVOUS SYSTEM

Introduction

THE NATURE AND THE POSITION of any lesion in the central nervous system are both extremely important factors in the life history and prognosis of diseases of the central nervous system. For instance, an obstruction may cause fluid to back up, a cortical lesion may cause convulsions; the cranial vault and vertebral canal are closed cavities, and therefore, edema of the brain may cause disability or death. There are no lymphatics present in the central nervous system. The spinal fluid possibly serves the function of the lymphatics. The blood vessels of the brain consist of elastic and muscular layers; however, the layers are smaller than corresponding layers in vessels of the same size found in other parts of the body. The parenchyma of the brain has no conscious innervation; therefore, a deep-seated lesion is not painful.

BASIC TISSUES OF THE CENTRAL NERVOUS SYSTEM

The ten basic tissues of the brain include the following: notochord, neuroglia (astrocytes, oligodendroglia), microglia, ependymal, choroid plexus, neuron, sheath cell, meninges, capsular cells, and spinal fluid.

The central nervous system originates from the ectoderm of the embryo. The ectoderm forms layers, and the layers fuse to form the neural tube. The neural tube consists of epithelial lined cells (ectodermal) surrounded by mesenchymal cells. Everything arises from the lining cells or primitive medullary epithelium. The primitive epithelium proliferates to form sheaths of cells. The sheaths differentiate into nerve cells and supporting cells. Some of the latter cells are neurons, others are cells undergoing glial differentiation into glial cells. The primitive glioblast forms the spongioblast with an elongated unipolar or bipolar process. Oligodendroglia have a few short processes. The cytoplasmic processes of the glial cells are not a product of the cell. The astrocytic glia have many processes forming cytoplasmic astrocytes and long, thin, fibrillar astrocytes. The primitive medullary epithelium forms the ependyma. The development of the leptomeninges is uncertain.

The neurons (nerve cells) of the central nervous system are incapable of regeneration. Glial cells and capillaries are capable of regeneration.

In the peripheral nervous system, regeneration proceeds when the proximal and distal end of a nerve are brought into opposition so that granulation tissue does not grow between the proximal and distal portion. The axis cylinder grows, and the sheath of Schwann grows as an empty sheath. Susbsequently, the axis cylinder grows into the empty sheath of Schwann. If a peripheral nerve fails to regenerate, a connective tissue scar develops. The axis cylinder has a great potential for growth and will grow into granulation tissue as well as grow freely into an empty sheath of Schwann. In an amputation neuroma pain is elicited and the axis cylinder with the sheath of Schwann grows out into a connective tissue scar.

In the central nervous system, the neurons are surrounded by myelin held by the glial cells. The oligodendroglia serve the function of the Schwann cells in the central nervous system. When the continuity of the central nervous system is broken, necrosis, softening, and cyst formation develop. Lysis occurs in the areas and, as if with the greatest care, a glial scar develops.

The neural ectodermal structures include the following: notochord, neuroglia, neuron, ependyma-sheath, capsule cells, and choroid plexus. The medullo-epithelium of the neural tube forms the neuroglia (astrocytes and oligodendroglia) and the ependyma. The mesoderm forms the microglia. There are no microglial tumors of the brain since microglia only proliferate as normal cells. All other cells and tissues of the brain may form neoplasms.

Notochord cells are found in choroidal rests near the pituitary gland. The notochord cell resembles a fat cell; however, it has a centrally located nucleus. Notochord cells have a mucinous stroma. Many notochord cells have a vacuolated cytoplasm. The notochord cell represents the cell of the intervertebral disc and chordoma.

The neuroglia consists of the astrocytes and oligodendroglia. The astrocytes form the supporting structure, i.e. a reactive and reparative structure. There are three types of astrocytes, i.e. gemistocytic, fibrillary, and protoplasmic. The fibrillary astrocyte is found in the white matter of the brain. This astrocyte contains an oval nucleus with a dusting of chromatin granules and eosinophilic granules. One process is long and thick and attaches the fibrillary astrocyte to blood vessels. The protoplasmic astrocyte is located in the cortex of the brain. It has an oval shaped, light- or dusty- colored nucleus, and its process are thicker and fewer in number compared to the fibrillary astrocyte. During pathologic processes, the protoplasmic astrocyte can react by shrinking and form gemistocytic cells. The latter cells develop around neoplasms or areas of softening of the brain. The astrocyte may also react by proliferation, i.e. gliosis (reparative scarring of the central nervous system). The gemistocytic astrocyte has an eccentric, oval, and dusty nucleus with abundant cytoplasm. This astrocyte is a large, round cell.

The oligodendroglia is located in the cortex and white matter of the brain. The nucleus is the only part of the cell that stains with hematoxylin and eosin. The nucleus of the oligodendroglia is approximately one-third smaller than the astrocyte nucleus. This cell contains plump chromatin granules, scant cytoplasm, and short processes that can only be seen with special stains. During pathologic processes, the oligodendroglia may undergo severe alterations and mucoid degeneration. Alterations in oligodendroglia are nonspecific and are part of a toxic reaction. Oligodendroglia probably represent the prime cell in satellitosis.

The microglia are of mesodermal origin. They are small, phagocytic, and polymorphic (many-shaped) cells. They are generally crescent-shaped cells with scanty cytoplasm, and only the nucleus is visible with hematoxylin and eosin stain. Special stains are required to demonstrate various alterations. During pathologic processes, microglia may have an eccentric nucleus, and the cytoplasm becomes filled with lipid. The latter alteration occurs during softening of the brain. Rod-cell formation, which is a thinning out of the cell with formation of a rod, also occurs in microglia. The rod cell is seen accompanying chronic infections and is in the cortex during paresis. However, the rod cell is not pathognomonic of those conditions.

The ependymal cells line all of the ventricles of the brain. They are cuboidal-columnar cells whose nuclei have an epithelial appearance. Their process extends into the parenchyma of the brain with the formation of a network similar to that formed by the astrocytes. In the immature, young ependymal cells, there are cilia and blepharoplasts, i.e. small oval bodies arranged in a line. The cilia and oval inclusions are absent in mature ependymal cells. During pathologic processes, the ependymal cell proliferates and reduplicates the cell layers. This is a normal occurrence during the aging process. During the inflammatory process, i.e. ependymitis, the ependymal cells are swollen, and erosion of an entire layer of ependymal cells may result. The inflammatory reaction may spread to the subependymal regions.

The choroid plexus resembles the ependymal cells. The choroid plexus is a villous structure composed of a preependymal membrane with a subarachnoid vascular core, i.e. the ependyma and prearachnoid invaginates (embryo). The choroid plexus is loose and highly vascular, and therefore, reacts to the inflammatory process. Neoplasms of the choroid plexus are rare. However, cysts are commonly present in this plexus. Brain sand occurs in the choroid plexus and represents calcified structures, which can be seen on the radiograph. Fibrosis may also take place in the choroid plexus.

The neuron is the functional unit of the brain. The neuron consists of a nerve cell body and processes; however, they represent extremely complex cells with tremendous metabolic activity and are highly sensitive to all changes in their environment. The neuron present in the outer cortex are termed Betz's cells or Golgi type I cells. The granular cell of the cerebellum is a neuron termed the Golgi type II cell. Neurons range from 5 to 30 microns in size and assume various morphologic patterns.

The Betz cell (Golgi type I neuron) has a centrally located nucleus. The abnormal Betz cell has an eccentrically located nucleus. The Betz cell has a dusty color with a definite nuclear membrane. Neurofibrils extend from the body into the axon. During pathologic processes, the following alterations may take place in the neurons: shrinkage, swelling, vacuolization, pigmented cells, degeneration, and chromatolysis. During shrinkage, the processes become tortuous. Shrinkage of neurons occurs during anoxia, chronic inflammation, and senility. Swelling of neurons produces a disappearance of the processes. Swelling of neurons occurs in pellagra. The swelling present in the neurons during the early stage of pellagra is reversible. Vacuolization of neurons may take place in any toxic state. Retrograde degenertion of neurons occurs during aging and in chronic disease states. Retrograde degeneration produces lipochrome granules in the neurons. Chromatolysis occurs in the neurons accompanied by peripherally located chromatin in the nucleus, diffuse Nissl substances in cytoplasm, and retrograde degeneration of the nerve cell body. The axons have already been damaged when chromatolysis takes place.

Satellite stasis is not necessarily a sign of nerve cell damage. It may represent a protective action of the brain for the nerve cell body. Satellite stasis indicates the ringing of the nerve cells with oligodendroglia. Astrocytes and microglia as well as oligodendroglia take part in satellite stasis.

Neuronophagia is the ringing of the nerve cell body with oligodendroglia and microglia accompanied by mononucleosis of the blood stream. Neuronophagia is present during poliomyelitis.

Degeneration may occur in the peripheral nerves of the body. During retrograde degeneration of peripheral nerves, the Nissl bodies become dispersed. In Wallerian degeneration the peripheral nerve undergoes retrograde degeneration distal to the site of the lesion. Lesions of peripheral nerves located close to the nerve cell body produce a tendency for the nerve cell to shrink. Retrograde degeneration may involve peripheral nerves as far back as the first node of Ranvier. During retrograde degeneration, pigment is present in nerve cells, there is dissolution of the myelin sheath, and the sheath cells of Schwann proliferate.

Sheath and capsule cells are neuroectodermal in origin. The sheath of Schwann encircles the periphery of the axis cylinders. Sheath and capsule cells are replaced by oligodendroglia. The capsule cells surround the ganglion cells. During ganglionitis, the capsule cells show proliferative changes.

CONGENITAL ANOMALIES OF THE CENTRAL NERVOUS SYSTEM

Rachischisis is a congenital defect (fissure) located in the dorsal arch of the spinal column. In the skull, it is similar to protrusion of the central nervous system. Meningocele is a hernial protrusion of the meninges through a defect in the skull or vertebral column. Meningoencephalocele is a hernial protrusion of the meninges and brain through a defect in the skull. Spina bifida occulta is the lack of fusion of the dorsal vertebral arch. Hydrocephalus is an abnormal accumulation of fluid in the cranial vault accompanied by enlargement of the head, prominence of the forehead, and sunset eyes. Meningomyelocele is the hernial protrusion of a part of the meninges and substance of the spinal cord through a defect in the vertebral column.

The Arnold-Chiari syndrome or deformity consists of meningomyelocele at the base of the brain. The bottom of the spinal cord is generally held stationary. The brain stem is, however, herniated through the foramen magnum and displaced caudally. The weight of the normal brain is 1,200 gms. However, when the weight of the brain is less than 1,000 gms, a congenital anomaly is present termed *microcephalus*. If the weight of the brain exceeds 1,700 gms, the congenital anomaly present is termed *macrocephalus*.

INFLAMMATORY DISEASES OF THE CENTRAL NERVOUS SYSTEM

Introduction

Inflammatory diseases of the central nervous system include encephalitis (inflammation of the brain), myelitis (inflammation of the spinal cord), leptomeningitis (inflammation of the leptomeninges), pachymeningitis (inflammation of the dura), radiculitis (inflammation of the nerve roots between the central nervous system and motor nerve), and neuritis (inflammation of the peripheral nerves).

Leptomeningitis and ganglitis are similar inflammatory lesions, which are dependent upon the site of involvement. The morbid anatomy of leptomeningitis and ganglitis reveals suppuration, hemorrhage, and necrosis. The etiologic agent in the inflammations is a microorganism. Meningoencephalitis is caused by a viral infection in certain instances and by a bacterial infection in other instances. Poliomyelitis is a viral infection that attacks the anterior horns. Leptomeningitis and encephalitis are generally present in a simultaneous fashion. The diagnosis of the latter infections depends on immunology, animal inoculation, and culture. Neuropathology reveals a proliferative process. The axon breaks down and inflammatory cells infiltrate into the parenchyma. Polymorphonuclear leukocytes are mobilized in an acute encephalitis, and lymphocytes are mobilized during chronic encephalitis. In severe inflammations, the glial elements proliferate and the nerve cell bodies degenerate.

Encephalitis

Encephalitis may be focal or general. Focal encephalitis indicates the presence of localized brain abscesses. The spinal cord, pons, and medulla are rarely involved by abscesses. On the other hand, the cerebral hemispheres are commonly involved by abscess formation. Abscesses develop toward the periphery of the cerebral hemispheres. Blood vessels and fibroblasts proliferate, and the edema develops in the tissues surrounding the abscess. Microglia proliferate following abscess formation in the cerebral hemispheres. Perivascular cuffing occurs as the inflammatory cells become mobilized in the Virchow-Robin spaces.

Hemorrhagic encephalitis or flea-bitten brain is a descriptive term rather than pathologic process. Lethargic encephalitis is a descriptive term for a symptom rather than a pathologic process. If the brain has a gross gray color, the diagnosis is probably polioencephalitis. If the brain has a white color, the diagnosis is probably leucoencephalitis. Diffuse, transverse, and disseminated are terms applied to encephalitis or myelitis. Encephalitis may be classified as follows: Wernicke's polioencephalitis, syphilitic encephalitis, and tuberculous encephalitis. The nomenclature for the various forms of encephalitis reveals the etiology or time factor, is descriptive, is related to a toxic agent, or utilizes the name of an individual.

Hemorrhagic encephalitis is generally due to a toxin or drug. Carbon monoxide poisoning primarily involves the globus pallidus bilaterally. Barbiturates and salvarsan may also produce a hemorrhagic encephalitis of the brain stem.

Necrotic encephalitis is a chronic inflammation resulting from tuberculosis, syphilis, and mycotic infections of the brain. Proliferative vascular encephalitis and local encephalitis accompany an acute bacterial infection of the meninges.

Postinfectional encephalitis (leukoencephalitis) occurs as a sequel to various acute virus diseases, i.e. measles, small pox vaccination, rubella, varicella, and antirabies inoculation. The lesions are inflammatory and produce demyelinating diseases. Leukoencephalitis involves the sub-pia mater and periventricular and perivenous demyelinization. The microglial cells undergo hypertrophy, and astrocytes are involved in the repair process. The myelin sheaths are destroyed, and the end stage of postinfectional encephalitis consists of formation of areas of demyelinization as the myelin is destroyed accompanied by destruction of axon cylinders. Typhus and Rocky Mountain spotted fever appear as similar diseases because both are accompanied by the presence of the glial nodule. Japanese B encephalitis affects only the base of pons without producing any inflammation of the upper portion of the pons. Infiltration of inflammatory cells is present only at the base of the pons, and neurophagia is prominent.

Inflammation of the Meninges

Inflammatory diseases of the meninges include pachymeningitis and leptomeningitis. The inflammation of the meninges involves the dura mater, arachnoid, and pia mater. The meninges are compised of mesothelial cells, fibroblasts, and fixed-tissue histiocytes. Injury to the dura mater, arachnoid, and pia mater results in the proliferation of mesothelial cells, histiocytes, and mononuclear cells. These three cell types may form a false membrane, which is characteristic of the subdural hematoma. During inflammation of the meninges, histiocytic and mononuclear cells are the most active cellular elements in the meninges. Following meningeal hemorrhage, the fibroblasts become the most reactive cellular element in the meninges. The base of the leptomeninges normally contains melanin; therefore, pigmentation in this region is not the result of inflammation or degeneration. The blood vessels passing inward from the surface of the meninges carry a layer of pia mater, which extends down to the perineuronal spaces. This is one route of divergence, i.e. from the parenchyma to the leptomeninges.

Leptomeningitis is an acute bacterial inflammation caused by invasion of streptococci and meningococci. Chronic leptomeningitis is due to tuberculosis, syphilis, and leprosy. Pseudotumors of the leptomeninges represent the primary and metastatic leukemias. The dura mater is primarily involved during an inflammation of the brain and during syphilitic pachymeningitis. The dura mater is secondarily involved in osteomyelitis, brain abscesses, and chronic infections.

Suppurative leptomeningitis is an inflammation of the leptomeninges. The leptomeninges become filled with polymorphonuclear leukocytes due to an infiltration of the subarachnoid spaces by leukocytes. The brain proper is not involved by the inflammatory process during suppurative leptomeningitis. The inflammatory process is the result of infection by pyogenic meningococci. The spinal cord and subarachnoid space contain an infiltrate of polymorphonuclear leukocytes, and macrophages with ingested polymorphonuclear leukocytes.

Inflammation of the central nervous system also encompasses brain abscesses, suppurative myelitis, as well as encephalitis.

When an abscess is located in the pons, it may prove to be fatal because no drainage exists from the entrapped abscess. An abscess of the brain may be surrounded by encephalitis consisting of perivascular infiltrations mobilized in the adventitial spaces.

Aseptic leptomeningitis may be present in which the abscess of the brain is sterile with no organisms present. The latter may be demonstrated following culturing of the purulent material removed from the abscess. An epidural abscess is commonly present following tuberculosis. The dura mater becomes hyperplastic, and there is degeneration of the spinal cord. In an extradural abscess the suppuration may be responsible for paralysis within a period of twenty-four hours; therefore, this abscess must be drained as soon as possible. Degeneration of the spinal cord may follow the extradural abscess. The extradural abscess may be due to a carbuncle.

Tuberculous meningitis results from pulmonary tuberculosis. Ninety-six percent of instances of tuberculous meningitis spread from a primary infection in the lungs to secondarily infect the meninges. A fibrinous leptomeningitis develops following pulmonary tuberculosis, which is characterized by small white nodules. Cortical caseation necrosis results with mobilization of abundant Langhans' giant cells. A tuberculoma forms in the meninges accompanied by destruction of adjacent tissue. Gummas similar to those of tertiary syphilis may develop during tuberculous meningitis. The reticulum persists in the meningeal gumma of tuberculous meningitis.

Ependymitis is a suppurative inflammation that accompanies poliomyelitis, herpes simplex, leptomeningitis, and chronic meningitis. There is, however, a relationship between the inflammatory process of ependymitis and demyelinization. Acute diffuse demyelinated myelitis produces a zone of demyelinization with cellular proliferation plus proliferation of microglia.

Syphilis of the central nervous system produces chronic leptomeningoencephalitis. During syphilitic leptomeningitis, the blood vessels become obstructed due to proliferation of cells from the vessel wall. Syphilis produces vasculitis of the blood vessels of the central nervous system, which is accompanied by pachymeningitis. Syphilitic infection of the meninges and brain results in general paresis. During general paresis, there is a thickening of the meninges, cortical atrophy of the brain, and dilatation of the ventricles. General paresis produces a cellular proliferation of the glia, microglia form red blood cells and perivascular cuffing is prominent. Iron is deposited in the parenchyma and walls of the blood vessels during general paresis.

Tabes dorsalis or locomotor ataxia is a disease of the lower sensory neurons and is a late manifestation of syphilis. There is degeneration of the posterior root fibers and their upward extensions into the spinal cord during tabes dorsalis. Lesions develop in the spinal cord, and leptomeningitis is present. The posterior roots and columns of the lumbosacral region are destroyed. The glia and astrocytes proliferate and produce glial scarring (isomorphic gliosis).

Acute Anterior Poliomyelitis

Acute anterior poliomyelitis indicates that the anterior gray matter of the spinal cord has undergone inflammation. Bulbar poliomyelitis indicates that the brain is affected by the virus of poliomyelitis.

Poliomyelitis produces an early and transient leptomeningitis. Poliomyelitis begins as a viral infection of the anterior gray matter of the spinal cord, motor cortex, and gray matter of the pons. In acute anterior poliomyelitis, the blood vessels and the anterior gray matter contain a perivascular cellular mobilization (infiltration) of inflammatory cells. There is destruction of the anterior gray matter, inflammation, hemorrhage, and softening of the brain, all of which result directly from the causative viral microorganism. A marked cellular proliferation occurs accompanied by proliferation of microglia in the affected region of the gray matter. The perivascular infiltration and edema present alter the proper functioning of nerve cells.

However, as soon as the edema is resolved, the nerve cells return to their normal function. Poliomyelitis occurs in the following forms: a nonparalytic poliomyelitis, a transient paralytic poliomyelitis, and a permanent paralytic poliomyelitis. Twenty years following the development of poliomyelitis, the spinal cord may contain a cavity and glial scars located on the diseased side. The motor neurons remain normal.

Ascending (acute) paralysis, i.e. Landry's paralysis may accompany poliomyelitis and neuritis. The blood vessels are surrounded by polymorphonuclear leukocytes and eosinophils during Landry's paralysis.

Neurotropic Viral Diseases

Herpes zoster (shingles) is a neurotropic virus affecting the aged (75 to 85 years of age). Herpes zoster is quite rare in young individuals. Herpes zoster produces a severe illness with pain due to involvement of the gasserian ganglion, sensory ganglion, and semilunar ganglion. The virus is not present in the herpetic vesicles located in the nervous system. The vesicles of herpes zoster develop following the release of histamine.

Herpes simplex produces vesicles, and the herpetic virus is present in the residue. Ophthalmic herpes simplex produces a corneal scar followed by viral encephalitis in the brain. Herpes simplex of the trigeminal nerve is extremely dangerous.

Measles is a viral infection that may develop in the spinal cord, producing areas of demyelinization. The measles virus is capable of producing paralysis. Measles encephalitis is accompanied by a cuff of inflammatory cells and areas of demyelinization. If the patient survives, the measles and the paralysis disappear. During measles, the spinal cord undergoes demyelinization of the gray matter and perivascular infiltration of the white matter.

Multiple Sclerosis (Disseminated Sclerosis)

Multiple sclerosis is a disease characterized by plaques of demyelinization and gliosis in the central nervous system. The demyelinization shows a predilection for the borders of the white matter and gray matter of the brain and spinal cord as well as in the periventricular areas.

The plaques are gray and translucent and fail to demonstrate a constant relationship to the blood vessels. The demyelinization traverses the white and gray matter of the brain and spinal cord. Sclerotic-appearing areas represent the regions of the plaques. The plaques vary in age due to the presence of the common exacerbations and remission that are very characteristic of this disseminated sclerosis, producing demyelinization and gliosis. The plaques of demyelinization commonly develop toward the periphery of the white and gray matter. The gitter cells are located in the periphery of the white and gray matter and are replaced by reparative astrocytes during multiple sclerosis. Perivascular cuffing is a prominent finding with lymphocytes mobilized during acute and subacute multiple sclerosis. During repair, the nucleus of the astrocyte disappears, and only the processes of the astrocyte are retained.

VASCULAR DISEASES OF THE CENTRAL NERVOUS SYSTEM

Venous drainage from the brain occurs through convergence of venous vessels to the sagittal sinus and then downward through the jugular vein to the heart.

A stroke or occlusion of blood vessels results in headache and vertigo, or it may be sudden and of insidious onset. Spasm of a blood vessel may precede occlusion. Symptoms described above may subside in a few days. Occlusion of vessels in the brain result in the following findings. There may be minimal change during the first twenty-four hours following occlusion of vessels. After twenty-four hours, polymorphonuclear leukocytes mobilize in the affected brain tissue, and there is chromatolysis of ganglion cells. The nucleus of the ganglion cells becomes darker than normal, and the cells become swollen. In three to four days, the cerebral cortex begins to soften, and gitter or scavenger cells begin to phagocytize the debris. Following recovery, the gitter cells disappear and astrocytes appear with scarring, or cysts develop. A fibroglial scar forms in two to three weeks. Proliferation of glial cells and fibrocytes begins in six to seven days following the occlusion.

The site of a cerebral infarct may be in the stem or base of the brain, where occlusion of blood vessels occurs very easily. Infarcts are due to occlusion of the posterior superior cerebral artery, producing the following symptoms: pain, vertigo, vomiting, hoarseness, unilateral disturbance in cerebral coordination. Infarcts also occur in the angle of the medulla oblongata and spinothalamic tract. The infarcts involve the facial nucleus, producing a self-limiting disorder. Ninety-five percent of affected individuals recover, and one to two percent may die from the occlusion. Five to ten percent of affected individuals have residual difficulties, i.e. vertigo and ataxia. Occlusion of the superficial vessels of the cerebral cortex causes a shrinkage of the gyri. Senile progressive vascular occlusion occurs in individuals in mental hospitals.

Bilateral infarcts occur at the basal ganglia. This is a common site for occlusion due to arteriosclerosis with infarcts developing in the white matter of the cerebral hemispheres.

Microscopically, infarcts of the brain show softening and necrosis, hemorrhage, and inflammatory cells. The cortical arch is disturbed and few ganglion cells are present in the infarct. Gitter cells and inflammatory cells are common, and gitter cells are mobilized in the leptomeninges. Fat-filled gitter cells and macrophages containing blood pigment are present at the infarct. An infarct is the site of a nonspecific response in the central nervous system.

Hemorrhage occurs from traumatic injury or arteriosclerosis in the basal ganglia, producing a lethal form of vascular disease. Fifty to seventy-five percent of patients succumb following cerebral hemorrhage due to trauma. Death may occur six days following the hemorrhage. The cerebral substance is softened, and a group of vessels may rupture. It may be difficult or impossible to find the specific point of leakage of blood.

Hemorrhage may be multiple in the brain stem during hypertension. Trauma may produce little hemorrhage elsewhere, but hemorrhage takes place at the brain stem. Eye signs indicate that hemorrhage is present in this basal area.

Superficial hemorrhage produces pressure on the cerebral cortex and the ventricular system. Hemorrhage may be deep seated or cortical and cause death because of the multiple nature of the brain stem. Superficial hemorrhages are generally dissolved.

Microscopically, hemorrhages are located perivascularly; however, the continuity of the blood vessels is maintained. It is difficult to determine the disruption of the vessels histologically. There is some loosening of blood vessel walls, and bleeding points occur at some distance from the main hemorrhage. The white matter is pale and deficient in its blood supply.

The cerebral aneurysm occurs at the junction point of the trunks of blood vessels at the base of the brain. A large, basilar aneurysm produces cerebellum findings, compression of the eighth nerve, and facial paralysis. Diffuse hemorrhage following a ruptured aneurysm produces stiffness of the neck or a rigid neck, temperature, severe pain, loss of consciousness, and neurological findings. An aneurysm into the ventricle system causes dilated walls. The blood clot may rupture through the ventricular system to the surface. Other aneurysms cause minimal bleeding. Aneurysms are congenital in nature and may originate from an arteriosclerotic origin following inflammation of the blood vessel wall. Thinning of the blood vessel wall results in eventual rupture. Thirty-five percent of individuals with a first hemorrhage arising from an aneurysm succumb. Eighty percent die from an aneurysm, if not corrected, in two years.

Vascular disease encompasses the following in the CNS: arteriosclerotic thrombosis and hemorrhage; hypertension; aneurysms; vasospasm, embolism; arteriovenous malformations; Sturge-Weber syndrome; vascular tumors; and trauma.

Cerebral vascular accidents include ischemia, arterial or venous thrombosis, hemorrhage, and emboli. Ischemia of the brain is due to anoxia, i.e. deficiency of oxygen as a result of interference with oxygenation. Ischemic attacks with vasospasms exist only when some pathology is present. Ischemia of the brain is associated with systemic hypotension, blood loss, surgical shock, syncope, and migraine variance.

The degree of damage during cerebral vascular accidents depends upon the following: rapidity of the alteration, place of central nervous system involvement, and the amount of collateral circulation to the area. Collateral circulation to the involved area is an extremely important factor in any vascular lesion of the brain. Any ischemic change will cause an alteration in the physiology and biochemistry of the nerve cell bodies. The morphologic effect is an increase in the eosinophilia (paleness) of the cytoplasm of the nerve cells. The nucleus of the nerve cell becomes pale and pyknotic along with the pale cytoplasm. There is a dropping out of nerve cell bodies in the cerebral cortex during ischemia. However, there is no reaction by the brain to this nerve cell alteration. Later on there is a proliferation of astrocytes and perivascular dropping out of tissue, which is grossly termed *aptat lacunaris*. Microscopically, the perivascular dropping out of tissue is termed *aptat crivale*.

The etiologic factors of arterial thrombosis include arterial disease, increased coagulability, and increased circulatory rate. There is an architectural difference in the vessels located in the brain compared to blood vessels throughout the rest of the body. The latter makes the cerebral vessels more susceptible to alterations. Arteriosclerosis occurs at the base of the brain, producing pipe stem arteries. Advanced ischemia of the cerebral cortex may occur during arteriosclerosis, producing granular atrophy of the cortex with narrow gyri and wide sulci. Lipids are deposited in the vessel wall during arteriosclerosis. During syphilis (cerebrovascular), the elastic membrane of blood vessels undergoes reduplication and fraying accompanied by endothelial proliferation.

Collagen diseases affect the blood vessels of the brain. Lupus erythematosus and periarteritis nodosa alter the cerebral vasculature. There is a thickening of the vessel wall and closing of the lumen and a marked perivascular infiltration of inflammatory cells. Senile blood vessels of the brain show hyalinization of the vessel wall. The etiologic factor in aneurysms in the brain is thrombosis and hemorrhage. Thrombosis is the most common etiologic agent. Alterations occur in the parenchyma of the brain during thrombosis. During the initial twenty-four to thirty-six hours, minimum necrosis develops. Complete thrombosis results in damage to all structures. Incomplete thrombosis causes damage to the mesenchymal tissues; however, the blood vessels are preserved. In early infarction of the brain, the blood vessels release

PMN leukocytes, which diffusely invade the parenchyma of the brain. The brain parenchyma becomes ischemic (anemic), and hemorrhage occurs in the form of discrete and confluent areas accompanied by congestion of cerebral vessels.

An early hemorrhagic infarct of the brain produces pale hemorrhagic brain tissue; however, the nerve cells are preserved. In thirty-six to forty-eight hours the stage of malacia occurs in the cerebral infarct, and the parenchyma of the brain breaks down. The destruction of tissue lasts from days to weeks or even months. When repair begins, the capillaries send out buds, and the histiocytes and microglia of the central nervous system are activated. At the forty-two to seventy-two hour stage, the astrocytes undergo proliferation. The astrocytes are larger than the microglia, and the area of proliferation appears more cellular than normal.

During the cystic stage of a hemorrhagic infarct, a gross softening and vacuolation becomes evident. The glial wall is composed of astrocytes. Astrocytes surround the vessels, and recanalization commences. There is an accumulation of lymph, i.e. symptomatic inflammation. Gitter cells are actively phagocytic and are transformed into microglia.

The gyrus area of the cerebral infarct is an area walled off by astrocytes with a darker periphery. Gitter cells are located inside the astrocyte layer. During symptomatic inflammation, the lymphocytes predominate and are mobilized in the area. Cavity formation develops after the gitter cells phagocytize the material and remove it from the area. The pigmentation located in the affected area of the hemorrhagic infarct is slowly removed by phagocytes. Old infarcts contain hemosiderin pigment (blue color) and hematoidin (yellow color). The end stage of the hemorrhagic infarct consists of depression and destruction of the middle cerebral artery due to thrombosis.

Venous thrombosis may occur in the major sinuses of the brain. The latter may be fatal when a damming back and hemorrhage occurs. Microscopically, a hemorrhagic infarct results accompanied by small hemorrhages and vascular engorgement. Venous sinus thrombosis is associated with infection, meningitis, and hemorrhagic diseases. Thrombosis of the great vein of Galen causes a backing up and hemorrhage of the vein.

HEMORRHAGE IN THE BRAIN

There are six categories of hemorrhage in the brain, i.e. extradural, epidural, subdural or intradural, subarachnoid, intraventricular, and intracerebral hemorrhage. *Hematomyelia* is a term indicating hemorrhage in the horns of the brain. A hemorrhagic syndrome is possible in the brain because all or a combination of the six hemorrhages may co-exist.

Epidural hemorrhages are due to laceration of an artery secondary to fracture of the parietal bone. Hemorrhage occurs between the internal tables of the skull and outer layer of the dura. The artery is the source of the bleeding and, therefore, the course is rapid. Subdural hemorrhages are either spontaneous or traumatic in etiology. The hemorrhage may occur intradurally, or the hemorrhage may be located subdurally with the formation of a neomembrane.

The dura consists of mesothelial cells and the neomembrane. The thicker the neomembrane the older the hemorrhage. A slow hemorrhage (subdural) produces insidious clinical findings. The cerebrospinal fluid is imbibed into the subdural hemorrhage, and late clinical symptoms develop.

The subarachnoid hemorrhage may occur primarily or secondarily and may be spontaneous or traumatic in origin. The spontaneous subarachnoid hemorrhage is primarily due to a ruptured aneurysm. The subarchnoid hemorrhage may be due to the following causes: congenital, arteriosclerosis, and a mycotic aneurysm. Congenital aneurysms are not present at birth but develop during life. The congenital aneurysm occurs in the circle of Willis at the bifurcation, or where a defect is present in the media of the vessel since less elastic and muscle tissue occurs at the defective site. An arteriosclerotic aneurysm occurs later in life and is due to a defect in the media of the vessel.

Syphilitic aneurysms are rare in the brain and are generally arteriosclerotic aneurysms. Mycotic or inflammatory aneurysm are associated with subacute bacterial endocarditis. The mycotic aneurysm is a secondary cause of subarachnoid hemorrhages. There is an extension of the intracerebral hemorrhage to the surface of the brain.

Intraventricular hemorrhages occur primarily or secondarily and are due to neoplasms and toxic and infectious stress. Direct rupture of the subappendimal veins is due primarily to an increase in pressure in the brain followed by a sudden drop in pressure.

Intracerebral hemorrhages are all caused by thrombosis in arteries, veins, or capillaries. There are three characteristics of intracerebral hemorrhages. Firstly, the hemorrhage destroys and dissolves the cerebral tissue. Secondly, the hemorrhage displaces the adjacent cerebral structures and also invades adjacent tissues. Thirdly, there is no topographical distribution of the hemorrhage The sites of the hemorrhage are lateral to the areas of putrom termed the *site of Charcot*. The area has numerous vessels, which are prone to arterial disease. The Charcot area is therefore a site of predilection to hemorrhage. All cerebral hemorrhages are not grossly visible. Small, grossly visible, petechial hemorrhages may occur in the parenchyma of the brain in toxic states. Blood vessels undergo necrosis in toxic states, leading to ring hemorrhages. A ring hemorrhage is a hemorrhage that localizes around a blood vessel that has become necrotic (perivascular hemorrhage).

Emboli may affect the cerebral tissue. Emboli may be aseptic in character arising from pulmonary or cardiac origins, or septic in subacute bacterial endocarditis, fat, air, and tumor cell. Aseptic emboli appear grossly similar to thrombosis of the hemorrhagic type. Emboli have an acute and repair stage. Septic emboli form aneurysms and abscesses. Fat emboli occur following a fracture of the long bones. The brain reacts markedly to fat emboli, showing a mobilization of a cellular exudate and a marked edematous reaction. Air emboli occur in individuals with emphysema and chronic pulmonary diseases. Therefore, it is essential to take a thorough clinical history in all instances of air emboli.

Hemorrhage is responsible for most of the edema of the brain. Glial neoplasms also cause edema. Hemorrhage within the pons is one cause of death.

Congenital anomalies develop in the circle of Willis. Arteriosclerosis develops in the larger basal, vertebral and internal carotid arteries.

The end stage of cerebral hemorrhages is a large cystic cavitation. The following represent the stages present in a cerebral infarct: necrosis, malacia, proliferation of astrocytes from forty-eight to seventy-two hours, and cystic cavitation.

Hematomyelia is hemorrhage into the spinal cord. Traumatic hemorrhage may be secondary to central neoplasia with a rim of the spinal cord located peripherally.

NEOPLASMS OF THE CENTRAL NERVOUS SYSTEM

In primary neoplasms of the central nervous system the actual cell type involved is of major importance. All central nervous system neoplasms may be considered malignant by virtue of their location in vital brain tissue.

Intracranial neoplasms comprise the following: gliomas, pituitary neoplasms, meningiomas, metastatic neoplasms, and neurinomas. The most prevalent intracranial neoplasms are the gliomas. The gliomas include the following: astrocytoma, glioblastoma multiforme, unclassified very malignant tumors, and the medulloblastoma. Neoplasms of the spinal cord include the meningioma, neurinoma, and intramedullary (intracord) ependymal ependymoma.

The benign neoplasms of the brain include the following: astrocytoma, ependymoma, astroblastoma, oligodendroglioma, hemangioblastoma, cavernous hemangioma, pinealoma, cholesteatoma, ganglion neuroma, and retinoblastoma. The malignant neoplasms of the brain include the following: glioblastoma multiforme, and medulloblastoma.

Benign neoplasms of the central nervous system, according to definition, may cause death because of their location. Neoplasms of the central nervous system cause edema, characteristically, in the cerebellum. There is widening and flattening of the gyri and a decrease in the sulci of the temporal lobe.

Microscopically, there is a loosening of the ground substance of the brain. Fluid is present in perivascular and perineural spaces. The presence of fluid in the perineural spaces is not always diagnostic of edema because artifacts of fixation may simulate edema. During edema there is a decrease in the stainability of the cerebral tissues, and cell responses occur with swelling of oligodendroglia.

Early alterations in the nerve cell body cause death of the cell. Edema occurs around or distant to a neoplasm of the brain. The actual cellular alterations occur close to the neoplasm.

There are no gitter cells present in the areas of edema of the brain. Gitter cells, however, are present during infarction of the brain. Metastatic neoplasms of the brain do not provoke very much edema. Metastatic neoplasms to the brain are generally fairly well circumscribed masses. Metastatic neoplasms to the brain arise from the following primary sources: one-third metastasize from neoplasms of the lungs, one-fourth metatasize from neoplasms of the gastrointestinal tract, and one-tenth metastasize from neoplasms of the breast and kidney. Seventy percent of metastatic neoplasms are multiple in the brain, and ninety-two percent of brain neoplasms occur in the cerebrum. Metastases to the cerebellum provoke a minimal reaction around the neoplasm. During metastases to the cerebellum, the granular cell layer may be preserved although it is quite susceptible to invasion by the neoplastic cells.

Metastases occur from neoplasms of the central nervous system. The medulloblast metastasizes along the cerebrospinal fluid. Central nervous system neoplasms may spread beyond the central nervous system to the ependyma and liver. However, some authors have stated that they have never seen neoplasms of the central nervous system metastasize beyond the central nervous system. Central nervous system neoplasms, however, may extend through the skull by direct extension.

HISTOGENESIS OF NEOPLASMS OF THE CENTRAL NERVOUS SYSTEM

The medullary epithelium of the neural tube gives rise to the pineal parenchyma, which gives rise to the pituitary, primitive spongioblast, medulloblast, and choroidal epithelium. The primitive spongioblast produces the ependyma, which gives rise to the ependymoma. The primitive spongioblast also gives rise to the astrocyte series, i.e. the astrocyte and astrocytoma. The primitive spongioblast further gives rise to the oligodendroglia (glial cell). The medulloblast gives rise to the nerve cell body. The microglia are of mesodermal origin. Kernihan proposed a dedifferentiation theory in which he believes that cerebral cells become mature then regress back to a more primitive form.

The medulloblastoma arises from the medulloblast originating from the neural tube. The medulloblast is related to the retinoblastoma and neuroblastoma. The medulloblastoma is a radiosensitive neoplasm composed of young and aplastic cells. The type of cell, the pattern of growth, and the clinical behavior pattern are similar for the medulloblastoma, retinoblastoma, and neuroblastoma. The medulloblastoma originates from the external granular layer of the cerebellum during the first decade of life prior to twenty years of age. The medulloblastoma is located in the midline of the primary cerebellum. Seeding of neoplastic cells occurs by means of the cerebrospinal pathway. There is no stroma, and minimal reticulum may be present. However, the cellular sarcoma shows a positive reticulum stain. The medulloblastoma forms rosettes composed of cells with hyperchromatic nuclei, uniform, small, oat-shaped cells with sparse cytoplasm arranged in a circular pattern. The blood vessels located within the neoplasm have thin walls with no stromal background and very little cytoplasm. A perivascular arrangement occurs with wheels of cells arranged around a central focus (rosette).

Astrocytomas arise from the astrocyte with its astrocytic nucleus (foremost), and fibrillary stroma from the glial processes. Cystic spaces develop, and cells pass from a uniform type to a pleomorphic variety. The cerebellar astrocytoma is highly cystic and contains numerous blood vessels. The blood vessels react by proliferation and endothelial thickening. The blood vessels react to the point of occlusion of the lumen. Microsopically, there is great cellularity, increased thickness of blood vessel walls, and a background network of glial fibers. Medullary astrocytomas contain oligodendroglia.

The malignant form of the astrocytoma is the glioblastoma multiforme. The type cell of origin is the spongioblast. The glioblastoma multiforme is composed of all types of cells. The latter is a pleomorphic neoplasm with areas of necrosis surrounded by spongioblasts. Pallisading of cells occurs around the areas of necrosis. The glioblastoma contains multinucleated tumor giant cells undergoing frequent mitosis, bizarre cell forms, hemorrhage, perivascular proliferation, and occlusion of blood vessels. Following irradiation, there is an increase in connective tissue in the glioblastoma. Cells surrounding the necrotic areas show pallisading of cells at right angles to the necrotic zones.

Oligodendroglioma occurs primarily in the cerebral hemispheres. It has the following characteristics: uniformity of cells; the cell type resembles normal, small, dark, round cells with clumping chromatin; and an indistinct cytoplasm. Pavementation occurs in sheets when the blood vessels react. This neoplasm is slow growing and contains calcium deposits.

Ependymomas consist of four cell types, i.e. ependymal, papillary, cellular, and malignant. The ependymal ependymoma contains wedge-shaped cells with cytoplasm at one end and processes from each pole, one process passing to the blood vessels. The cellular elements of the ependymoma form rosettes. The ependymoma of the spinal cord contains cells arranged in chords, and blood vessel rossettes. The papillary ependymoma contains peripheral cells and stroma.

The meningiomas arise from the arachnoid or are attached to the dura. They invade the dura and cranium. Noninvasive cerebral tumors simply displace the surrounding tissue. There are many types of meningiomas, in which all elements of the mesenchyme are produced. The two common types of the meningiomas are the meningothelial and fibroblastic meningiomas. The fibroblasts are the basic cell of the neoplasm. The meningioma causes bilateral paralysis of the lower limbs and is generally located over the cerebral convexity and sphenoid ridge.

Grossly, the meningioma has a gray brown color and is located in the leptomeninges. The meningioma has a gritty surface when cut due to the presence of calcification throughout the neoplasm. Microscopically, the neoplastic cells have a large, pale, oval nucleus; abundant cytoplasm; and often indistinct cell borders. The cellular elements produce a whorled pattern particularly in the meningiomatous meningioma. Surrounding the whorled pattern are trabeculations of connective tissue. When the meningioma has a predominantly fibroblastic appearance it is termed a *fibroblastic meningioma*. Psammoma is a variety of the meningioma that arises from arachnoid granulations. The centers of the whorls form radiopaque psammoma bodies in this meningioma.

The undifferentiated neurogenic tumors are the medulloblastoma located in the cerebellum in children, the retinoblastoma located in the retina in children, and the neuroblastoma located in the adrenal medulla in children. The chordoma is a rare neoplasm of the central nervous system. It consists of a loose stroma with minimal swollen cells. The cells appear similar to fat cells.

VASCULAR NEOPLASMS OF THE BRAIN

Vascular neoplasms of the brain include the angiomas that develop in vessels of various sizes and shapes. The angioma is, however, generally a single lesion in the arteries, veins, and capillaries. The hemangioblastoma develops in the midline of the cerebellum, produces occlusion on one side of the brain, and is a rare lesion in the cerebral cortex. The hemangioblastoma may be associated with malformations of the retinal arteries. Von Lindahl's disorder consists of an angioma in the brain accompanied by eye and cerebellum symptoms. A mass is located in the back of the head, and the neoplasm occludes the ventricular system. The hemangioblastoma is difficult to remove *in toto*. The ocular lesion in this disorder may be asymptomatic and familial in nature.

NEOPLASMS OF THE PERIPHERAL NERVOUS SYSTEM

Peripheral nervous system neoplasms include the neuroma (amputation or traumatic neuroma) located superficially in the subepidermal tissues, neurinoma (neurilemmoma, Schwannoma) located in the subcutaneous tissues, and the neurofibroma located on the sheath of deep nerves. The amputation or traumatic neuroma consists of a proliferation of Schwann's cells, mesodermal proliferation, and proliferation of axis cylinders. The amputation neuroma is characterized by trabeculations and axis cylinders proliferating in the local area.

The neurinoma (neurilemmoma or Schwannoma) replaces the older term *acoustic neuroma*. The origin of the neurinoma is not known; however, they may possibly arise from the Schwann's cells of the nerve sheath. The neurinoma develops in the spinal cord with one-half of the neoplasm outside and the other half inside the spinal cord. It has been termed the *dumbbell tumor* of the acoustic nerve. The neurinoma is an encapsulated tumor. Microscopically, palisaded nuclei are arranged into an organoid pattern or body termed the *Verocay body*. It may be composed of interlacing bundles and cystic spaces. If the interlacing bundles are solid without cystic spaces, the area consists of Antoni type A tissue. When cystic spaces are present, the area consists of Antoni type B tissue. Pigment and hemorrhage may be present in the neurinoma. Large cells are present, which contain fat. However, no axis cylinders are present in the neurinoma.

Multiple neurofibromatosis or Von Recklinghausen's disease produces nonencapsulated tumors. The neurofibromatosis fails to contain palisading of cells or Verocay bodies, which are so prevalent in the neurinoma. However, the neurofibroma (multiple) consists of interlacing bundles arranged in a haphazard pattern with axis cylinders. The axis cylinders may be demonstrated with silver stain.

The malignant neurinoma or malignant Schwannoma possibly arises from Schwann's cells. The Schwann's cells proliferate and may undergo a malignant change, forming the malignant neurinoma.

Blood vessel tumors develop in the peripheral nervous system. Angiomatous malformations of the peripheral nerves are differentiated from true neoplasms of blood vessels. The malformations include capillary telangiectasis, venous angiomas, arteriovenous angiomas or fistulas. The latter do not bleed or undergo degenerative changes.

The capillary hemangioma is a true neoplasm due to endothelial proliferation, which occurs in the peripheral nervous system. The hemangioendothelioma and hemangiosarcoma are true neoplasms arising from endothelial proliferation in the peripheral nervous system. In the venous angioma, the blood vessels are abnormal and the surrounding tissue is destroyed by the angioma. However, if the venous angioma occurs in the brain, the surrounding brain tissue is not reactive. Capillary hemangiomas occur in the cerebellum. The cystic hemangioma may also develop in the cerebellum.

References

Adams, R.D. and Richardson, E.P.: In Folch-Pi, J. (Ed.): *Chemical Pathology of the Nervous System*, Oxford, Pergamon Press, 1961.
Asbury, A.K., et al.: *Medicine, 48:*173, 1969.
Bailey, F.W.: *Bull Los Angeles Neurol Soc, 26:*32, 1961.
Bailey, O.T.: *J Neuropathol Exp Neurol, 20:*170, 1961.
Blackwood, W., et al. (Eds.): *Greenfield's Neuropathology,* 2nd ed. London, Edward Arnold and Co., 1963, p. 520.
Bowsher, D.: *Cerebrospinal Fluid Dynamics in Health and Disease,* Springfield, Thomas, 1960.
Breutsch, W.L.: In Baker, A.B. (Ed.): *Clinical Neurology,* 2nd ed. New York, Hoeber-Harper, Inc., 1962.
Broman, T., Edstrom, R., and Steinwall, O.: *Acta Psychiatr Scand, 36:*69, 1961.
Courville, C.B.: *J Forensic Sci, 7:*431, 1962.
Dastur, H.M., Desae, A.D., and Dastur, D.K.: *J Neurol Neurosurg Psychiatry, 25:*370, 1962.
Dean, G.: *The Porphyrias,* Philadelphia, Lippincott, 1963.
Duma, R.J., et al.: *N Engl J Med, 281:*1315, 1969.
Fazio, C.: Proceedings of the Seventh International Congress of Neurology, Rome, Vol. 2, p. 317, 1961.
Feigin, I. and Popoff, N.: *Arch Neurol, 6:*151, 1962.
Freytag, E.: *Arch Pathol, 75:*402, 1963.
Greenhouse, A.H. and Neubuerger, K.T.: *Arch Neurol, 10:*47, 1964.
Harkins, J.C. and Reed, R.J.: Tumors of the Peripheral Nervous System, Fasc. 3. 2nd Series, *Atlas of Tumor Pathology.* Washington, D.C., Armed Forces Institute of Pathology, 1969.
Hicks, S.P., Cavanaugh, M.C., and O'Brien, E.D.: *Am J Pathol, 40:*615, 1962.
Hirano, A. and Zimmerman, H.M.: *Arch Neurol, 7:*227, 1962.
Hoeprich, P.D. (Ed.): *Infectious Diseases.* Hagerstown, Har-Row, 1972.
Kepes, J.: *Am J Pathol, 39:*499, 1961.
Kernohan, J.W. and Uihlein, A.: *Sarcomas of the Brain,* Springfield, Thomas, 1962.
Klatzo, I., Jajdusek, D.C., and Zigas, V.: In Van Bogaert, L., Rademaker, J., Hozay, J., and Lowenthal, A. (Eds.): *Encephalitides,* Amsterdam, Elsevier Press, Inc., pp. 172-190, (kuru) 1961.
Klatzo, I.: *J Neuropathol Exp Neurol, 26:*1, 1967.
Klosovskjy, B.N.: Hydrocephalus. In *Manual of Neurology,* vol. 8, 1963.
Litvak, J., Yahr, M. and Ransohoff, J.: *J Neurosurg, 17:*945, 1960.
Malamud, N., Hirano, A. and Kurland, L.T.: *Arch Neurol, 5:*401, 1961.

Manno, N.J., Uihlein, A. and Kernohan, J.W.: *J Neurosurg, 19*:754, 1962.
McAlpine, D., et al.: *Multiple Sclerosis: A Reappraisal.* Baltimore, Williams and Wilkins, 1972.
Menkes, J.H.: *Neurology, 12*:860, 1962.
Meyer, A.: In Blackwood, W., et al. (Eds.): *Greenfield's Neuropathology,* 2nd ed. London, Arnold, 1964, p. 621.
Meyer, A.: In Blackwood, W., et al. (Eds.): *Greenfield's Neuropathology,* 2nd ed. London, Arnold, 1964, p. 235.
McCaughey, W.T.E.: *J Nerv Ment Dis, 133*:91, 1961.
Neumann, M.N.: *J Neuropathol Exp Neurol, 22*:148, 1963.
Plum, F. and Posner, J.B.: *Diagnosis of Stupor and Coma.* Philadelphia, Davis Co, 1962.
Poser, C.M.: *Arch Neurol, 4*:323, 1961.
Roizin, L.: *J Neuropathol Exp Neurol, 19*:591, 1960.
Rubinstein, L.J.: Tumors of the Central Nervous System. Fasc. 6, 2nd Series. *Atlas of Tumor Pathology.* Washington, D.C., Armed Forces Institute of Pathology, 1972.
Russell, D., Rubinstein, L.J., and Lumsden, C.E.: *Pathology of Tumors of the Nervous System,* 2nd ed. London, Arnold, 1963.
Schulman, S. and Barbeau, A.: *J Neuropathol Exp Neurol, 19*:591, 1960.
Scott, T.R. and Netsky, M.G.: *Int J Neurol, 2*:51, 1961.
Shy, G.M.: *World Neurol, 3*:144, 1962.
Smith, W.T., et al.: *Brain, 88*:137, 1965.
Spain, D.M.: *The Complications of Modern Medical Practices.* New York, Grune, 1963.
Swartz, M.N. and Dodge, P.R.: *N Engl J Med, 272*:842, 1965.
Van Cleave, C.D.: *Irradiation and the Nervous System.* New York, Rowman, 1963.
Verhaart, W.J.C.: *Acta Neuropathol, 1*:107, 1961.
Weiner, L.P., et al.: *N Engl J Med, 288*:1103, 1973.
Weiss, P. and Scott, B.I.: *Proc Natl Acad Sci USA, 50*:330, 1963.
Zeman, W. and Dyken, P.: *Pediatrics, 44*:570, 1969.
Zeman, W., et al.: *Neurology (Suppl), 18*:Part 2, January, 1968.

INDEX

A

Abnormalities in septation of the heart, 225, 228
Abscess, 48, 95, 148, 357, 401, 423
  Brodie's, 401
  cold, 134
  of liver, 281
  paravertebral, 401
  perinephritic, 258
  retropharyngeal, 95
Achlorhydria, 301
  gastric, 301
Achondroplasia, 407, 408
Achylia, 302
Acid-base disturbances, 55
Acidosis, 258
Acromegaly, 312, 404
ACTH, 15, 163, 193, 309, 314
Actinic radiation, 177
Actinomycosis, 143, 147
  bovis, 143
  israeli, 143, 147, 148
  of the liver, 281
  lumpy jaw, 147
Adaptation of living agents, 126
Addison's disease, 56, 82, 315
Adenocarcinoma, 202, 207, 346
  of colon and rectum, 276
    annular constrictive, 276
    metastases from, 276
    polypoid, 277
  of gall bladder, 289
  of lung, 254
  of small intestines, 272
  of stomach, 270
  of urinary bladder, 265
Adenoma, 202
  of pituitary gland, 313
Adenomyosis, 340
Adenosis (breast), 362

Adenovirus infection, 154
Adhesions, 100
Adrenal gland(s), 310
  carcinoma, and Cushing's syndrome, 316
  cortex, 316
    adenoma of, 316
    function of, 314
    hemorrhage, 314
    hyperfunction, 315
    hyperplasia in, 315
    lesions in, 315
      destructive, 315
      regressive, 315
    necrosis, 314
    tumors of, 316, 317
  medulla, 316
    function of, 316
    lesions of, 316
    tumors of, 316
  myelolipoma of, 317
  neuroblastoma, 317
  paraganglioma of, nonchromaffin, 316
  pheochromocytoma of, 316
  tumors of, 316, 317
Adrenocorticotropic hormone (ACTH), 309, 314
Adrenogenital syndrome, 315
Aedes algypti, 282
Agenesis, 198, 257, 268, 319
  of kidney, 257
Agglutins, cold, 105
Aging, 26, 118
Agranulocytosis, 303
Air embolism, 9, 87
Albers-Schönberg disease, 407
Albright's syndrome, 408
Alcoholism, 284
  and portal cirrhosis, 284

Aleukemic leukemia, 304
Alkaline phosphatase of blood, 382, 405
Allergic diseases, 215
Allergy (hypersensitivity), 107, 215
Alterations in white blood cells, 298, 303
  acute leukemia, 304
  agranulocytosis, 303
  aleukemic leukemia, 305
  chronic lymphatic leukemia, 304
  chronic myeloid leukemia, 304
  cyclical neutropenia, 305
  infectious mononucleosis, 292, 303
  leukemia, 305
  leukocytosis, 306
  leukopenia, 306
  monocytic leukemia, 305
  plasma cell leukemia, 305
Amyloidosis, 40, 280, 294, 314
  associated with multiple myeloma, 294
  of liver, 280
  macroglossia due to, 40
  of spleen, 294
  types of, 40, 280
Anaphylactic shock, 246
Anaphylaxis, 216
Anaplasia, 202
Anaplastic carcinoma of lung, 254
Anasarca, 51
Anemia, 65, 300
  osteosclerotic, 300
  pernicious, 302
Anemias due to blood loss, 300
  congenital hemolytic anemia, 300
  Cooley's anemia, 301
  erythroblastosis fetalis, 301
  hemoglobinuria, 301
  hemolytic anemia, 116, 301
  sickle-cell anemia, 302
  spherocytic anemia, 302
Anemias due to decreased red blood cell production, 301
  aplastic anemia, 302
  hypochromic anemia, 302
  idiopathic hypochromic anemia, 303
  myelophthisic anemia, 303
  pernicious anemia, 302
Aneurysms, 74, 237, 428

  dissecting, 74, 238
  fusiform, 74, 237
  mycotic, 238
  syphilitic, 238
Angioneurotic edema, 62, 216, 387
Ankylosis, 411
  of joints, 42
Anomalies of the kidney, congenital, 257
  agenesis, 50, 257
  congenital hypoplasia, 258
  congenital polycystic kidney, 258
  dysplasia, 258
Anomalies of the stomach, 268
Anthracosilicosis, 43
Anthracosis, 43, 247
Antibodies, 105, 219
Antigen, 106, 219
Antihemophilic globulin (AHG), 307
  deficiency of, 307
Aortic valvulitis, syphilitic, 235
Aplasia, 50, 198
Aplastic anemia, 302
Appendiceal stasis, 273
Appendicitis, 272
  acute, 273
  chronic lymphoid, 273
  gangrenous, 273
  hemorrhagic, 273
  left-sided acute, 274
  obliterative, 273
  suppurative, 273
Argyrosis, 42
Arteriolar sclerosis, 70, 77, 229, 232
Arteriosclerosis, 69, 229, 239, 429
Arteritis, 90
  necrotizing, 90
Arthritis, 417
  acute, 411
  associated with gout, 412
  gonococcal, 412
  staphylococcal, 412
  streptococcal, 412
  suppurative, 412
  syphilitic, 412
  tuberculosis, 412
Arthus phenomenon, 34, 106, 219
Asbestosis, 150
Aschoff body, 219
Ascites, 59, 285

due to malnutrition, 197, 285
Aseptic necrosis of bone, 401
Aspergillosis, 143
Aspirin, hypersensitivity to, 107, 215
Astroblastoma, 433
Astrocytoma, 433
Atelectasis, 247
Atherosclerosis, 229
Atresia, 272
 of appendix, 272
 of stomach, 270
Atrophy, cellular, 36, 37, 49, 197
Atypical interstitial pneumonia, 250
Azotemia, 66

B

Bacillary dysentary, 275
 in sigmoid colon and rectum, 275
Bacillus coli, 273
Bacteremia, 124, 127
 in infections, 125
Bacterial diseases, 126
 acute, 126
 staphylococcus infections, 126
Bacterial endocarditis, 90, 233
 acute, 90, 233, 234
 subacute, 233
Bacterial pericarditis, 233
Bacterial specificity, 125
Banti's syndrome (splenic anemia), 295
Basal cell carcinoma, 206
Basosquamous cell carcinoma, 206
Behcet's disease, 393
Beriberi syndrome, 195
Berylliosis, 150
Bile plugs in canaliculi, 279, 285
Bile stasis, 279
Biliary cirrhosis, 285
 extrahepatic type, 285
 hypertrophic, 286
 intrahepatic type, 286
 posthepatic, 286
Bilirubin, 67, 283, 287
Biotin deficiency, 195
Blastomycosis, 145
 North American, 145
 South American, 145
Blood clotting mechanism, 83
Body water and electrolytes, 53

Bone deformity, 406
 due to fibrous dysplasia, 406
Bone disorders of obscure etiology, 405
 Albright's syndrome, 405
 fibrous dysplasia, 406
 osteoporosis, 406
 Paget's disease of bone, 406
Bone pain, 405
 in fibrous dysplasia, 406
 in Paget's disease, 405
Bone remodelling, 400
Bone tenderness, 400
Bone tissue, 400
 mosaic pattern in, 405
 reaction to neoplasms, 408
Bowen's disease of vulva and vagina, 349, 395
Brain, 414
 abscess of, 415
 hemorrhages of, 420
 infarct of, 421
 tumor, metastatic, 433
Breast, 354
 abscess of, 357
 adenosarcoma of, 364
 cancer, 364
  spread of, 365
 carcinoma of, 365
 carcinosarcoma of, 366
 comedocarcinoma, 360
 dysplasia, 360
 fibroadenoma of, 362
 hypertrophy, 360
 infection in, 357
 lactating, 355
 lymphangiosarcoma and, 366
 myoepithelial cell proliferation in, 354
 necrosis of, fat, 357
 papilloma of, duct, 362
 sarcoma of, 367
 tumors of, 362
Brenner tumor (Ovary), 329
Brill's disease, 157
Brodie's abscess (chronic bone abscess), 401
Bronchial adenoma, 254
Bronchial asthma, 217
 and emphysema, 217
Bronchiectasis, 247

Bronchiolar carcinoma, 255
Bronchogenic carcinoma, 255
  anaplastic carcinoma, 256
  squamous cell carcinoma, 256
Bronchopneumonia, 248
Bronzed diabetes, 286
Brown atrophy of the heart, 226
Brucellosis, 128, 141, 142, 291
  of liver, 281
Buerger's disease (thromboangitis obliterans), 240
Burn, 176
Burn shock, 176
Burning feet syndrome, 183, 184

C

Caisson disease, 167
Calcific pericarditis, 236
Calcification, disturbances of, 185
Calcium, 185
Calculi, 258
Cancer, 200, 241, 346
Candida albicans, 143, 349
Candidiasis, 143, 349
Capillary dilatation, 94, 95
Capillary hemangioma, 241
Capillary permeability, 95
Carbuncle, 126
Carcinoid neoplasm of appendix, 274
Carcinoma, 202, 364
  cholangiocarcinoma, 287
  hepatocarcinoma, 287
  in situ, 202, 346
  of the large intestines, 275
  in the liver, 287
Cardiac cirrhosis, 286
Cardiac edema, 51
Cardiac failure, 235
Cardiac shock, 82
Cardiomyopathy, 236
Cardiovascular syphilis, 235
Carotenemia, 42
Carotid body tumor, 212
Caseation necrosis, 133, 333
Cat-scratch disease, 291
Cavernous sinus thrombosis, 241
Cavitation of reinfection tuberculosis, 253
Cell injury, pathology of, 24, 30, 197
Cellulitis, 127, 291

Cerebral
  arteriosclerosis, 426
  artery, thrombosed aneurysm of, 426
  embolism, 427
  hemorrhage, 427
  infarction, 428
  sclerosis, diffuse, 429
  thrombosis, 428
  tissue, petechial hemorrhages in, and carbon monoxide poisoning, 429
Cerebral, vascular accident, 428
Cerebroside lipoidosis, 188,
  Gaucher's disease, 188
Cervicitis, 342
  acute, 342
  chronic, 342
  tuberculous, 343
Cervix, 341, 346
  carcinoma of, 346
  epidermidization of, 344
  erosion of, 346
  metaplasia in, squamous, 346
  mucosa, dysplasia of, 346
  polyp, 346
Chancre, 138, 359
Cheilitis venenata, 387
Chemical
  injury, 160
  poisons, 160, 167
Chemotaxis, 95
Chickenpox, 15
Chloasma, 401
Cholangiocarcinoma, 200
Cholangioma, 289
Cholangitis, 280
  primary, 280
Cholecystitis, 287
  acute, 288
  chronic, 288
Cholelithiasis, 288, 289
  complications of, 288
  metabolic stones, 288
  mixed stones, 288
  pure calcium bilirubinate gallstones, 288
  pure calcium carbonate gallstones, 288
  pure cholesterol gallstones, 288
Cholesterol lipoidosis, 279

Cholesterolosis, 288
Chondroma, 207, 409
Chondromatous metaplasia, 208
Chondrosarcoma, 209, 409
Chorea, 23
    Huntington's, 23
Choriocarcinoma, 324, 341
    ovarian, primary, 324
    testicular, 325
    uterine, 340
Choriomeningitis, lymphocytic, 423
Choristoma, 200
Christian's disease, 188
Christmas disease, 307
Christmas factor, 307
Chromoblastomycosis, 146
Chromophobe, 311
    adenoma, pituitary, 311
Chromosome, 20
Chronic irritation, 197
Chronic passive congestion, 280, 295
    of liver, 280
    of small bowel, 280
    of spleen, 295
Cirrhosis of the liver, 280, 284
    biliary, 284
    with hemochromatosis, 285
    portal (laennec's), 284
    postnecrotic, 284
    Valley fever, 144, 253
Cold abscess, 134
Cold agglutinins, 154, 249
Cold, common, 154
Collagen diseases, 219, 429
Condyloma Acuminatum, 348
Congenital anomalies, 16, 198, 257, 419
    agenesis, 198, 257
    syphilitic, 284
Cirrhosis with hemochromatosis, 285, 286
Cloaca, 401
Clostridium tetani, 128
Clostridium welchii, 39, 128
Cloudy swelling, 31, 32
Coagulation necrosis, 31
Coarctation of aorta, 228
Coccidioidomycosis, 143, 253
    of lungs, 144, 253
    atresia, 272
    diverticuli, 270

Congenital anomalies of the heart, 18, 225
Congenital atresia of small intestines, 270
Congenital diseases, 16, 257
Congenital hemolytic anemia, 116, 298
Congenital hypoplasia of kidney, 257
Congenital polycystic kidney, 257
Congenital stenosis, 112
Congenital syphilis, 140
Connective tissue, diseases of, 221, 429
Contracture, 112
Cooley's anemia, 300
Cor biventriculare, 235
Cor triloculare, 235
Coronary arteriosclerosis and myocardial infarction, 230
Corynebacterium diphtheriae, 127
Coxsackie virus group A, 154
Cretinism, 404
Crush syndrome, 81
Cryptococcosis, 143
Cushing's syndrome, 311, 404
Cyclical neutropenia, 303
Cystadenoma, 202, 326, 363
Cystic basal cell carcinoma, 206
Cystic disease of the breast, 361
    adenosis of breast, 361, 362
    cysts of breast, 361
Cystitis, inflammatory, 265, 360

D

Darier's disease, 389
Defensive responses, 7, 9
Deficiency diseases, 183, 184
Degenerative diseases, 8, 31
Degenerative joint disease, 411
Delayed hypersensitivity, 107
Dermatitis, 220, 385
    atopic, 385
    contact,
        allergic, 220, 386
    irritant, primary, 386
    neurodermatitis, 388
    radiation, 177
Dermatofibroma protuberans, 207
Dermatomyositis, 218, 222
Dermatotrophic viruses, 154
Dermoid cyst, 213, 327
Desmoid tumor, 197, 200

Developmental abnormalities of bone tissue, 405
  achondroplasia, 405
  osteogenesis imperfecta, 405
  osteopetrosis, 405
Diabetes, bronzed, 312
Diabetes insipidus, 312
Diabetes mellitus, 121, 312
Diabetic gangrene, 37
Diapedesis, 66, 95
Diphtheria, 291
Diplococcus, 127
Diplococcus pneumonia, types 1, 2 and 3, 127
Discoid lupus erythematosus, chronic, 222, 390
Disease, etiology of, 3, 4
Diseases associated with elevated whie blood cell counts, 298, 303
  lymphocytosis, 304
Diseases associated with lowered white blood cell counts, 298, 303, 306
  leukopenia, 304, 306
  lymphopenia, 305, 306
  neutropenia, 305, 306
Diseases due to increased red blood cells, 298
  polycythemia (erythemia), 298, 300, 301
Diseases of aging, 118
Diseases of the appendix, 272
  carcinoid tumor, 274
  congenital anomalies, 273
  inflammatory disease, 273
  mucocele, 274
Diseases of the arteries, degenerative, 229
  arteriolar sclerosis, 229
  arteriosclerosis, 230
  atherosclerosis, 230
  coronary arteriosclerosis and myocardial infarction, 231
Diseases of the arteries, inflammatory, 230
  arteritis, 85, 90, 139
  Buerger's disease (thromboangitis obliterans), 240
  polyarteritis nodosa (periarteritis nodosa), 219, 222
  syphilitic arteritis, 225

Diseases of the biliary tract, 287
  cholelithiasis, 287
  empyema of gall bladder, 288
  hydrops of gall bladder, 289
  inflammation of gall bladder, 289
  lithiasis, 289
  neoplasms, 289
Diseases of the blood and bone marrow, 300, 301, 306
  alterations in the red blood cells, 300
  alterations in the white blood cells, 304
  hemophilias, 306
  purpuras, 305
Diseases of the esophagus, 267
  circulatory disturbances, 268
  congenital anomalies, 267
  infections, 268
  neoplasms, 268
  Plummer-Vinson syndrome, 268
  scleroderma, 268
Diseases of the heart, 225
  congenital anomalies, 225
    abnormalities in septation, 226
    coarctation of the aorta, 227
    patent dutctus arteriosus, 28
    patent foramen ovale, 228
    transposition complexes, 229
Diseases of the kidneys
  congenital abnormalities, 257
  glomerulonephritis, 258
    acute, 258
    chronic, 259
    subacute, 259
  uremia, 258
Diseases of the large intestines, 274
  congenital anomalies, 274
  inflammatory diseases, 275
  neoplasms, 275
  vascular disturbances, 275
Diseases of the liver, 279
  cirrhosis, 284
  degenerative changes, 280
  infections, 281
  jaundice, 283
  neoplasms, 287
Diseases of the lymphatics, 306
  lymphangitis, 306
  lymphedema, 306
Diseases of the lymph nodes, 291

inflammatory diseases, 292
metastatic neoplasms to lymph
   nodes, 293
Diseases of the peritoneum, 276, 277
   inflammatory, 277
Diseases of the respiratory system, 246
   Atelectasis, 247
   infectious diseases of the lung, 247
   pulmonary edema, 248
   pulmonary embolism and infarction, 248
Diseases of the skeletal system, 405
Diseases of the small intestines, 270
   congenital anomalies, 271
   inflammation, 271
   intestinal obstruction, 272
   neoplasms, 272
   vascular disturbances, 272
Diseases of the spleen, 294
   anomalies, 294
   circulatory disturbances, 295
   inflammation, 295
   neoplasms, 296
   retrograde changes, 294
Diseases of the stomach, 268
   anomalies, 268
   circulatory disturbances, 269
   inflammatory lesions, 269
   neoplasia, 270
   peptic ulcer, 270
Diseases of the urinary bladder, 265
   inflammatory cystitis, 360
Diseases of the veins, 86, 240
   phlebitis, 86
   phlebothrombosis, 240
   thrombophlebitis, 240
   varicose veins, 86, 91, 241
Disorders of bones due to vitamin deficiency and excess, 402
   hypervitaminosis D, 402
   osteomalacia, 403
   rickets, 403
   scurvy, 403
   vitamin C deficiency, 402
   vitamin D deficiency, 402
Dissecting aneurysm, 74, 238
Disseminated lupus erythematosus, 222
Disseminated sclerosis, 425
Dissemination of disease, 46
Diverticuli, 324, 370

   of appendix, 324
   of esophagus, 324
   of stomach, 324
Ductus arteriosus, patent, 225
Duodenal peptic ulcer, 274
Duodenal stasis, 275
Dwarfism, hypophyseal, 50
Dynamic ileus, 272
Dysentary endamoebic, 275
Dyspepsia, 269
Dysphagia, 257
Dysplasia of kidney, 257
Dyspnea, 246
Dystrophic calcification, 36, 39
   in the heart, 225
Dystrophy, 49, 197
Dysuria, 258

E

Ecchymosis, 67
   causes of, 67
Eclampsia, 351
Eczema, 216
Edema, 56
   pulmonary, 59
   of small intestines, 271
Edema producing factor, 56
Eisenmenger's complex, 225
Electrolyte disturbances, 53
Eletcrolytes in exudate, 57
Elephantiasis, 143, 371
Emboli or thrombi in mesenteric arteries, 87
Embolic spread of neoplastic cells, 202
Embolism, 9, 87, 202
Embolus, septic, 87, 281
Embryoma, 200, 212
Emphysema, 250
Empyema of gall bladder, 288
Encephalitis, 420
Enchondroma, 406
Endamoebic dysentary, 275
Endarteritis obliterans, 139
Endemic typhus, 157
Endocarditis, 219
   associated with disseminated lupus erythematosus, 219
Endocrine, 309
   adenomatosis, multiple, 310
   atrophy, 309

disturbances, skeletal lesions in, 407
neoplasia, 310
syndromes, 309
Endometriosis, 324, 339
Endometritis, 320
  puerperal, 320
  syncytial, 320
Endometrium, 320
  adenoacanthoma of, 320
  adenocarcinoma of, 321
  carcinoma of, polypoid, 321
  cyclic changes, 320
  cysts, 320
  hyperplasia,
    endometrial, 321
  in menstrual phase, 320
  polyp, 320
  in proliferative phase, 320
  sarcoma of, stromal, 320
  in secretory phase, 320
Endosteal fibrosarcoma of bone, 209
Endotoxins, 126
Enteritis, regional, 275
Epidemic hemorrhagic fever, 157
Epidemic pneumonia of newborn, 249
Epidemic typhus, 157
Epidermoid cyst, 213
Epidermolysis bulbosa, 394
Epididymitis, 368
Epidural
  abscess, 415
  hemorrhage, 420
Epithelial neoplasms, 201
Epithelioid histiocytes, 132, 252
Erysipelas, 126
Erythema multiforme, 392
Erythema multiforme exudativum, 393
Erythemia, 300, 302
Erythroblastosis fetalis, 300
Esophageal varices, 91
Esophagitis, 267
  acute, 268
  subacute, 268
Esophagomalacia, 268
Etiology of systemic diseases, 3, 4
Ewings sarcoma, 209, 211
Exfoliative cytology, 346
Exotoxins, 126
Exudate, 57

F

Fallopian tubes, 332
  pregnancy in, 333
  tumors of, 334
Fallot, tetralogy of, 228
Fat necrosis, 31
Fatty change, 31, 279
  of the heart, 228
  of the liver, 279
Fatty degeneration in the heart, 226
Fatty infiltration of the myocardium, 226
Fatty ingrowth, 31, 228
  of the myocardium, 228
Fecaliths (stones) in the appendix, 272
Felty's syndrome, 295
Female
  genitalia, 318
  anomalies, 318
  diseases of the ovaries, 324
  menstrual cycle, 319
  neoplasms of the ovaries, 326
  uterus, diseases of, 334
Fever, 103
Fibrinoid necrosis, 41, 219
Fibrinolysin factor, 76, 89
Fibroadenoma, breast, 360, 362
Fibrocystic disease, 357
Fibroid (Leiomyoma, uterine), 337
Fibroma, 207
Fibrosarcoma, 209
Fibrosis of breast, 365
Fibrous dysplasia of bone, 406
  monostotic, 406
  polyostotic, 407
Filariasis, 371
Foramen ovale, patent, 228
Foreign bodies in appendix, 272
Fracture, classification of, 160, 165
Fractures of bones, 160
  delayed healing of, 166
Frei test, 347
Friedländer's bacillus, 128
Fröhlich's syndrome, 31
Frostbite, 176
Fungal diseases, 143
Fungal infections, 143
  of the liver, 281
  of the lungs, 253

Index

actinomycosis, 254
coccidioidomycosis (Valley fever), 254
histoplasmosis, 254
moniliasis, 254
Fungi, 143
  deep, 143
  superficial, 143
Furuncle, 126
Fusiform aneurysm, 237

G

Gall bladder, inflammation of, 287
  acute cholecystitis, 288
  chronic cholecystitis, 288
Ganglioneuroma, 316
Gangrene, 37
Gangrenous cellulitis, 37
Gangrenous inflammation, 37
Gartner's cyst, 350
Gas gangrene, 40, 128
Gastric malrotation, 268
Gastric mucosal changes in pernicious anemia, 267
Gastritis, 269
  acute, 269
  atrophic, 269
  chronic, 270
    atrophic, 270
    hypertrophic, 270
Gastroenteritis, 270
Gaucher's disease, 188, 296
Gene(s), 20
General adaptation syndrome, 102, 162
Genitalia
  female, 318
  male, 368
    chancroid, 369
    diseases of the urethra, 370
    penis, diseases and neoplasms of, 377
    prostate gland, 378
    scrotum, diseases and neoplasms of, 371
    testes, diseases and neoplasms of, 372
Genotype, 20
Geriatric diseases, 119
German measles, 155
Ghon complex, 134, 359

Ghon tubercle, 134, 359
Giant-cell tumor of hyperparathyroidism, 403
Giant-cell tumors of bone, 403
Gigantism, 211, 312
Glander's disease, 128
Glioblastoma multiforme, 435
Glomerulonephritis, 219, 258
  acute, 219
  chronic, 258, 259
  subacute, 258, 259
Glomus tumor, 242
Glossitis venenata, 387
Gonococcal arthritis, 347
Gonorrhea, 332, 347
Gouty arthritis, 411
  sodium biurate deposits, 411
Grading of squamous-cell carcinoma, 200
Granular cell myoblastoma, 202
Granulation tissue, 101
Granulocytopenia, 142
Granuloma inguinale, 348, 369
Granulomatous diseases, 101, 130, 149
Granulomatous inflammation, 100, 130, 149
  chronic, 100, 130, 149
  of the liver, 279
Granulomatous lymphadenitis, 131, 291
  etiology of, 130, 291
Granulosa cell tumor, 330
Gumma, 139, 359
Gummatous necrosis, 139, 359
Gummatous periostitis, 402
Gynecomastia, 285, 360

H

Hamartoma, 200
Hand-Schüller-Christian syndrome, 188, 296
  of the spleen, 296
Hansen's disease, 136
Healing, 7, 11, 110, 166
  of bone tissue, 166
  essentials for wound, 110
  factors preventing, 110
  of fractures of long bones, 166

Heart
  congenital anomalies of the, 225, 228
    abnormalities in septation, 226
    coarctation of the aorta, 227
    patent ductus arteriosus, 227
    patent foramen ovale, 228
    transposition complexes, 228
  degenerative diseases of the, 60, 226
  disturbances
    of calcification, 227
    in carbohydrate metabolism, 226
    of fat metabolism, 225
    of protein metabolism, 225
  nutritional deficiencies, 226
  postmortem changes, 226
Hemangiectasia, 208
Hemangioma, 208
Hemarthroses, 307
Hematin pigment, 283
  malarial pigment, 283
Hematocrit, decreased, 65
Hematogenous pigmentation, 43
Hematoidin, 43
Hematoma, causes of, 67
Hematomyelia, 433
Hematopoiesis, extramedullary, 300, 301
Hematoporphyrin, 44
Hematuria, 258
Hemochromatosis, 43, 185
Hemoconcentration, 56, 176
Hemoglobin
  adult, 65, 299
  fetal, 299
Hemoglobin S, 299
Hemoglobinuria, 300
Hemolysin, 105
Hemolytic anemias, 116, 299
  congenital, 298
Hemolytic disease of the newborn, 300
Hemolytic jaundice, 284
Hemophilia, 84, 307
  Christmas disease (hemophilia B), 307
  classic hemophilia A, 307
  hemophilia C, 307
  von Willebrand's disease, 307

Hemophilia A, classic, 307
Hemophilia B, 307
Hemophilia C, 307
Hemophilus influenza, 128, 233, 247
Hemophilus pertussis, 128
Hemorrhage, 66, 84, 163, 431
  causes of, 67, 431
  in large intestines, 67
  in small intestines, 270
  superiosteal, 163
Hemorrhagic shock, 80, 107
Hemorrhoids of colon, 91
Hemosiderin, 43
Hemosiderosis, 43, 185
Hepar lobatum, 282
Hepatitis, infectious, 280
  jaundice and, 283
Hepatization, 282
  gray, 282
  red, 282
Hepatocarcinoma, 287
Hepatocellular damage, 280
Hepatolenticular degeneration, 280, 286
Hepatomegaly, 282
Hepatotoxic agents, 280
Hereditary diseases, 16, 19, 218
Heredity, 16
  cancer and, 197
  nephritis and, 258
Hernia, 277
  diaphragmatic, 277
Herpangina, 155
Herpes simplex, 155, 425
Herpes zoster, 155, 425
Herpetic gingivostomatitis, 155
Heterophile agglutinin titre, serum, 155
Heterophile antibodies, 157
Heterozygote, 20
Histamine, 52
Histamine stimulation, 52
Histiocytosis-X, 188, 296
Histoplasma capsulatum yeastlike fungi, 143, 283
Histoplasmosis, 143, 283
  of the liver, 283
  of the lungs, 247
Hodgkin's disease, 149, 293
  early, 149

granuloma, 149, 293
late, 293
paragranuloma, 293
sarcoma, 293
of the spleen, 295
Hodgkin's granuloma (disease), 293
Hodgkin's paragranuloma, 293
Hodgkin's sarcoma, 293
Homozygote, 20
Hormone(s), 309
adrenocorticotropic (ACTH), 309
ovarian, 324
pituitary gonadotropic, 311
of pregnancy, 325
relationships, 309
Horseshoe kidney, 257
Huntington's chorea, 23
Hutchinson's triad, 138, 281
Hyaline
change, 40
degeneration, 40
droplet degeneration, 38
membrane disease of infancy, 250
necrosis, 40
Hyalinization, 40
Hydatidiform mole, 340
Hydroarthrosis, 51
Hydrocele, 420
Hydrocephalus, 420
Hydrochloric acid, 268
loss of, 268
Hydronephrosis, 258
Hydropericardium, 237
Hydropic degeneration, 30, 31
Hydrops of gall bladder, 288
Hydrosalpinx, 332
Hygroma colli cysticum, 209
Hypercholesterolemia, 184
Hyperemia (congestion), 51, 63
of small intestines, 270
Hyperestrogen, 285, 331, 359
Hyperglycemia, 185
Hyperlipemia, 184
Hypernephroma (renal cell carcinoma), 264
Hyperparathyroidism, 403
Hyperplasia, 114, 198
Hyperproteinemia, 183
Hypersensitivity, 107, 215
Hypertension, essential, 75, 78, 231, 315

Hypertensive heart disease, 230
Hyperthyroidism, 15, 309, 404
Hypervitaminosis A, 188
Hypervitaminosis D, 189, 402, 403
Hypochromic anemia, 300
idiopathic, 300
Hypogonadism, 313
Hypokaliemia, 184
Hypoplasia, 49, 114, 198
Hypoproteinemia, 122
Hypoproteinemic edema, 61, 122
Hypoxia, 50, 64

I

Icterus (jaundice), 283, 300
regurgitation, 284
retention, 284
Idiopathic hypochromic anemia, 301
Ileitis, regional, 272
Immediate hypersensitivity, 107, 215
Immobilization osteoporosis, 403
Immunity, 102, 105
Impairment, 8, 34, 46, 183
Inclusion bodies, 38, 154
Infarction, 9, 37, 88, 279
of large intestines, 90
of liver, 90, 279
of small intestines, 90
of spleen, 90
Infection, 124
bacterial specificity, 124
complications of, 125
definition of, 124
disturbances in healing, 125
factors related
to host, 124
to microorganisms, 125
to tissues, 125
incidence of bacteremia, 125
infectious diseases, 27, 124
organisms' influence on tissues, 125
spread of, 125
systemic antibiotic and salivary flora, 125
systemic effects of, 125
virulence and adaptation, 124
Infections of bone tissue, 400
acute osteomyelitis, 400
Pott's disease, 401
syphilis of bone, 402

tuberculosis of bone, 402
Infectious diseases of the lungs, 246
  bronchiectasis, 246
  bronchopneumonia, 247
  epidemic pneumonia of newborn, 248
  emphysema, 248
  interstitial pneumonia, 248
  lobar pneumonia, 248
  pneumonitis, 248
  primary atypical pneumonia, 248
Infectious granulomas, 130, 149
Infectious hepatitis, 282
Infectious mononucleosis, 156, 291, 292, 303
Inflammation, acute, 9, 94
  beneficial effects, 95
  cardinal signs of, 94
  cellular elements in, 95
  cellular responses in, 95
  fluid exudation in, 96
  fluid responses in, 96
  local clinical features, 97
  lymphatic blockage, 98
  pain in, 99
  purpose of exudate, 100
  sequence of events, 101
  systemic effects of, 102
  vascular responses, 103
Inflammation of joints, 411
  acute arthritis, 411
  gonococcal arthritis, 412
  staphylococcal arthritis, 412
  streptococcal arthritis, 411
  suppurative arthritis, 411
  syphilitic arthritis, 411
  tuberculous arthritis, 411
Inflammatory cystitis, 265
Inflammatory edema, 51
Influenza viruses, 154
Influenzal pneumonia, 249
Inherited diseases, 16, 19
Interstitial pneumonia, 249
Intersussception, 272, 277
Intestinal lipodystrophy, 274
Intestinal malrotation, 272
Intestinal obstruction, 272
Intestinal polyposis, 277
Intracranial neoplasms, 433
Intrinsic factor, deficiency of, 270

Involucrum, 401
Iodine deficiency, 187
Ionizing radiation, 178, 179
Iron deficiency, 185, 301
Iron dust, 43
Iron metabolism, disturbances in, 184
Irradiation, 176, 178
Irritation, chronic and neoplasia, 197, 250
Irritational fibroma, 199
Ischemia, 64, 66

J

Jaundice (icterus), 283, 360
  hemolytic, 284
  regurgitation, 284
  retention, 284
Joints, inflammation of, 411, 412

K

Karyolysis, 30
Karyorrhexis, 30
Keloid, 198
Keratosis follicularis, 389
Kidney, 257
  abscesses of, 257
  adenoma of, 263
  amyloid, 258
  anomalies, 257
  aplasia, 257
  arteriosclerosis in, 258
  artery, stenosis, 260
  atrophy of, hydronephrotic, 261
  calculi, 263
  cancer of, 264
  contracted, 264
  cyst of, 264
  in cytomegalic inclusion disease, 265
  degeneration of, hydropic, 258
  disease
    classification of, 260
  polycystic, congenital, 258
    in adult, 258
    in newborn, 258
  pyemic, 401
  sarcoma of, 263
  thrombosis, venous, 264
  tuberculosis of, 260
  tumors of, 263
Klinefelters' syndrome, 360

Index

Koch's phenomenon, 106
Kraurosis vulva, 349
Kveim skin test, 149
Kwashiorkor, 183, 190
Kyphosis, 120

L

Laboratory aids in diagnosis of infectious diseases, 250
Laboratory diagnosis of the pneumonias, 250
Lactation mastitis, 357
Laennec's cirrhosis, 284
Langhan's giant cells, 132, 252
Lead, 172
L. E. cell, 221
Leiomyoma, 208
Leiomyosarcoma, 209
Leishmania donovani, 158
Leishmaniasis, 158
Leonine face, 136
Lepromas, 136
Lepromatous leprosy, 136
Lepromin positive, 136
Leprosy, 136
Leptomeningitis, 420
Leptospirohemorrhagica (Weil's disease), 280
Leukemia, 67, 304
  acute, 304
  aleukemic, 305
  chronic lymphatic, 304
  chronic myeloid, 304
  monocytic, 305
  plasma cell, 306
Leukemia, lymphatic, 305
Leukocytosis, 15, 102, 104, 157, 163, 273, 303, 400
Leukopenia, 142, 302, 303
Leukoplakia of vulva, 349
Lichen planus, 388
Liebman Sachs endocarditis, 219
Lipidosis of reticuloendothelial system, 188
  Gaucher's disease, 188
  Niemann-Pick disease, 188
Lipochromes, 44
Lipoma, 207
Liposarcoma, 209
Lipping of joints, 411, 412

Liquefaction necrosis, 31
Liver, 275
  abnormalities of, congenital, 275
  abscess of, 275
  adenoma of, 287
  amyloidosis of, 276
  autolysis, 275
  cancer of, mesodermal, 287
  carcinoma of, 287
    primary, 287
  cirrhosis, 276
  cloudy swelling in, 276
  congestion of, passive, 276
  degeneration, 277
  disease, 275
  eclampsia in, 277
  edema in, 276
  fatty metamorphosis of, 275
  glycogen in, 275
  hamartoma of, 288
  hemangioma of, 288
    cavernous, 288
  hemochromatosis of, 280
  hemorrhage in, 276
  histoplasmosis of, 278
  hyaline substances in, 276
  infarction of, 277
  infiltrations in, 280
    amyloid, 280
  injury to
    chemical, 281
    drug, 282
  in juandice, chronic idiopathic, 285
  necrosis of, 276
  nutmeg, 276
  pigmentation of, 277
  tumors of, 287
  in typhoid fever, 280
Lobar pneumonia, 127, 248
Ludwig's angina, 127
Lumpy jaw, 147
Lung abscess, 249
Lupus erythematosus, 219, 221
  disseminated, associated with endocarditis, 219
Lupus vulgaris, 134
Lymphadenitis, 221, 273, 291
  acute, 273, 291
  chronic, 273, 291
  chronic granulomatous, 291

Lymphadenopathy, 96, 221, 305
  causes of, 96, 305
  cervical, 96
  generalized, 96, 305
Lymphangioma, 208
Lymphangitis, 290, 365
Lymphedema, 51, 61
Lymphocytes, 98, 157
Lymphocytosis, 98, 157, 303
Lymphogranuloma venereum, 141
Lymphoid appendicitis, chronic, 273
Lymphoid hyperplasia, 273
Lymphomas, malignant, 210, 294
  lymphatic leukemia, form of, 294
Lymphopathia venereum, 291, 347
  369
Lymphopenia, 293, 306
Lymphosarcoma, 209, 293
  giant follicle, 293
Lymphosarcoma, 209, 210, 293
Lysin, 105

M

McBurney's point, rigidity at, 273
McCallum's plaque, 226
Malaria, 283
Malarial pigmentation, 283
  hematin, 283
Male
  breast, carcinoma of, 360
  genitalia, 368
    tuberculosis of, 370
Malignant, 197, 200
Malignant (accelerated) hyptertension, 231
Malignant teratoma, 328
Malignant transformation, 197, 212, 275
Malnutrition, 122, 197
Margination, 95
Mastitis, 354
  chronic cystic, 356
  plasma cell, 357
  tuberculous, 357
Measles, 155, 425
  German measles, 155
Meckel's diverticulum, 271
  of small intestines, 271
Mediterranean anemia, Cooley's, 300
Megacolon, congenital, 274
  in large intestines, 274
Meig's syndrome (Ovary), 329
Melanoma, malignant (Melanocarcinoma), 212, 350, 395
Melanosis, 42
Melena, 67
Meningitis, 420
Mesenchymal neoplasms, 199, 202, 209
Metabolic diseases, 55, 121
Metachromatic staining for amyloid, 40
Metaplasia, 198, 383
  gastric carcinoma and, 270
  of gastric mucosa, 270
Metastases to bone tissue, 204, 276, 410
  osteosclerotic, 410
  osteosclerotic anemia due to, 410
Metastatic calcification, 36
  causes of, 36
Metastatic neoplasms, 47, 202, 204, 276, 316
Methemoglobin, 299
Microcytosis, 300, 301
Midline lethal granuloma, 212
Miliary tuberculosis, 134
Miner's lung (anthracosilicosis), 43, 247
Mole, hydatidiform, 340
Molluscum contagiosum, 154
Mönckeberg's medial calcification or sclerosis, 70
Mongoloid facies (Mongolism), 313
Monilia infection of esophagus, 254
Moniliasis, 254, 349
Monocytic leukemia, 304
Mononuclear leukocytes, 98
Mononucleosis, 304
Moon face, 315
Mucin, secretion of, 34
Mucoepidermoid carcinoma, 197
Mucocele of the appendix, 273
Mucoid degeneration, 35, 36
Mucoid fluid, 34
Mucous patch, 138, 281
Multiple myeloma, 305
Multiple sclerosis, 425
Mumps, 156
Muscular hypertrophy, 114, 198
Mycobacterium leprae, 136

Index

Mycobacterium tuberculosis, 133
Mycosis, 143
  actinomycosis, 143
  blastomycosis, North American, 143
  chromoblastomycosis, 143
  coccidiodomycosis, 143
  dermatomycosis, 143
  fungoides, 143
  phycomycosis, 143
Mycotic aneurysm, 238
Mycotuberculosis bovis, 138
Mycotuberculosis hominis, 133
Myeloma, 408
  bone, multiple, 408
Myelophthisic anemia, 302
Myoblastoma, 208
Myocardial infarction, 230
Myocarditis, 233, 235
  uremic, 235
Myoglobin, 44
Myxedema, 35, 51
Myxoma, 208
Myxomatous change, 35
Myxosarcoma, 209

N

Necrosis, 8, 31, 37, 280
Necrosis of the liver, 280
  central zonal, 280
  diffuse, 281
  focal, 281
  midzonal, 280
  peripheral zonal, 281
Necrotizing inflammation (arteriolitis), 77, 261
Neisseria gonorrhea, 127
Neisseria meningitides, 127
Neisseria meningococci, 127
Neoplasia, 197, 200, 241
  etiology of, 197, 200
  treatment of, 198
Neoplasms, 197, 202
  benign angiomatous, 241
  benign epithelial, 202
  benign mesenchymal, 202
  benign myogenic, 202
  of head and neck, 212
  malignant epithelial, 199
  malignant mesenchymal, 199, 209
  midline lethal granuloma, 212
  of peripheral nervous tissue, 210
Neoplasms of bone tissue, primary, 408
Neoplasms of bone which may progress to malignancy, 408
  enchondroma, 409
  giant-cell tumor, 409
  neurofibroma, 410
  osteocartilagenous exostosis, 409
  solitary plasmacytoma, 410
Neoplasms of the esophagus, 268
  esophageal carcinoma, 268
Neoplasms of the gall bladder, benign, 289
  adenomas, 289
  adenomyomas, 289
  papillomas, 289
Neoplasms of the kidney
  benign, 263
    adenomas, 263
    fibroma, 263
    leiomyofibroma, 264
    leiomyomas, 264
    lipomas, 264
    papillomas, 264
  malignant, 264
    hypernephroma (renal cell carcinoma), 264
    Wilm's tumor, 264
Neoplasms of the large intestines, 275, 276
  adenoma, 276
  adenomatous polyps, 276
  benign polyposis of colon and rectum, 276
Neoplasms of the liver, benign, 287, 289
  adenoma, 287
  hemangioma, 288
Neoplasms of the lung, 254
  bronchial adenoma, 254
  bronchiolar carcinoma, 255
  bronchogenic carcinoma, 255
    anaplastic carcinoma, 255
    squamous cell carcinoma, 255
Neoplasms of the lymph nodes, 292
  giant follicle lymphosarcoma, 292
  Hodgkin's disease, 293
  lymphatic leukemia, 293
  lymphosarcoma, 293
  malignant lymphoma, 294

reticulum cell sarcoma, 294
Neoplasms of the pelvis and ureter, 264
   infiltrating squamous cell carcinoma, 264
   papillary carcinoma, 265
   papillomas, 265
   transitional cell carcinoma, 265
Neoplasms of the small intestines, benign, 272
   benign polyps, 272
   fibroma, 272
   leiomyoma, 272
   lipoma, 272
Neoplasms of the spleen, 296
   Hodgkins' disease, 296
   leukemia, 296
   lymphosarcoma, 296
Neoplasms of the stomach, 270
   benign, 270
      fibroma, 270
      gastric adenomatous polyp, 270
      leiomyoma, 270
      lipoma, 270
      neurofibroma, 270
   malignant, 209, 270
      adenocarcinoma, 270
      fibrosarcoma, 270
      leiomyosarcoma, 270
      lymphosarcoma, 270
Neoplasms of the urinary bladder
   benign, 265
   malignant, 265
      adenocarcinoma, 265
      epidermoid carcinoma, 265
      papillary transitional cell carcinoma, 265
Neoplastic diseases, 202
Nephritis, 258
Nephrosclerosis, malignant, 259
Nephrosis, lower nephron, 83, 258
Nephrotic edema, 61, 258
   renal edema, 61, 258
Nerve cells, 414, 415
   peripheral, diseases of, 415, 437
Nervous system, 414, 437
   anomalies, 419
   anoxia and, 419
   central, viral diseases of, 425
   degeneration, subacute combined, 419

demyelinating diseases, 426
diabetic coma and, 430
hemangioblastoma, 433
hemangioma of, 434, 437
in hypoglycemia, 431
infection of, 419
intoxications and, 430
lymphoma of, malignant, 433
in malaria, 430
poisons and chemical, 430
reaction to injury, 419
sarcoma of, 433
in syphilis, 421
tumors of, 434
vascular diseases, intramedullary, 426
Neuralgia, 415
Neurilemmoma, 212
Neuroblastoma, sympathicoblastoma, ganglioneuroma (Adrenal), 316
Neurofibroma, 211
Neurofibromatosis, generalized, 212
Neurogenic shock, 176
Neuroma, amputation, 211
Neurotoxin, 156
Neurotrophic viruses, 156
Neutropenia, 293, 306
Nevi, 212, 350, 395
   blue, 395
   compound, 212, 395
   intradermal, 212, 396
   junctional, 212, 396
   pigmented, 212, 396
Nicotinic acid deficiency, 192
Niemann-Pick disease, 188
Night blindness, 190
Nocardosis, 149
Noma, 212
Noncaseous granuloma, 135, 149
Normocytic anemia, 65, 300
North American blastomycosis, 145
Nutritional diseases, 183, 184

O

Obliterative appendicitis, 273
Ochronosis, 42
Ocular infectious diseases, 124
Oophoritis, 324
Orchitis, 383
   acute, 383
   granulomatous, 384

Index

Organization, 109
Osler-Weber-Rendu disease, 208
Osseous xanthomatosis, 188, 296
  Hand-Schüller-Christian syndrome, 188, 296
Osteitis, 400
  fibrosa cystica, 401
  syphilitic, 400
Osteoarthritis, 120, 411
Osteocartilagenous exostosis, 402
Osteochondritis of bone, 407
Osteodystrophy, chronic, 407
Osteogenesis imperfecta, 407
Osteogenic sarcoma, 409
  and Paget's disease, 405
Osteolytic osteosarcoma, 209, 409
Osteoma, 200, 408
Osteomalacia, 403
Osteomyelitis, 126, 400
  acute, 400
  complications of, 401
Osteoptrosis, 402, 407
Osteoporosis, 120, 405
  disuse atrophy, 405
  generalized, 405
  immobilization, 405
  localized, 405
  senile, 405
Osteoradionecrosis, 204
Oseteosarcoma, 209, 409
Ovaries, 324
  cancer of, 326
  carcinoma of, 326
    embryonal, 325
  choriocarcinoma, primary, 326
  cyst of, 325
  cystadenoma of, 325
  development of, 324
  dysgerminoma of, 326
  fibroma of, 326
  hormones, 324
  inflammation of, 325
  mesonephroma of, 326
  tumors of, 326

P

Pachymeningitis, 422
Paget's disease of bone, 405
Paget's disease of breast (nipple), 366
Pancarditis, 230
Pancreatitis, 309
Pannus, 412
Pantothenic acid deficiency, 189, 195
Papanicolaou smear (exfoliative cytology), 346
Papillary cystadenoma, 202
Papillary transitional cell carcinoma of urinary bladder, 265
Papilloma, 204, 265
  of urinary bladder, transitional, 265
Papillomatous hyperplasia, 204
Paracoccidioidomycosis, 146
  (South American Blastomycoses), 146
Paralytic ileus, 272
Parasitic cirrhosis, 286
Parasitic infections of the liver, 281
Parathyroid, 403
  adenoma, 404
  diseases of, 405
  hyperplasia, primary, 403
Parenchymatous degeneration, 8, 31
Paronychia, 126
Passive hyperemia, chronic, 51, 64
Pasteurella tularensis, 142
Patent ductus arteriosus, 228
Pathogenicity, 124
Pathologic fractures, 160, 165
Pathophysiology of shock, 79, 80, 176
Pavementation, 95
Pellagra, 192, 418
Pelvis and ureter, abnormalities of, 348
  pyelitis, 348
  ureteritis, 349
Pemphigus, 390
Pemphigus vulgaris, 391
Penicillin, hypersensitivity to, 215
Penis, 377
  carcinoma of, squamous cell, 378
  venereal lesions of, 379
Peptic ulcer
  duodenal, 268
    acute perforation, 268
  of the stomach, 269
    chronic, 269
    malignancy and, 270
    perforation of, 270
    theories of, 270
Periarteritis nodosa (polyarteritis no-

dosa), 220, 222
Pericardial effusions, 58
Pericarditis, acute, 236
  chronic, 233, 236
Pericolitis, 272
Perienteritis, 272
Periostitis, 400
  gummatous, 401
  syphilitic, 401
Peritonitis, acute, 272
  generalized, 272
Pernicious anemia, 192, 295
Petechiae, 66
  causes of, 66
Peutz-Jeghers syndrome, 277
Phagocytosis, 37
Pheochromocytoma, adrenal, 316
Phlebitis, 91
Phlebolith, 241
Phlebosclerosis, 91
Phlebothrombosis, 86, 91, 240
Phlegmon, 126
Phlegmonous inflammation, 126
Phosphorus poisoning, 172
Pigment metabolism, 42
Pigmentation, 6, 42
Pinocytosis, 72
Pinta, 141
Pituitary cachexia, 42, 311
Pituitary gland, 311
  adenoma of, 313
  anterior lobe, 312
  diseases of, 311
  function of, 311
  hormones, gonadotropic, 312
  posterior lobe, 311
  Rathke's pouch in, epithelial
    remnants of, 311
  structure of, 311
  syndromes, 311
Pityriasis rosea, 388
Plasia, 198
Plasma cells, 98, 304
Plasma cell leukemia, 304
Plasma thromboplastic antecedent
  (PTA or factor XI), deficiency of,
  307
Plasma thromboplastic component,
  deficiency of, 307
Platelet, factor, 307

Platelet thromboses, 9, 85
Pleomorphic adenoma, 204
Pleomorphism, cellular, 199
Plexiform neuroma, 211
Plumbism, 168, 172
Plummer-Vinson syndrome, 185, 267
  of esophagus, 185, 267
  neoplasia associated with, 185, 267
Pneumococcal pericarditis, 236
Pneumoconiosis, 251
  anthracosilicosis (Miner's lung), 252
  anthracosis, 251
  asbestosis, 252
  berylliosis, 252
  siderosilicosis, 252
  silicosis, 252
Pneumonia, primary atypical, 250
Pneumonitis, 247
Poisoning, 167, 170, 172
  alcohol, 168, 175
  arsenic, 168, 170
  barbiturate, 175
  beryllium, 170
  cadmium, 170
  carbon
    monoxide, 170, 173
      hemorrhages and petechial, 170
    tetrachloride, 168, 175
  chemical, 167
  chloroform, 168
  classification of, 169
  corrosive, 169
  cyanide, 168
  drug, 168, 170
  halogens, 172
  intestinal inflammations and, 170,
    172, 173
  lead, 168
  mercury, 168
  mushroom, 173
  nephrosis and, toxic, 168
  nitrogen dioxide, 168
  petroleum products and, 168
  phosphorus, 170, 172
  stomach and, 170, 172
Poliomyelitis, 154, 156, 420, 424
  spinal cord in, 154, 424
Polyarteritis nodosa, 85, 90, 219, 220
  periarteritis nodosa, 85, 219, 222
Polycystic kidney, 258

Index

Polycythemia, 85, 302
  rubra, 302
  vera, 302
Polymorphonuclear leukocytes, 15, 102
Polyposis of colon and rectum, benign, 275
  diffuse, 275
  intestinal, 275
  Peutz-Jeghers syndrome, 276
  solitary, 276
Polystasis of bile ducts, 285
Porphyrins, 44
Porphyrinemia, 44
Portal (Laennac's) cirrhosis, 284
Portal hypertension, 59, 285
Posthepatic cirrhosis, 283, 285
Postmortem changes in the heart, 225
Postnecrotic cirrhosis, 282
Pott's disease, 401
Primary atypical pneumonia, 250
Progeria, 121
Prostate, 119, 378
  adenocarcinoma of, 379
  carcinoma of, 380
  hypertrophy, benign, 380
    anatomic changes due to, 380
  inflammation of, 379
  sarcoma of, 380
  tuberculosis in, 378
  tumors of, 380
Prostatitis, 380
Protein metabolism, disturbances of, 187
Prothrombin time, 84
Protoporphyrin, excretion of, 44
Protozoal infections, 158
Pruritis, 284, 349
  in regurgitation juandice, 284
Pseudoepitheliomatous hyperplasia, 199
Pseudohermaphroditism, 22, 315, 318
Pseudomonas aeruginosa, 127
Psoriasis, 388
Ptomaine poisoning, 128
Pulmonary edema, 246
Pulmonary embolism, 246
Pulmonary infarction, 247
Pulmonary tuberculosis, 251
Purpura, 67, 303, 306
  thrombocytopenic purpura, 84, 306
  thrombotic thrombocytopenic purpura, 84, 306
Purulent, 95
  inflammation, 95
  meningitis, 420
Pustule, 126
Putrefaction, 39
Pyelitis, 264
Pyelonephritis, 261
  hypertension accompanying, 261
  supurative, 262
  tuberculosis, 262
Pyemia, 401
Pyknosis, 30
Pyridoxine deficiency, 193

Q

Q fever, 157
Queyrat, erythroplasia of, 395
Quincy sore throat, 126

R

Rabies, 156
Rachitic rosary, 403
Radiation cachexia, 176, 177, 179
Radiation dermatitis, 178
Radiation injury to tissues, 25, 122, 176, 177
Radiation, interstitial, 122, 177
Radiation, secondary, 176, 177
  reduction of, 177
Radiation sickness, 176, 177, 179
Radiation, systemic, 176, 177
  effects of, 176, 177
Radioactive contamination, 176
Radioactive isotopes, 28
Radioisotopes, 25
Radioresistant tissues, 180
Radioresponsive tissues, 180
Radiosensitive tissues, 180
Radium, 25
  needle implant, 25
Raynaud's phenomenon (disease), 240
Reed-Sternberg cells, 293
Regeneration of tissues, 12, 41, 113
Regional ileitis, 272, 275
Reiter's syndrome, 389
Renal calculi, 263
  staghorn, 263
Renal cell carcinoma (hypernephroma), 264

Renal failure, chronic, 258
Renal threshold, 54
Repair, 11, 109
  fracture, 112
  by scar formation, 112
Resolution, 11, 97, 109
  of lobar pneumonia, 247
Respiratory allergy, 216
Respiratory viruses, 154
Reticuloendotheliosis, 188, 296
  of spleen, 296
    Hand-Schüller-Christian syndrome, 188, 296
Reticulum cell sarcoma, 209, 292
Retropharyngeal abscess, 126
Rhabdomyoma, 200
Rhabdomyosarcoma, 209
Rhagades of congenital syphilis, 138, 281
Rh-agglutinins, anti-, 300
Rheumatic arthritis, 197
Rheumatic endocarditis, 219, 232
Rheumatic fever, 219, 232
Rheumatic heart disease, 232
Rheumatoid
  arthritis,
    subcutaneous nodule of, 411, 412
Rh factor, 300
  anti—Rh agglutinins, 300
  Rh—negative mother, 300
  Rh—positive father, 300
Riboflavin deficiency, 187
Rickets, 186, 403
Rickettsial diseases, 26, 157
Rickettsial pox, 157
Rigor mortis, 41
Ringworm infection, 143
Rocky Mountain spotted fever, 157
Rubella, 155
Rupture of internal viscus, 167

S

Sago spleen, 269
Salpingitis, 332, 347
  acute, 333
  chronic, 333
  tuberculous, 333
Sarcoid granuloma, 135, 149
Sarcoid syndrome, 149
Sarcoidosis, 135, 149

Sarcoma, 209
  osteogenic, 405
Scarlet fever, 127
Schistosomiasis, 286
Schwannoma, benign, 211
Scleroderma, 219, 222, 386
  of esophagus, 267
Sclerotic osteosarcoma, 209
Scoliosis, 313
Scrofula, 134
Scrotum, diseases and neoplasms of, 370
Scrub typhus, 157
Scurvy, 194
Senile atrophy, 49
Senile gangrene, 37
Senile osteoporosis, 405
Sensitivity to tuberculosis, 107, 215
Septicemia, 125
  generalized, 125
Sequestrum, 400
Serum hepatitis, 280
Serum sickness, 223
Sheehan's syndrome, 311
Shingles, 155
Shock, 79, 80, 107, 176
  blood volume and, 79
Shwartzman phenomenon, 216
Sickle cell anemia, 299
Sickle cell trait, 299
Siderosilicosis, 43
Siderosis, 43
Silicosis, 28, 150
Simmond's disease, 42, 311
Skeletal lesions in endocrine disorders, 406, 409
  acromegaly, 406
  cretinism, 406
  Cushing's syndrome, 407
  hyperthyroidism, 408
Skin hypersensitivity (allergy), 218, 386
Skin, 385
  cancer, 395
    appendages, 396
  carcinoma, 395
  fibrosarcoma of, 395
  hemangioma of, capillary, 386
  infections of, 386
  inflammations of, 386

Index

melanocarcinoma, 395
melanoma of, juvenile, 395
precancerous lesions of, 386
structure of, 385
in syphilis, 386
tuberculosis of, 386
tumorlike conditions of, 386
wounds, healing of, 386
Skin test for tuberculosis, 134
Skin tuberculosis, 134
Smallpox, 155
Somatic death, 41
South American blastomycosis, 145
Spherocytes, 295, 299
Spherocytic anemias, 295, 299
Sphingomyelin in reticuloendothelial cells, 296
Niemann-Pick disease, 296
Spina bifida occulata, 16, 198
Spirochaeta pallida, 138, 282
Spirochetal diseases, 138, 282
Spirochetal infections of the liver, 138, 282
Spirochetemia of primary syphilis, 138, 281
Spleen, accessory, 258
rupture of, 258
spotted, 258
Splenic anemia, 295
Splenic disease, primary, 295
Splenic tumor acute, 295
Splenitis, acute (acute splenic tumor), 295
Splenomegaly, 293, 295, 305
Sporotrichosis, 146
Sporotrichotic chancre, 146
Spotted fever (Rocky Mountain), 157
Squamous cell carcinoma, 204
of esophagus, 268
of gall bladder, 289
grading of 205
of lung, 254
Squamous metaplasia, 199, 336
Staghorn renal, calculi, 263
Staphylococcal arthritis, 411
Staphylococcal flora, resistant, 126
Staphylococcus albus infection, 126
Staphylococcus aureus, 126, 400
Staphylococcus infections, 126
Stein-Leventhal syndrome, 326

Stenosis, 49, 112
Sternberg-Reed cell in Hodgkin's disease, 293
Stevens-Johnson syndrome, 393
Stomach, 268
adenocarcinoma of, 270
carcinoma of, 270
leiomyoma of, 271
leiomyosarcoma of, 271
mucosa of pernicious anemia, 269
poisons and, 268
polyps of, benign, 270
sarcoma of, 271
tumors of, 270
ulcer, 270
Strawberry tongue, 127
Streptococcal arthritis, 126
Streptococcal infections, 126, 233
Streptococci, 126, 233
Streptococcus pyogenes, 127
Stress, 102, 309
Stroke, 426
Subarachnoid hemorrhage, 431
Subdural, 431
abscess, 423, 432
hematoma, 432
Suppuration, 94
Suppurative arthritis, 411
Suppurative cellulitis, 94
Syncope, 81
Synovial tumors, 409
benign giant-cell tumor of tendon sheath, 410
synovial sarcoma, 410
Syphilis, 138, 281, 368, 373, 402, 423
acquired, 138, 281, 373
of bone tissue, 402
cardiovascular, 225
central nervous system, 402, 423
congenital, 281, 402
meningovascular syphilis, 402, 423
primary, 138, 268, 373
secondary, 138, 368
tertiary, 138, 368
Syphilitic aortic valvulitis, 229
Syphilitic arteritis, 229
Syphilitic arthritis, 411
Syphilitic cirrhosis, 280
Syphilitic glossitis, 368
Syphiloma, 347

Systemic effects, of local inflammation, 13

T

Tabes dorsalis, 424
Temporal, pericardial, 58
Telangiectasia, 208
Temporal arteritis, 240
Tensile strength of wounds, 110
Teratoma, 200, 212, 327
Testis(es), 372
  atrophy of, 372
  carcinoma of, embryonal, 373
  choriocarcinoma of, 374
  emboli in, atheromatous, 372
  gumma of, 374
  seminoma of, 375
  syphilis and, 374
  teratocarcinoma, 377
  teratoma of, 376
  tuberculosis of, 374
  tumors of, 377
Tetralogy of Fallot, 228
Theca-lutein cysts, 329
Thecoma, ovary, 330
Thermal injury, 176
Thirst, 54
Thromboangitis obliterans, 240
Thrombocytopenia, 304
Thrombocytopenic purpura, 84, 306
  thrombotic, 84, 306
Thromboembolism, 87
Thrombophlebitis, 56, 86, 240
Thrombosis, 9, 85
Thrombotic thrombocytopenic purpura, 84, 306
Thrombus, 86, 87, 240
Thyroid, 309, 404
  adenoma of, 404
  carcinoma of, 404
  diseases of, 309, 404
  hyperplasia, in Graves' disease, 404
  inflammation of, 405
  in myxedema, 405
  tumors of, 406
    Hürthle cell, 406
Thyroiditis, 406
Toxemia, 351
  of pregnancy, 351
Toxins, bacterial and zootic, 174

Transposition complexes, 227
  Eisenmenger's complex, 228
  Tetralogy of Fallot, 228
Transudate, 57
Trauma, 160
Traumatic diseases, 160
Traumatic fracture, 160
Treponema pallidum, 138, 323
Trichomonas vaginalis, 348
Trigeminal ganglion, herpes zoster of, 155
Tsutsugamushi fever, 157
Tubercle, 133
Tubercular pericarditis, 236
Tuberculoid leprosy, 136
Tuberculosis, 134, 359, 401, 423
  human, 134, 359
  of bone, 401
  of the intestines, 274
  of the kidney, 258
  of the liver, 280
  of the lungs, 246
    reinfection, 253
  pulmonary, 246
    primary type, 247
    reinfection type, 247
  reinfection (superinfection), 253
    cavitation of, 253
  of the vertebrae, 401
Tuberculous arthritis, 401, 411
Tuberculous cavitation, 253
Tuberculous lymphadenitis, 306
Tuberculous meningitis, 423
Tuberculous osteomyelitis, 401, 411
Tuberculous pyelonephritis, 259
Tularemia, 141, 142
Tumor, 200
Tumor cell emboli, 87
Turner's syndrome, 318
Typhoid fever, 128
  of terminal ileum, 274
Typhus group, 157
  rickettsial diseases, 157

U

Ulcer, 275
Ulcerative colitis, chronic, 275
  complications of, 275
  malignant transformation in, 275
Ultraviolet irradiation, 178

Undulant fever, 128, 142
Uremia, 164, 258, 275
  ulcers in the colon during, 259, 275
Uremic frost, 258
Uremic myocarditis, 258
Uremic pericarditis, 258
Ureteral cholic, 264
Ureteritis, 264
Urobilinogen, 44
Urticaria, 216
Uterus, 334
  adenoacanthoma of, 335
  adenocarcinoma of, 336
  choriocarcinoma of, 336
  endometriosis of, 336
  fibroid of, 337
  leiomyoma of, 335
  myoma of, 335
  sarcoma of, 335
  tumors of, 336

V

Vagina, diseases and neoplasms of, 346, 349
Vaginal tuberculosis, 348
Vaginitis, 291, 348
Valley fever, 144, 253
Varicella, 154
Varicose veins, 91, 241
Vasa vasorum of aorta, 228
  proliferation of, 228
Vascular disease of the kidney, 259
  arteriosclerosis, 260
  glomerulonephritis, 261
  infarction, 261
  necrotizing arteriolitis, 77, 261
  nephrosclerosis, 262
  thrombosis, 262
Vascular disease, peripheral, 239
Vascular responses in inflammation, 95, 100
Vasodilatation, 95
Vegetations, 85
Viral diseases, 154
Viral hepatitis, acute, 280
Viral inclusion bodies, 154
Viral infections of the liver, 280
  infectious hepatitis, 280
Viral theory of neoplasia, 197
Virulence, 125

Viruses, 154
Vitamin, 189, 195, 301
  A, deficiency of, 190
  B complex, deficiency of, 191
  B_1, deficiency of, 192
  B_2, deficiency of, 192, 301
  B_6, deficiency of, 192
  B_{12}, deficiency of, 116
  C, deficiency of, 193, 402
  D, deficiency of, 194, 402
  D resistant rickets, 195, 402
  E, deficiency of, 190
  K, deficiency of, 190
Voluntary muscle, diseases of, 412
  bacterial myositis, 412
  parasitic myositis, 412
  traumatic myositis ossificans, 412
  viral myositis, 412
  Zenker's degeneration, 40, 412
Volvulus, 277
von Recklinghausen's disease of bone, 402, 438
Von Willebrand's disease, 307
Vulva, 346
  carcinoma of, 350
  gonorrheal inflammation of, 346
  in granuloma inguinale, 348
  hidradenoma of, 348
  leukoplakia of, 349
  in lymphogranuloma venereum, 348
  in syphilis, 347
  tumors of, 350
  venereal lesions, 346

W

Wallerian degeneration, 166
Wassermann test (syphilis), 359
Water, 53
  body disturbances of, 53
Waterhouse Friderichsen syndrome, 314
Weil's disease (leptospirohemorrhagica), 280
Wet gangrene, 37
Whooping cough, 128
Wilm's tumor, 264
  of kidney, 264
Wilson's disease, 286
Wire loop renal lesions, 258
Wound shock, 107, 176

X

Xanthomatoses, 188, 286, 296
X-chromosome, 22
Xeroderma pigmentosum, 121

Y

Yaws, 141
Y-chromosome, 22

Yellow atrophy, acute (liver), 280
Yellow fever, 157, 282
   midzonal necrosis and, 280

Z

Zenker's degeneration of voluntary muscle, 410
Zenker's hyaline degeneration, 40
Zoster, Herpes, 155

616.0702 G17   108545

GARDNER

SYNOPSIS OF PATHOLOGY FOR THE ALLIED
HEALTH PROFESSIONS

College Misericordia Library
Dallas, Pennsylvania 18612